COMMUNICATION *and*

EDUCATION *Skills for*

Dietetics PROFESSIONALS

THIRD EDITION

COMMUNICATION *and* EDUCATION *Skills for* *Dietetics* PROFESSIONALS

THIRD EDITION

Betsy B. Holli, EdD, RD, LD
Professor
Department of Nutrition Sciences
Dominican University
River Forest, Illinois

Richard J. Calabrese, PhD
Director
Master of Science in Organization Management
Dominican University
River Forest, Illinois

WITH A CONTRIBUTION BY
Ann B. Williams, PhD
Associate Professor of Psychology
Dominican University
River Forest, Illinois

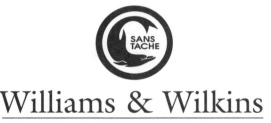

Williams & Wilkins
A WAVERLY COMPANY

BALTIMORE • PHILADELPHIA • LONDON • PARIS • BANGKOK
BUENOS AIRES • HONG KONG • MUNICH • SYDNEY • TOKYO • WROCLAW

Editor: Donna Balado
Managing Editor: Jennifer Schmidt
Production Coordinator: Marette Magargle-Smith
Project Editor: Karen Ruppert
Designer: Diane Buric
Cover Designer: Graphic World Inc.
Typesetter: Maryland Composition Inc.
Printer & Binder: McNaughton & Gunn, Inc.

Printed in the United States of America

First Edition,

Library of Congress Cataloging-in-Publication Data

Holli, Betsy B.
    Communication and education skills for dietetics professionals / Betsy B. Holli, Richard J. Calabrese ; with a contribution by Ann B. Williams.
    —3rd ed.
        p.   cm.
    Prev. ed. cataloged with title: Communication and education skills : the dietitian's guide.
    Includes index.
    ISBN 0-683-30015-6
    1. Communication in diet therapy.   2. Patient education.   3. Interpersonal communication.   I. Calabrese, Richard J.
RM214.3.H65   1997
615.8′54—dc21
                                                                                                97-6053
                                                                                                CIP

The publishers have made every effort to trace the copyright holders for borrowed material. If they have inadvertently overlooked any, they will be pleased to make the necessary arrangements at the first opportunity.

To purchase additional copies of this book, call our customer service department at **(800) 638-0672** or fax orders to **(800) 447-8438**. For other book services, including chapter reprints and large quantity sales, ask for the Special Sales department.

Canadian customers should call **(800) 268-4178**, or fax **(905) 470-6780**. For all other calls originating outside of the United States, please call **(410) 528-4223** or fax us at **(410) 528-8550**.

Visit Williams & Wilkins on the Internet: **http://www.wwilkins.com** or contact our customer service department at **custserv@wwilkins.com**. Williams & Wilkins customer service representatives are available from 8:30 am to 6:00 pm, EST, Monday through Friday, for telephone access.

98 99 00
2 3 4 5 6 7 8 9 10

To Melvin and Steven Holli and

Susan H. Swinford

and to

Kay

preface

Effective communication skills are essential for competent dietetics practice. The communication skills are not ends in themselves, but are the basis for strengthening interpersonal relationships, for shaping people's food choices, and for impacting on the nutritional status of the public. Skills related to educating others and to communicating with patients, clients, employees, other health care professionals, the public, and the media are of increasing importance to dietetics professionals.

One aim of medical nutrition therapy is to facilitate change in the clients' or patients' eating behaviors. Poor communication skills can directly affect patient/client adherence to dietary recommendations, patient understanding and satisfaction, and for the manager, relationships with employees and staff. A great deal of literature is now available on methods and interventions to improve communication and education and to enhance dietary change. While there is no one unified model or theory to follow, this book offers numerous theoretical and practical ideas and strategies for practitioners to incorporate into their professional practices. A combination of educational (what to do) and behavioral (how to do it) interventions provides a comprehensive approach to effective food and health behavior change.

Dietetics education emphasizes not only scientific and technical knowledge and skills but also communication and education skills. The publication of the original American Dietetic Association (ADA) role delineation studies, determining what practitioners were doing in their work in the 1980s, brought attention to the need for communication skills. Based on the original and subsequent studies, the ADA Standards of Education for educational programs include knowledge and performance skills in effective communication and education in the required competencies for dietitians and dietetic technicians. The contents of the registration examinations are also based on the role delineation studies. Results of updated role delineation studies published in 1996 confirmed specific job responsibilities of dietetics professionals involving communication with and education of patients, clients,

groups, the public, other health professionals, students, and staff.

The purpose of this edition of the book remains the same. The book is intended to help both current practitioners and students improve their communication with patients, clients, employees, and others, and thus improve their professional practice. One does not develop these skills by only reading about them, however. The mastery of any skill depends on practice and actual experience. Besides the suggested activities that have always been included, this edition adds review and discussion questions to each chapter, as well as a short case study. We hope that these will further enhance learning.

We appreciate the feedback we have received on earlier editions of the book and encourage readers to continue it. Many suggestions have been incorporated into this edition. In attempting to make each chapter able to stand alone, a small amount of repetition may be noticed by some readers. We have broadened the title and chapters by using the term "dietetics professional," as does the American Dietetic Association and the *Journal of the American Dietetic Association.*

In addition to revising and updating all the chapters based on the current literature, four chapters have been added. Because clients and employees come from diverse groups, a new chapter includes multicultural counseling and counseling throughout the life span. Most professionals enhance their communication interactions visually. "Planning, Selecting, and Using Media" is a new chapter dealing with these topics. For those who asked for material on educational principles and theories, more has been added and reorganized into a separate chapter. Finally, nutrition counseling is covered in a chapter of its own, separate from the counseling chapter that precedes it.

Special thanks are due to many people for their assistance or suggestions. We express our appreciation especially to Judith Beto, PhD, RD, FADA; Jane Allendorph, MS, RD; Kathleen Prunty, MBA; the nutrition and dietetics majors at Dominican University; and the library staff, including Ken Black. We are grateful to anonymous reviewers selected by the publisher who labored chapter by chapter to provide suggestions to improve the quality of the final manuscript. We are indebted to Steven Beto for photography and to Spencer Phippin for sketches that enhance the visual aspects of the book. The staff at Williams & Wilkins encouraged us frequently. Our family members supported us during the long hours of research-ing, writing, and rewriting, for which we are very grateful.

Betsy B. Holli
Richard J. Calabrese
River Forest, Illinois

contents

one

COMMUNICATION AND EDUCATION SKILLS FOR DIETETICS PROFESSIONALS

American consumers have concerns about foods, nutrients, and health. Today the dietetics professional can be expected to field questions concerning dietary fat, cholesterol, saturated fatty acids, trans fatty acids, weight control, phytochemicals, vegetarianism, antioxidants, food safety, food labeling, irradiation, fiber, bioengineered foods, and more.

Dietetics practitioners need good communication skills. As a profession committed to building a healthier nation by bridging the gap between nutrition knowledge and eating behaviors, our challenge is to connect people's nutrition knowledge with action and change (1). Beyond enhancing normal growth and development, optimal nutritional status is "an integral part of health promotion and disease prevention" (2). Dietary changes by the public could reduce the risk for several major chronic diseases.

Interpersonal skills were identified by participants in a survey as one of three sets of crucial competencies needed by dietetics practitioners. From focus groups and personal interviews, a study found that professionals must be able to "communicate persuasively with team members, patients, policy makers, customers, and the public, all in their own frames of reference and language" (3). They must achieve results in counseling and educating patients and clients as well as manage others by hiring, coaching, and motivating employees.

Administrative dietitians, dietetic technicians, and managers, who communicate with and manage subordinate employees, discover that communication skills are an important key to leadership and managerial effectiveness. Communication is considered an important skill for dietetics, and a strengthening of such skills for dietetics practitioners at all levels is strongly recommended (4).

The United States is an ethnically and racially diverse nation. The number of minorities in the population has risen, especially in urban areas. As a result, it is important for dietetics professionals to be able to communicate effectively with various groups of clients and employees.

In recent years, all health professionals have become more aware of the need to acquire skills in interpersonal relations because their jobs require frequent interaction with others, including clients, patients, employees, colleagues, the public, and other health professionals. In addition to having the requisite scientific and technical skills, professionals must be able to relate effectively to others.

Human relationships are the foundation through which one's scientific and technical skills are practiced. Thus there is a need to focus on the process of delivering nutrition services in treating illness, injury, and chronic medical conditions through medical nutrition therapy. The two phases of medical nutrition therapy are (a) "assessment of the nutritional status of the patient or client" and (b) "treatment, which includes diet therapy, counseling, or use of specialized nutrition supplements" (5). In addition, coordination of team efforts for patient care clearly requires communication and cooperation. Communication is a link connecting all health team members, including the patient.

The American Dietetic Association (ADA) is the world's largest organization of food and nutrition professionals. In defining the nutrition goals for the nation, the ADA recommended that most routine contacts with health professionals should include some nutrition education and counseling (6). Concerning nutrition education for the public, it is the position of the ADA that for the public to achieve optimal nutritional health, "nutrition education should be an integral component of all health promotion, disease prevention, and health maintenance programs, through incorporation into all appropriate nutrition communications, promotion, and educational systems" (7).

The scope of dietetics is broad. Dietitians and dietetic technicians are accepting positions in diverse new areas as health care moves beyond hospitals. They are employed in a variety of positions and in a number of different work settings. While the majority are employed in food service, inpatient care, or outpatient clinics in health care systems (acute-care hospitals, medical centers, and long-term care facilities), others work in food service for students, restaurant/hotel guests, or employee cafeterias; food and pharmaceutical companies; commu-

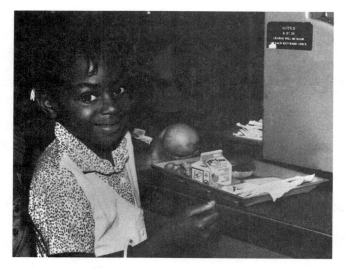

FIGURE 1.1. Taste is a major determinant of people's food choices.

nity and public health agencies; or private practice as entrepreneurs who are self-employed doing individual client counseling or consulting with health care facilities or other organizations. Others are in advertising, marketing, sales, journalism, research, and home health care.

In a survey, practitioners reported engaging in a wide range of professional activities and functions. These activities included most commonly clinical services, followed by nutrition information/communication, public health/community nutrition, wellness/disease prevention, and food services (8). Job functions and activities varied with the work setting and dietetics practice roles are changing as the health care system changes.

The ADA Council on Practice identifies five divisions of dietetics practice including the divisions of clinical nutrition, food and nutrition management, education and research, community nutrition, and consultation and business practice (9). Each of these areas of practice is divided further into subspecialty groups for those who wish to network within their area of interest. Within the ADA are a number of special interest groups. While new ones are formed often, as of 1997, they included the following:

Public Health Nutrition

Gerontological Nutritionists

Dietetics in Developmental and Psychiatric Disorders

Vegetarian Nutrition

Hunger and Malnutrition

Environmental Nutrition

Oncology Nutrition

Renal Dietitians

Pediatric Nutrition

Diabetes Care and Education

Dietitians in Nutrition Support

Dietetics in Physical Medicine and Rehabilitation

Dietitians in General Clinical Practice

Perinatal Nutrition

Nutrition Entrepreneurs

Consultant Dietitians in Health-Care Facilities

Dietitians in Business and Communications

Sports, Cardiovascular, and Wellness Nutritionists

Management in Health-Care Systems

School Nutrition Services

Clinical Nutrition Management

Technical Practice in Dietetics

Dietetic Educators of Practitioners

Nutrition Educators of Health Professionals

Nutrition Education for the Public

Nutrition Research

Food and Culinary Professionals

HIV/AIDS

All of these specialists use communication skills and education skills in daily practice.

Practitioners need to be professionally active in a communication network to have ongoing dialogue with other professionals in one's area of expertise. One way to participate in such a dialogue is to join one of the dietetic practice groups and to attend professional meetings. Although sharing information is the primary purpose of networking, the contacts that networks provide are invaluable. Electronic networks are also available. The ADA's World Wide Web site, for example, can be visited at http://www.eatright.org. Many other web sites are also available.

The ADA has focused on the knowledge base necessary for professional practice and defined the requisite skills and competencies needed by practitioners. Since 1973, the ADA has been assessing and defining, through role-delineation studies, the meaning of competence in the field of dietetics. Information from role-delineation studies, which identify major and specific responsibilities of the dietetics practitioner and the knowledge needed to practice, is helpful in the education of practitioners, in the credentialing process, and in the process of assurance of quality service and practice.

Role delineation studies have identified the major and specific job responsibilities of entry-level dietetic technicians and registered dietitians as well as beyond-entry-level registered dietitians in relation to communication and education skills and the knowledge needed for practice (8, 10). Clinical dietitians, for example, are expected to plan, organize, implement, and evaluate nutrition education for clients and patients, give classes to groups, counsel individuals concerning nutrition concepts and

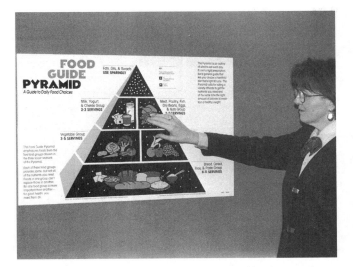

FIGURE 1.2. Dietetics professionals teach clients about nutrition.

desired changes in eating habits, and educate health team members on nutrition-related topics.

A study of 180 practitioners involved in direct patient care found strong correlations between dietitians' confidence in their counseling skills and their estimates of the likelihood of client compliance. Thus confidence in their counseling skills was correlated with the intensity of their counseling efforts (11). Communicating plans for medical nutrition therapy to individuals or families, as well as health team members, with documentation in the medical record, is a major responsibility.

A study of clinical dietitians found that the four activities consuming the largest amount of work time were conducting individual diet instructions, conducting nutrition assessments, reviewing and recording in medical records, and supervising support personnel (12). The clinical dietitians surveyed reported the need for continuing education topics, such as patient counseling and education, behavior modification and change, interpersonal communication, and patient compliance strategies (13).

In public health and community nutrition, responsibilities include providing nutrition education to groups and to individual clients for health promotion, health maintenance, and rehabilitation. Developing orientation and training programs for support personnel is also required (14). A study of members of the Public Health Nutrition dietetics practice group examined the knowledge and skill members applied on the job. High-ranking competencies needed included applying skills in communicating scientific information at a level appropriate to different audiences and in selecting and/or developing nutrition education materials and approaches appropriate for target groups (15).

In food-service systems management, the professional is expected to interview applicants for identified positions, to orient, train, and develop staff, and to counsel subordinates. She provides educational programs (on-the-job training, in-service training, and continuing education) that meet the needs of employees (16). One study ranked communication skills as essential (17).

The consultant is a dietetics professional in private practice who confers with health care facilities and other institutions, providing advice, instructions, or recommendations for obtaining organizational objectives. Home health care is a growing career opportunity (18). Dietitians working in home health care gave high ratings to the following needed skills: patient counseling, caregiver education, documentation, diet histories, and developing a nutrition care plan (19).

Dietetic technicians are expected to use effective oral and written communication skills in dietetics practice and to participate in the education of clients and other personnel. They need knowledge of basic concepts of effective oral and written communication and documentation, basic techniques of interviewing and counseling, and effective methods of teaching.

Common knowledge and skills needed by all professionals for interpersonal relations include being able to apply the principles of verbal and nonverbal communication, public speaking, principles and techniques of interviewing and counseling, theories and strategies for behavior modification and motivation, principles and theories of learning, teaching methods and techniques, knowledge about using media, and knowledge of working with diverse groups. These are skills that are not innate, but they can be learned and improved with practice.

The Future Search Conference forecasts new diverse and nontraditional practice roles that cross several disciplines (20). Expanded opportunities in a variety of practice settings will be available for dietitians who are cross-trained in several areas. One priority identified for immediate action was to enhance people's skills in research, leadership, counseling, communication, multiple competencies, management, and partnerships.

HELPING OTHERS

Dietetics is a "helping" profession concerned primarily with providing services beneficial to individuals and society, and dedicated to improving the nutritional status of people. Helping professions can be described as process professions that do something with knowledge, such as communicating, interpreting, and applying nutritional science to the language and lifestyles of people to benefit their health. The helping approach may also be used in managing subordinate staff. The professional seeks to guide others in converting knowledge into actions that bring about change.

Helping is a process involving a conversation or series of conversations with another person. Whether in social work, nursing, or dietetics, the professional seeks to answer the question, "What is helpful?"

A great deal of helping involves problem solving. Resolving the person's problem may entail arriving at a decision; developing knowledge, insights, or mutual understanding; setting goals for change; or venting feelings. Clients and patients require the assistance of professionals in overcoming and solving their problems when they are unable to do so alone. The individual may be incapable of problem resolution owing to lack of information, knowledge, skill, motivation, or resources, or because of emotional feelings, such as anxiety.

Helping offers the potential for an individual's growth and development, and for achieving change. Helping another person is a process of enabling that person to grow in the direction he or she chooses. Thus, the clients, not the professional, determine whether they want help at all, and if they do, it is they who make the decisions about their needs and select the goals for their own change or growth. Although the individual seeks the assistance of the professional, the ultimate responsibility in making decisions regarding nutrition and health and in self-management rests with the client. The locus of control, or responsibility for controlling the medical problem, is internal in the client rather than external in the medical team.

Clients and patients should not be perceived as passive recipients of services. They are active participants in their treatment, working with the professional to restore or optimize their health. Ultimately, clients or patients are responsible for managing their own nutrition and health. The acceptance of help is voluntary, and the aim of the professional is to make people self-sufficient so that eventually they can manage on their own, solving future problems alone. In reporting determinants of patient satisfaction with diet counseling, one study found that patients were not passive participants in the counseling process, but that they wanted to participate in decisions regarding their diets (21).

Since helping is future oriented, counseling of both clients and employees focuses on what can be done to improve actions and performance; it does not dwell on the failures of the past. When focusing on what is acceptable to and possible for the individual, rather than on the individual's failure to comply with previous recommendations, helpers avoid labeling people as "uncooperative," "unmotivated," or "disinterested."

Helping is far more than providing information on nutrition and related topics. Books, magazines, newspapers, television, computer software, the world wide web, family, and friends can supply information; one does not need a professional to provide it. The resolution of problems, however, and the personal discovery of the meaning of solutions for one's life come from the interaction between the helper and the individual. Problem solving involves listening, communicating, and educating and is fundamentally a learning experience for the individual. The interaction between the helper and the individual is a goal-oriented process through which change occurs in the form of learning new information, knowledge, or skills; gaining new insights and perspectives; modifying feelings; changing behaviors; and developing new resources as decisions are made and problems resolved.

The professional and the client should engage in problem solving as partners, joining forces and interacting in seeking solutions to ensure an effective learning experience. Providing pat answers and quick solutions that may be obvious to the professional does not help the person learn to solve his problems, and this approach should be avoided. Through engaging in the problem-solving process and exploring alternatives with the guidance and encouragement of the professional, the client gains insight into the situation, makes decisions, sets goals, learns to manage resources, and brings about the salutary and desired changes that problem resolution entails. Another benefit of involving individuals in solving their own problems is that it greatly increases self-motivation. People implement their own solutions, while often rejecting those provided by others.

The helping process takes place in the relationship developed between the helper and the individual client. The relationship is a key to the effectiveness of helping and problem solving. The professional strives to create an environment of respect and trust by arranging and maintaining conditions in which individuals perceive themselves as accepted, warmly received, valued, and understood. If the individual feels inferior, dependent, unappreciated, misunderstood, or manipulated, distrust can result, and the individual resists assistance.

Trust must be earned; without it vital self-disclosure on the part of the patient may be limited. The single most important element in interpersonal communication has been described as sender credibility or "the attitude the receiver of a message has toward the sender's trustworthiness" (22). Trust in this sense means "the expectation that self-disclosure will be treated with respect and that feedback from the other can be relied on" (2). Respect and trust can be conveyed by avoiding labeling the individual's responses "right" or "wrong," by providing privacy, by showing concern and understanding through careful listening, and by providing nonjudgmental verbal and nonverbal responses, including, when necessary, accurate paraphrasing of the meaning of the individual's comments and feelings.

The relationship between the professional and client is probably easiest to establish when the client is similar to the professional in educational level and socioeconomic status. There may be a potential problem when the client is very different. For example, professionals must deal with clients who are aged, illiterate, uneducated, hearing-impaired, alcoholic, or disabled, and who may be of various religious, cultural, and ethnic groups, or from lower socioeconomic groups. They may be individuals with critical injuries resulting from automobile accidents and burns, or people with life-threatening diseases, such as cancer and AIDS.

Professionals may need to examine their own values

and personal attitudes toward others in developing effective interpersonal relationships. This self-awareness provides some insurance against prejudice, or judging others by one's personal values, and enables the professional to function out of concern and respect for those who are different.

A number of skills are needed by helping professionals. They include techniques of interviewing and counseling; ability to relate to groups, individuals, and communities; effectiveness in bringing about change; capacity for self-understanding; establishment of professional, interdisciplinary relationships; and knowledge of personality, group, and societal dynamics. With these skills, the helper can assist others to assess all dimensions of a problem, to explore alternative solutions, and to stimulate action toward positive change and problem resolution.

The helper's proficiency in specific communication and helping skills directly affects the success or failure of helping transactions. Since considerable responsibility for desired outcomes of treatment must be assumed by the health professional, it is imperative that helpers develop and improve their counseling skills. The chapters in the book are intended to assist in developing these skills.

PROMOTING CHANGE

The solutions discovered through the problem-solving process, whether used with clients or employees, require some kind of action and change from people. The client who is learning dietary changes, for example, may be expected to know and remember lists of foods that can or should not be consumed, to read and understand food labels, to select a different restaurant menu, to shop for and prepare different foods, or to use different cooking methods. An employee may need to learn and to follow new work methods and procedures. Two basic questions to consider include (a) what sort of change do we wish to bring about, and (b) how can this be accomplished.

The successful professional may be viewed as a "change agent" who needs the ability to intervene to promote change in behavior. Knowledge of the social, cultural, psychological, and other forces affecting motivation for change in individuals or in groups, either positively or negatively, is necessary.

The professional is expected to use a variety of intervention strategies to promote desired change. To be an effective agent of behavioral change, four categories of necessary skills were identified: (a) relationship-building skills, (b) interviewing and assessment skills, (c) problem-diagnosis skills, and (d) behavioral intervention skills (23). Before applying change strategies, the professional should establish that the individual is an informed and willing partner and determine what knowledge he or she brings to the counseling session.

Some people are more resistant than others to making changes in lifestyles, and such resistance to modifying their old patterns of behavior is normal. Change upsets the established ways of doing things, creates uncertainty and anxiety, and forces the need for adjustments. Because attitudes are thought to be the predisposing agents of practice, they should be explored as well.

Every problem has two aspects—what the person **thinks** about it and how he or she **feels** about it. A client may **think,** for example, that a dietary regimen would be beneficial, but **feel** that it would be too difficult to follow. An employee may **think** that a new work procedure is interesting, but **feel** that the current methods are preferable. Both thoughts and feelings must be considered and dealt with for problem solving and change to occur.

Although helpers may see exactly what needs changing, they should bear in mind that the client is the one who decides which changes to make and who ensures that they continue. Thus, the client's priorities take precedence over those of the professional. Those being counseled should be given an opportunity to discuss changes and to ask questions, because the more they internalize the new ideas and solutions, the greater is the likelihood of their being committed to them.

Stages of Change

Prochaska and colleagues have proposed a model with progression through six stages of intentional change: precontemplation, contemplation, preparation, action, maintenance, and termination (24, 25). It is estimated that fewer than 20% of clients are at the "action" stage. Yet 90% of the programs are designed as if people are at the action stage (25). The key to successful interventions, including education and counseling, is to plan them around the stage the individual is in currently to enhance motivation and desired outcomes. Treatment approaches that are effective in one stage may be ineffective in another.

In stage one, **precontemplation,** people are unaware or less than fully aware that a problem exists, deny they have a problem, or are not interested in change, and thus have no intention of changing behavior in the near future (24, 25). They may have tried a change previously and failed, and be resistant to one's efforts to suggest changes. To identify this stage, one may ask: "Are you seriously intending to change (name the problem behavior) in the next six months?" For example, with people ignoring the relationship between a high-fat diet and coronary heart disease, one may ask, "Have you thought about eating less fat (or more fruits and vegetables) in the next six months?" (See Table 1.1 for other questions and interventions at each stage.)

In the second stage, **contemplation,** people are aware that a problem exists, such as needing to eat differently or exercise more, but they have no serious thought or commitment to making a change (24, 25). People may remain in this stage for months or years. They may be mentally struggling with the amount of energy, effort, and cost of overcoming a problem or may be discouraged

TABLE 1.1.

Stages of Change

STAGE	QUESTIONS FOR CLIENT	INTERVENTIONS
Precontemplation	"What can I do to help?" "Do you ever read articles about . . .?" "What do you know about the relationship between . . .?" "Does anyone in your family have this problem?" "Are you aware of the short- and long-term effects?"	Consciousness raising Assess knowledge Increase awareness Give information Assess values Assess beliefs Cognitive restructuring Discuss benefits and risks
Contemplation	"What have you been thinking about making a change?" "What are the pros and cons?" "How do you feel about it?" "What would make it easier or harder to do?" "What would be the results of the change?"	Assess knowledge Assess values Assess beliefs Assess thoughts Assess feelings Motivation Self-evaluation Cognitive restructuring
Preparation	"Are you intending to act in the next 1–6 months?" "How will you do it?" "What changes have you made already?" "What plans have you made?" "How will your life be improved by changing?"	Self-efficacy Commitment Discuss beliefs about ability Plan goals
Action	"What are you doing differently?" "What problems are you having?" "Who can help you?" "How can I help?" "What do you do instead of (the former behavior)?"	Stimulus control Self-reinforcement Social support Self-management Commitment Contracting Goal setting Group sessions Relapse prevention
Maintenance	"How do you handle small slips and lapses?" "What problems are you having?" "What are your future plans?" "Have you solved the problem?"	Coping responses Relapse prevention Self-management Commitment Goal setting Control environment
Termination		Self-efficacy Self-management

Note that the interventions at one stage can be continued during the next stage.

by previous failures. One may ask, "What have you been thinking about making a change?" "What are the pros and cons of doing it?" "How can you change your environment?" For example, "What do you think about eating less fat? What are the barriers to doing it?"

In the third stage, **preparation,** individuals are more determined to change and intending to take initial action soon, or in about 30 days (24, 25). They may report small changes in the problem behavior, such as reading a few food labels or buying fat-free ice cream. One may ask, "What, if any, changes have you planned or made in the past few weeks?"

Action, the fourth stage, is one in which people overcome the problem by actively modifying their habits, behaviors, environments, or experiences (24, 25). It is important to remember that a majority of clients are not in the action stage when referred for counseling. Considerable commitment of time and energy is required for the action stage when individuals are trying to change. One may ask, "What are you doing differently?"

The fifth stage, **maintenance,** is one in which people consolidate and stabilize gains made over several months in order to maintain the new, healthier habits and prevent relapse (24, 25). For some people, this stage continues for months, years, or a lifetime. One may ask, "How do you handle small lapses?"

The ultimate goal is the **termination** stage. However some types of problems, such as eating changes, require a lifetime of maintenance instead. People, for example, tend to become more sedentary and overweight as they age, contributing to continual problems.

Prochaska et al. proposed that people proceed through the stages in a spiral, rather than linear, fashion (24, 25). Because lapses and relapse are common problems, regression to an earlier stage may be expected several times as people struggle to modify or cease behaviors. Lapse and relapse and the negative emotional reactions (guilt, shame, failure) that may occur are discussed in more detail in a chapter on cognitions. Hopefully, people learn from their mistakes with the help of the counselor.

A second dimension of the model examines the processes of change when there are shifts in behaviors, attitudes, and intentions. When and how shifts occur has been studied. In a behavioral weight control program, the processes used early in treatment were the single best predictors of outcome (25, 26).

The processes of change should be integrated into the stages of change so that the treatment intervention matches the client's stage of change. In the early stages, focusing on the benefits of making a change and how that change can improve the individual's life is suggested. In precontemplation, consciousness-raising techniques, such as about the individual's risk for chronic disease based on dietary habits, and reevaluation of values, problems, self, and environment are appropriate. In the Seattle "5 A Day" worksite intervention to encourage employees to consume more fruits and vegetables, for

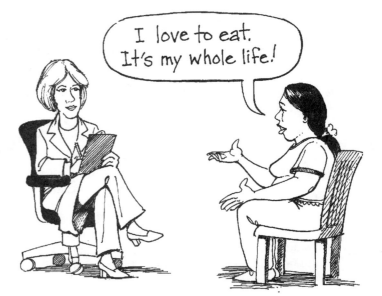

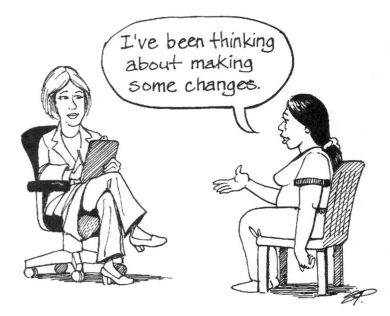

FIGURE 1.3. The dietetics professional's intervention should be matched to the client's stage of change.

example, a number of communication methods were used to move people from precontemplation to contemplation. They included posters, flyers, paycheck inserts, table tents in the cafeteria, and electronic mail (27).

Cognitive and affective self-reevaluation, in addition to consciousness raising, is suggested in the contemplation stage and self-liberation (a belief that one can change) and behavioral goals in the preparation stage. In action and maintenance stages, behavioral techniques of stimulus control, reinforcement management, recipe modification, coping responses during conditions when relapse is likely, and support from helping relationships are useful (28).

In counseling and education programs, to assume that everyone is at the action stage may lead one to plan an inappropriate intervention. The majority are likely to be at an earlier stage. Thus it is important to assess and identify the client's readiness to change and match the treatment intervention to it in order to achieve desired outcomes and success (29).

The stages of change model was used in defining the energy level of dietary fat in people's diets and was found to be effective in characterizing people by relative fat intake (29). Those in the stages of precontemplation to preparation may be expected to have higher intakes of fat than those in the action or maintenance stages (30). One study assessing stages of change in relationship to fat and fiber found that those on a higher fat intake were in the earlier stages (precontemplation, contemplation, and preparation) and those consuming less fat and more fiber, in the later stages (action and maintenance) (31).

The common approach of professionals who dispense more and more information to get people to change to more healthful eating behaviors is useless and needs modification. Giving out information does not always result in gains in knowledge, and nutrition knowledge does not necessarily lead to healthy food choices (32).

Using the stages of change model to achieve *Healthy People 2000* objectives of decreasing dietary fat and increasing fruit and vegetable consumption, Campbell et al. individually tailored messages using a computer and the individual's current dietary intake and self-reported stage of change (33). Changes in dietary fat intake were less affected by messages based on dietary guidelines than on those individually tailored to a person's stage of change. A variety of nutritional intervention strategies are needed at each stage.

When an individual deals with the necessity of change in food patterns and behaviors, knowledge and education are not in themselves sufficient to motivate change. Many people already know what they should eat! But they do not always act on their knowledge. The health professional cannot assume that recommendations will be followed just because the patient or client knows what to do. Why should any person change a lifetime of unrestricted eating that may be pleasurable? Wanting to make changes is a key point to consider in adopting changes in dietary practices. The person's motivation for change should be examined since people can be expected to resist change.

Several other factors influence success in planned change. Important characteristics of the regimen influencing adherence include complexity, effect on values and lifestyle, and cost. The more communicable something is (i.e., the easier to describe), the more clearly it is understood. Simplicity is an advantage, as increasing complexity of a regimen is associated with less readily adopted changes. The change must be compatible with the person's existing values and beliefs. If divisible into parts, a change may be tried out on a small scale so that any barriers can be worked out. For individuals who immigrated from another country, the eating habits of the new culture are one of the last factors to be assimilated (34). The change should have a relative advantage, or be perceived as preferable in efficiency, health, pleasure, economics, prestige, and the like. People want food that tastes good.

Pleasure or the absence of it may change the rate of acceptance of new practices. One problem is that many of the less nutritious foods, such as rich desserts, snack foods, and alcoholic beverages, have the highest prestige value. The influence of each factor on change is a relative one. Pleasure may be a major factor in some cases while cost or ease of food preparation is an important factor in another.

Group sessions are often used for nutrition education and for employee communication and training. The effect of support groups on change can be either positive or negative. Face-to-face communication with someone who has successfully altered a behavior can be effective in promoting the adoption of changes by others. While increasing knowledge and growing awareness may be developed in such groups, the actual change occurs through an individual's decision making.

DIETARY ADHERENCE

Dietetics practitioners are expected to promote good dietary adherence or compliance. Compliance may be defined as the extent to which the individual's food and dietary behaviors coincide with the dietary recommendations and prescriptions. It tells the extent to which individuals have been successful in integrating dietary changes and self-care behaviors into their day-to-day activities. In measuring compliance, some health professionals also consider whether or not appointments are kept. Human noncompliance dates back to the Biblical story of the Garden of Eden, where Eve ate the forbidden apple from the tree of knowledge, thus associating temptation and noncompliance with guilt and sin (35).

The term "compliance" has authoritarian overtones of a counselor deciding what is best for the individual, who is passive and compliant. The word "adherence" may suggest greater participation by the client in problem solving and decision making regarding dietary changes, which are voluntary behaviors. These terms, however, seem to be used interchangeably.

The individual must adopt dietary changes and sustain them over a period of time, often a lifetime if the condition is a chronic one such as diabetes mellitus, cardiovascular, or renal disease. The person is expected to make permanent changes to remain in optimum health. Diet may be only one of several changes the individual is expected to effect; additional changes related to smoking, drinking, or exercise habits, together with the need to take medications, may be seen as overwhelming.

Some responsibility for noncompliance rests with the professional. Although noncompliance may be viewed as failure on the patient's part to cooperate with recommendations, counselors are not excused from responsibility for other variables that are under their control, such as the quality of the client-counselor relationship and the use of appropriate influence strategies.

Noncompliance with medical advice has been well documented. Adherence to long-term medical regimens averages about 50% and to dietary regimens about 30%, with a range of 13 to 75% (35, 36). The figures suggest that some individuals abandon prescribed diets totally. In one report, only 2% of dietitians thought that most of their patients adhered to a prescribed diet following hospital discharge (37). Part of the problem was that dietitians did not aggressively pursue dietary counseling while patients were in the hospital, or did not take much initiative in planning for follow-up.

It is probably unrealistic to expect 100% adherence to dietary changes every day of the week. How many people have never been tempted to stray from eating nutritionally balanced meals every day of every month, including holidays and social occasions? The fact is that most have. Thus, short-term goals, such as following the diet two out of three meals daily or 4 days a week, may promote better adherence early in the counseling process; later, the regimen can be extended. Dietetics professionals know exactly what should be done and are steeped in the important reasons for dietary changes. Because they want the patient or client to be just as knowledgeable, they run the danger of setting unrealistic goals for change or giving too much information at one time, accomplishing less than they would by parceling out the recommendations over time.

Factors Influencing Adherence

The many factors influencing adherence to a prescribed dietary regimen are often reported and analyzed in terms of five sets of characteristics, those belonging to (a) the patient or client, (b) the relationship between the health care provider and the patient, (c) the clinical setting, (d) the treatment regimen, and (e) the features of the disease (38).

Some studies investigating demographic variables, such as age, sex, socioeconomic status, marital status, and the like, have not found that these variables predict compliance, although better comprehension of the regimen tends to be associated with higher educational levels. Recall and comprehension by the patient decrease in direct proportion to the amount of information given, probably because of supersaturation of the client with recommendations, or because of excessive anxiety on the client's part, which interferes with cognitive processes. Dispensing information over a period of time in small and manageable amounts, with repetition, should enhance recall. An imaginative combining of educational techniques, such as verbal and written instructions intermixed with visual aids, should also improve results (39).

Satisfaction with the level of care and with the attitude of the counselor have been reported to influence adherence. Problems may result if good rapport is not developed between the counselor and the client, with the counselor taking into consideration the person's concerns and expectations (40). The individual's interest level may be perfunctory, or appointments may be missed. Adherence may be more satisfactory if the patient sees the same counselor at each visit, and if clear-cut communication occurs so that the individual fully understands what is best and what is expected.

The characteristics of the clinic are also important. People kept waiting for long periods of time often fail to return for future appointments. A warm and caring environment, created by not only the counselor but also the entire office staff, puts clients into a frame of mind that enables them to benefit from their counseling.

The characteristics of the regimen are the most important factors in adherence. Of these, complexity is the most significant. Complexity of a regimen has been negatively associated with adherence, perhaps related to the difficulty of fitting the regimen into one's daily routine (41). Diets encompass many of the factors associated with a higher incidence of noncompliance. They include required changes in lifestyle, which tend to be restrictive, last a long duration or for a lifetime, and interfere with family habits (36). If other barriers exist, such as high cost of the diet, lack of access to the proper foods, or extra effort, time, and skill required in preparing the diet, the likelihood of nonadherence increases.

The nature of the illness is another variable. A serious, life-threatening problem, such as a heart attack, may convince an individual to make dietary and exercise changes, at least in the near term. A person with few overt symptoms, as in hypertension, may not see the need for adherence to a dietary regimen (38).

Assessing Adherence. Often assessment of adherence is difficult because it is based on indirect or subjective measures. Self-reports of the number of changes made with their frequency and duration, daily self-monitoring records of food intake, interviews such as diet histories and 24-hour recalls, and the professional's subjective judgment are used to collect data. All of these methods tend to be biased or inaccurate and may overestimate adherence. As a result, interviewing techniques that develop good rapport and are not threatening or judgmental to the client must be used if the practitioner is to receive honest, accurate information about adherence to dietary regimens. No completely reliable method of assessing adherence is available although clinical improvement may suggest it.

Strategies

What strategies can a counselor use to enhance client adherence along the path to long-term change and a

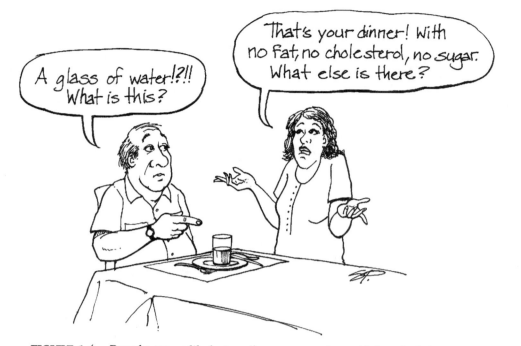

FIGURE 1.4.   People are unlikely to adhere to a regimen if they feel deprived.

healthy outcome? For long-term dietary change, one study recommended "goal setting and contingency contracting with goals and a time frame set by both parties, reminder calls, follow-up visits, self monitoring, and engaging in social support" (42). Using the stages of change model discussed earlier, as well as relapse prevention strategies and self-efficacy, discussed in later chapters, were also recommended.

The MDRD study (Modification of Diet in Renal Disease) found that the most effective element of intervention in producing dietary adherence to goals was the process of "self monitoring" of daily protein intake. It enhanced patient self-management by allowing individuals to identify targeted nutrient sources in their diets and then to develop strategies for modifying their eating behaviors to achieve desired goals (43). Psychosocial factors related to adherence included knowledge, attitudes, support, satisfaction, and self-perceptions of success. Adherence was measured on the basis of dietary protein intake data from self-reports and urinary excretion (44).

A third study also recommended self-monitoring along with goal setting and behavioral self-management (41). When areas in need of improvement are identified by self-monitoring, they can be translated into short-term, attainable goals for change. Social support by family members included in counseling sessions was also suggested.

Health Belief Model

People hold various beliefs about their health that may influence adherence to a dietary regimen more than their state of knowledge. The "Health Belief Model," which

attempts to explain preventive health behavior, was developed originally to interpret the decisions of people not currently suffering disease, but wishing to prevent health problems (45). It has been extended to more general adherence. It is one of several theories attempting to explain dietary behavior change.

The model postulates that the person's beliefs about health are determinants of his or her readiness to take action. The three key beliefs are (a) the extent to which the person believes that he is "susceptible" to contracting a specific disease, "has the disease" now, or is "resusceptible" in the case of an illness from which he has recovered; (b) how serious he thinks the disease is or its consequences are in having a negative effect on his life; and (c) what he perceives are the benefits of changing health behaviors in terms of reducing susceptibility to or severity of the disease, as compared to the psychological costs and barriers to taking action (38).

A woman with diabetes, for example, should believe that she has diabetes and is susceptible to serious complications, such as retinopathy; that adherence to the dietary and medical regimen will reduce the likelihood of serious complications; that she has the ability to comply; and that the benefits of adherence outweigh the costs. Of course, many individuals use denial as a defense mechanism and do not acknowledge that these consequences can happen to them. A man diagnosed with a high serum cholesterol level and made aware of its relationship to coronary heart disease may or may not decide to reduce the amount of fat and cholesterol in his diet, based on his health beliefs.

If the individual views taking action as time consuming, difficult, unpleasant, expensive, inconvenient, destroying quality of life, or upsetting, denial and avoidance motives may serve as barriers to change. If there are destructive beliefs, it is necessary to understand them and to facilitate more constructive ones. Best results are obtained when readiness to act is high and when physical, psychological, financial, and other barriers are low. The model has been used to study compliant behavior.

A study of individuals with diabetes found that those adhering to dietary plans were more health oriented, and they believed that diabetes was a threat to their health (46). Not everyone makes food choices based solely on health beliefs, however.

A Survey of American Dietary Habits found that Americans' primary reason for concern about diet and nutrition was general health maintenance (47). The gap between perceived importance of nutrition and care in selection of foods for a healthful diet widened between 1991 and 1993, however, showing that people were implementing their beliefs less frequently.

The pleasure of eating, perceived quality of life, cost considerations, accessibility, and social and cultural practices are examples of other factors affecting food choices. One needs to ask, "What does the individual value?" "Does the individual believe that personal actions can modify the threat?" "Does the individual feel capable of carrying out the recommended actions?" Self-efficacy is discussed in a later chapter.

In the Multiple Risk Factor Intervention Trial (MRFIT), groups of middle-aged men received nutrition counseling to alter food behaviors in an attempt to reduce the risk of coronary heart disease. In promoting adherence and assessing dietary compliance, two methods utilized were a food score and food diaries (48, 49).

Nutritionists developed a food-scoring system for participant behavioral self-monitoring based on the cholesterogenic composition of foods. Participants became versed in assessing their own food scores and could evaluate their food choices, thus providing a tool for positive reinforcement of proper food behaviors. Effective change in participants' food behaviors depended on the ability to recognize proper foods with low scores and substitute them for foods with higher scores, a process providing awareness and insight. Individual counseling encouraged achievement of a specific guideline score. The scores became an objective means of assessing dietary adherence and understanding (48).

In summary, no one intervention is successful all of the time in promoting dietary adherence. Feelings of personal control, self-efficacy, social support, self-monitoring, perceived threat of a disease, perceived benefits from changing behaviors, and other factors should be included in one's intervention strategies as well as into the stages of change (50). Goal setting, relapse prevention, stimulus control, and cognitive restructuring may be helpful. A comprehensive approach by the professional considering many of these factors is more likely to be successful.

ADMINISTRATIVE/MANAGEMENT DIETETICS

Those with administrative and managerial responsibilities need effective communication and education skills for personal relationships with subordinates and others on the management team in the administration of increasingly complex food-service systems. The manager deals extensively with employees and is expected to build good human relationships. Communication is described as "the key" to every relationship with each employee, and the quality of the relationships "largely determines the performance level of that employee" (51). Although one may "develop" human relations skills, there is no substitute for sincerity. A fundamental factor in interpersonal relations is the trust between the superior and the subordinate.

There are a number of interrelated management functions in which communication is important. They include hiring and staffing; conducting staff orientation and training; leadership, including motivation; performance appraisals; morale and productivity; handling employee dissatisfaction; and managing change in the organization.

The manager is expected to develop communication networks and to maintain effective horizontal and vertical lines of communication within the organization and the surrounding community. The manager needs to be skillful in verbal and nonverbal communication, in both speaking and listening, and in recognizing and eliminating barriers to effective communication. A study of members of the Dietitians in Business and Industry practice group and prospective and current employers of dietitians found that both employers and dietitians identified communication skills as "the most influential attribute affecting the employment of dietitians in business and industry" (52).

Education skills are important in the planning, implementation, and evaluation of training programs designed to help achieve the employee's personal goals as well as organizational objectives. In staffing the organization, identified positions are filled by the use of structured interviews with applicants. The new employees selected must be oriented and trained. The manager is also responsible for continuous education of current employees and for in-service education.

Increasingly, the autocratic leadership styles of the past have been replaced by more participative approaches. Employee-centered supervisors recognize the importance of allowing more subordinate participation in decision making. One advantage is that people are more likely to accept decisions that they have participated in making. In addition, supportive and participative approaches may produce better results in terms of productivity, morale, motivation, and lessened absenteeism. Management is concerned not only with what employees can do, but with what they will do, which depends on several forces in the work environment that influence motivation.

Effective communication skills are essential in day-to-

CASE STUDY

John Miller, aged 48 years, was referred by his physician to Joan Stivers, RD, as a result of a serum cholesterol level of 320 mg/dl. He is 6'0" tall and weighs 250 pounds.

Mr. Miller has a family history of heart disease. His older brother died of a heart attack. He is married with two children aged 20 and 24 years. His wife is employed full-time and so did not come to the appointment with him.

During the interview Mr. Miller stated, "I know I have a bad family history. I also know that I have put on a few pounds in recent years and should try to lose them. But after a day at work, I enjoy my dinner."

1. What stage of change is Mr. Miller in?
2. How would you match your nutritional intervention to his stage of change?

day dealings with peers and subordinates. This type of communication is utilized, for example, in discussing with employees the goals of the organization, work that needs to be done, policies, procedures, changes, problems that may be resolved through employee counseling, and performance appraisals. One-on-one communication with employees can have an important effect on employee attitudes and behavior.

The manager works not only with individuals, but also with groups. Communication may be facilitated through the use of meetings and conferences. Meetings may be used to dispense or collect information and for problem solving and decision making. Understanding the nature of groups and group process is essential. Knowledge of the social groupings of employees is necessary for creating conditions that will elicit cooperation, thus maximizing the attainment of organizational goals.

SUMMARY

All dietetics practitioners need to be confident of their abilities in patient/client and employee interactions. In addition to their scientific and technical competence, professionals are expected to be skilled in interpersonal relations. With patients and clients, a comprehensive approach considering psychological, cultural, environmental, and behavioral factors is needed in influencing dietary changes for the betterment of the individual's health (50). Clearly, information about proper diet is insufficient in changing dietary behaviors. The professional must be able to use a number of intervention strategies, including the helping process model, the health belief model, and stages of change in promoting adherence.

The following chapters offer a number of interventions including counseling theories and principles, behavior modification including stimulus control and reinforcement, family and social support, goal setting, self-monitoring, cognitive restructuring, self-efficacy, relapse prevention, motivation, and education. While nutrition education gives important information on **what** to do, other interventions are necessary in assisting people in **how** to make successful lifestyle changes.

REVIEW AND DISCUSSION QUESTIONS

1. How do dietetics professionals use communication skills?

2. What are the major divisions of dietetics practice?
3. What dietetics practice groups are of interest to you?
4. What is a helping profession?
5. What does helping involve?
6. What should be the relationship between the helper and client or helpee?
7. What are Prochaska's six stages of change?
8. What processes of change should be integrated at each of the six stages of change?
9. What five factors influence dietary adherence?
10. What strategies can be used to promote better dietary adherence?

SUGGESTED ACTIVITIES

1. Divide the group into pairs for a 10-minute walk. For the first 5 minutes, have one person close his eyes and permit himself to be guided by his partner without speaking. After 5 minutes, reverse roles and have the other person become the helper. Discuss the feelings of the helper and those of the person being helped. What were the attitudes toward helping and the feelings of trust?

2. From the dietetic practice areas mentioned in the chapter, select a subspecialty area of practice, and interview a dietitian or nutritionist about his or her responsibilities, including the use of communication skills and education skills. Share this information with peers.

3. With someone trying to make changes in food practices (such as dieting), discuss the changes and the factors influencing change, including barriers. What are the factors influencing the person's adherence?

4. Select a dietary regimen, such as increased fiber, restricted sodium, low calorie, or low fat and cholesterol, and follow it for 7 days. Keep a daily record of all foods eaten. How easy or difficult was it to comply with the diet for a week? What factors helped or hindered your adherence?

REFERENCES

1. Parks SC, Schwartz NE. National nutrition month—focus on healthy eating and fitness. J Am Diet Assoc 1994;94: 329.

2. Position of the American Dietetic Association: nutrition services in health maintenance organizations and other forms of managed care. J Am Diet Assoc 1993;93:1171.

3. Balch GI. Employer's perceptions of the roles of dietetics practitioners: challenges to survive and opportunities to thrive. J Am Diet Assoc 1996;96:1301.

4. Sullivan BJ, Schiller MR, Horvath MC. Nutrition education and counseling: knowledge and skill levels expected by dietetic internship directors. J Am Diet Assoc 1990;90:1418.

5. Identifying patients at risk: ADA's definitions for nutrition screening and nutrition assessment. J Am Diet Assoc 1994;94:838.

6. ADA is proactive on mid-course review of promoting health/preventing disease: objectives for the nation. J Am Diet Assoc 1986;86:378.

7. Position of The American Dietetic Association: nutrition education for the public. J Am Diet Assoc 1996;96:1183.

8. Kane MT, Cohen AS, Smith ER, et al. 1995 Commission on dietetic registration dietetics practice audit. J Am Diet Assoc 1996;96:1292.

9. Council on practice announces name changes. J Am Diet Assoc 1992;92:154.

10. Kane MT, Estes CA, Colton DA, et al. Role delineation study for entry-level registered dietitians, entry-level dietetic technicians, and beyond-entry-level registered dietitians. Chicago: American Dietetic Assoc, 1989; Vols. 1-3.

11. Martin JB, Holcomb JD, Mullen PD. Health promotion and disease prevention beliefs and behaviors of dietetic practitioners. J Am Diet Assoc 1987;87:609.

12. Meyer MK, Olsen MS. Productivity of the clinical dietitian: measurement by a regression model. J Am Diet Assoc 1989;89:490.

13. Klevans DR, Parett JL. Continuing professional education needs of clinical dietitians in Pennsylvania. J Am Diet Assoc 1990;90:282.

14. Baird SC, Sylvester J. Role delineation and verification for entry-level positions in community dietetics. Chicago: American Dietetic Assoc, 1983.

15. Hess AN, Haughton B. Continuing education needs for public health nutritionists. J Am Diet Assoc 1996;96:716.

16. Baird SC, Sylvester J: Role delineation and verification for entry-level positions in foodservice systems management. Chicago: American Dietetic Assoc, 1983.

17. Cluskey M, Messersmith AM. Instructional model for building qualitative management skills. J Am Diet Assoc 1990;90:1271.

18. Hahn NI. Home is where the jobs are. J Am Diet Assoc 1996;96:332.

19. Arensberg MBF, Schiller MR. Dietitians in home care: a survey of current practice. J Am Diet Assoc 1006;96:347.

20. Parks SC, Fitz PA, Maillet JO, et al. Challenging the future of dietetics education and credentialing—dialogue, discovery, and directions: a summary of the 1994 future search conference. J Am Diet Assoc 1995;95:598.

21. Trudeau E, Dube L. Moderators and determinants of satisfaction with diet counseling for patients consuming a therapeutic diet. J Am Diet Assoc 1995;95:34.

22. Henderson G. Physician-patient communication. Springfield: Charles C. Thomas, 1981.

23. Schlundt DG, Quesenberry L, Pichert JW, et al. Evaluation of a training program for improving adherence promotion skills. Pat Educ Counsel 1994;24: 165.

24. Prochaska JO, DiClemente CC, Norcross JC. In search of how people change: Applications to addictive behaviors. Am Psychol 1992;47:1102.

25. Prochaska JO, Norcross JC, DiClemente CC. Changing for good. New York: William Morrow, 1994.

26. Prochaska JO, Norcross JC, Fowler JL, et al. Attendance and outcome in a work-site weight control program: processes and stages of change as process and predictor variables. Addict Behav 1992;17:35.

27. Thompson B, Shannon J, Beresford SA, et al. Implementation aspects of the Seattle "5 a Day" intervention project: strategies to help employees make dietary changes. Top Clin Nutr 1995;11:58.

28. Greene GW, Rossi SR, Reed GR, et al. Stages of change for reducing dietary fat to 30% of energy or less. J Am Diet Assoc 1994;94:1105.

29. Sandoval WM, Heller K, Wiese WH, et al. Stages of change: a model for nutrition counseling. Top Clin Nutr 1994;9:64.

30. Sigman-Grant M. Stages of change: a framework for nutrition interventions. Nutr Today 1996;31:162.

31. Glanz K, Patterson RE, Kristal AR, et al. Stages of change in adopting healthy diets: fat, fiber and correlates of nutrient intake. Health Educ Q 1994;21:499.

32. Cronin FF, Achterberg C, Sims LS. Translating nutrition facts into action: helping consumers use the new food label. Nutr Today 1993;28:30.

33. Campbell MK, DeVellis BM, Strecher VJ, et al. Improving dietary behavior: the effectiveness of tailored messages in primary care settings. Am J Public Health 1994;84: 783.

34. Brownell KD, Cohen LR. Adherence to dietary regimens 1: An overview of research. Behav Med 1995;20:149.

35. Haynes RB. Introduction. In: Haynes RB, Taylor DW, Sackett DL, eds. Compliance in health care. Baltimore: Johns Hopkins Univ Pr, 1979.

36. Glanz K. Trends in patient compliance. Chicago: American Dietetic Assoc, 1981.

37. Schiller MR. Current hospital practices in clinical dietetics. J Am Diet Assoc 1984;84:1194.

38. Meichenbaum D, Turk DC. Facilitating treatment adherence: a practitioner's guidebook. New York: Plenum, 1987.

39. Wedman B, Kahan RD. Diabetes graphic aids used in counseling improve patient compliance. J Am Diet Assoc 1987;87:1672.

40. Hogan SE, Gates RD, MacDonald FW, et al. Experience with adolescents with phenylketonuria returned to phenylalanine-restricted diets. J Am Diet Assoc 1986;86: 1203.

41. McCann BS, Retzlaff BM, Dowdy AA, et al. Promoting adherence to low-fat, low cholesterol diets. Review and recommendations. J Am Diet Assoc 1990;90:1408.

42. Gilboy MB. Compliance-enhancing counseling strategies for cholesterol management. J Nutr Educ 1994;26:228.

43. Snetselaar L. New directions in nutrition for the renal patient. Perspect Appl Nutr 1994;1:3.

44. Milas NC, Nowalk MP, Akpele L, et al. Factors associated

with adherence to the dietary protein intervention in the Modification of Diet in Renal Disease Study. J Am Diet Assoc 1995;95:1295.

45. Rosenstock IM. Historical origins of the health belief model. Health Educ Monographs 1974;2:328.

46. Kouris A, Wahlquist ML, Worsley A. Characteristics that enhance adherence to high-carbohydrate/high-fiber diets by persons with diabetes. J Am Diet Assoc 1988;88:1422.

47. Morreale SJ, Schwartz NE. Helping Americans eat right: developing practical and actionable public nutrition education messages based on the ADA survey of American dietary habits. J Am Diet Assoc 1995;95:305.

48. Remmell PS, Gorder DD, Hall Y et al. Assessing dietary adherence in the Multiple Risk Factor Intervention Trial (MRFIT). J Am Diet Assoc 1980;76:351.

49. Remmell PS, Benfari RC. Assessing dietary adherence in the Multiple Risk Factor Intervention Trial (MRFIT). J Am Diet Assoc 1980;76:357.

50. Brownell KD, Cohen LR. Adherence to dietary regimens 2: components of effective interventions. Behav Med 1995;20:155.

51. Matejka JK, Dunsing RJ. Opening doors: good relationships as good management. Personnel J 1988;65: 74.

52. Kirk D, Shanklin CW, Gorman MA. Attributes and qualifications that employers seek when hiring dietitians in business and industry. J Am Diet Assoc 1989;89:494.

two

COMMUNICATION

American education has traditionally emphasized two communication skills, reading and writing, and ignored two others, speaking and listening. Consequently, many people today have grown up with the false assumption that speaking and listening are natural, that because one hears, one listens, and that because one speaks, one has speaking skills.

In all of the "helping professions," speaking and listening skills correlate with the professionals' effectiveness with clients and staff. Regardless of the physicians', nurses', or dietetics practitioners' desire to help, if they are unable to relate well on a one-to-one basis with clients and staff, they are likely to be perceived as ineffective. The trust, cooperation, and confidence of helpees are positively related to their perceptions of the caring and interest, as demonstrated through the helpers' interpersonal communication.

During the last five years a spate of studies has been done in the health professions to examine the "communication variable" as it relates to the myriad of other variables in the health care environment (1–18). Recent research reported that both employers and dietitians ranked communication skills as essential to success in business and industry positions (19). Other studies in the literature have stressed the need for professionals to develop communication skills, pointing out that individuals who develop these skills are able to establish better relationships with both clients and staff (20, 21). The need for contemporary managers and their employees to learn how to problem-solve, resolve conflicts, think creatively, listen, and, above all, communicate effectively has been well documented (22–24).

Communication Defined. The term "**communication**" is something of an enigma. Although everyone communicates, the concept is so expansive that it is difficult to define. In a broad sense, communication includes all methods that can convey thought or feeling between persons. The *Journal of Communication* has published no less than 15 working definitions of human communication (25). From among the definitions, two common elements emerge: *(a)* communication is the process of sending and receiving messages, and *(b)* for a transmission of ideas to be successful, a mutual understanding between the communicator and the listener must occur.

Effective communication can be operationally defined for dietetics practitioners as the ability to use language that is appropriate to the clients' and staffs' level of understanding, making sure that they have enough knowledge but are not overwhelmed; the ability to develop a relationship between themselves and their clients and staff; the ability to talk to them in a way that relieves anxiety; the ability to communicate to them in a way that assures their being able to recall information actively; and the ability to provide them with feedback.

This chapter discusses communication as a process, examines its components, and points out applications for practitioners. A model of the communication process is presented and discussed, followed by an explanation of the implications of the process for the verbal, nonverbal, and listening behaviors of the dietitian and dietetic technician. The topics of negotiating and communicating with legislators are also discussed, with the chapter concluding in a discussion of the barriers to communication.

Possessing only an intellectual appreciation of the various communication skills is of little use. Some sciences, such as mathematics, physics, chemistry, and biology, can be mastered by learning principles; the applied social sciences cannot. Being able to pass a test by explaining how one ought to interact with clients and staff, how to defuse their hostility, and how to create a supportive communication climate with them is not the same as actually being able to do it. Putting the principles into practice requires a conscious effort, repeated attempts, and months of trial. With practice, in a relatively short time, people can notice a difference in the way others respond to them. Honing the skills, however, needs to be an ongoing process, beginning with an understanding of the many elements included in the interpersonal communication transaction.

INTERPERSONAL COMMUNICATION MODEL

Complicated processes are easier to grasp when they can be visualized in a model. A model, however, is not the same as the actual phenomenon; rather, it is a graphic depiction to aid understanding. The elements included

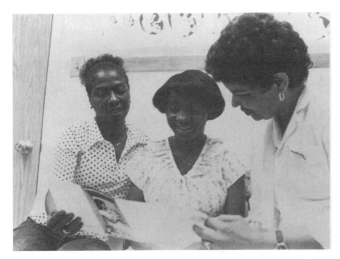

FIGURE 2.1. Communicating with clients requires both verbal and written skills.

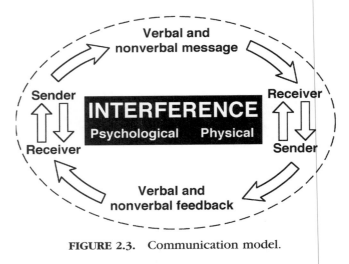

FIGURE 2.3. Communication model.

in the human communication model are the following: sender, receiver, the message itself—verbal and nonverbal—feedback, and interference. They are depicted graphically in Figure 2.3.

Components of the Communication Model

Sender. Senders of the messages are the first persons to speak, the ones who initiate the communication.

Receiver. Receivers of the message, listeners, usually interpret and transmit simultaneously. They may be listening to what is being said and thinking about what they are going to say when the senders stop talking. Even when silent, it is impossible for receivers in a two-way communication transaction not to communicate. They may be reacting physiologically with a flushed face or trembling hands, or in some other way, depending on their inferences from the message. Senders make infer-

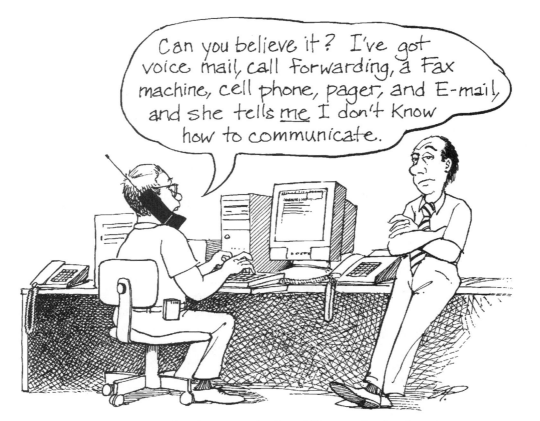

FIGURE 2.2. Good communication skills must be developed.

ences based on the receivers' appearance and demeanor and adjust subsequent communication accordingly.

Message. The receiver interprets two messages simultaneously: the actual verbal message and the nonverbal message inferred from the sender and the environment. Nonverbal inferences arise from the perceived emotional tone of the sender's voice, facial expression, dress, choice of words, diction, and pronunciation, as well as from the communication environment.

Feedback. The term "feedback" refers to the process of responding to messages after interpreting them for oneself. It is the key ingredient that distinguishes two-way from one-way communication. In two-way, face-to-face communication, the sender is talking, while looking at the other. The other's reactions to the sender's message, whether agreement, surprise, boredom, or hostility, are examples of feedback. Unless the communication channel is kept clear for feedback, distortion occurs, leaving the sender unable to detect accurately how the message is received (26).

In written communication, writers cannot clarify for readers because they do not see them. Even when writers carefully select words for the benefit of their intended readers, written communication is generally less effective than one-to-one verbal communication because of its inability to re-explain and adjust language in response to the feedback from receivers.

Interpersonal communication, after the first few seconds, becomes a simultaneous two-way sending and receiving process. While senders are talking, they are receiving nonverbal reactions from receivers. Based on these reactions they may change their tone, speak louder, use simpler language, or in some other way adjust their communication so that their message is better understood.

Interference. This term is used to denote multiple factors of the communicators (sender and receiver) and of their environment that affect the interpretation of messages. These factors include the unique attributes inherent in each individual; the room size, shape, and color; temperature; furniture arrangement; and the physiological state of each communicator at the moment. The sophisticated communicator needs to understand these contingencies and to compensate for them, when possible, so that the intended message is the one received.

A crying baby, the sound of thunder, and low-flying planes, for example, not only can hinder the receiver in hearing the sender's message, but also can generate messages and interpretations in the receiver that were never intended by the sender. Another source of interference is the physiological state of the communicators at the moment. No two bodies are exactly alike. Because no one has shared in the exact life experience of another, no two people understand language in precisely the same way.

Distortions can stem from psychological interference as well, including bias, prejudice, and being closed-minded. Psychological interference in health care pa-

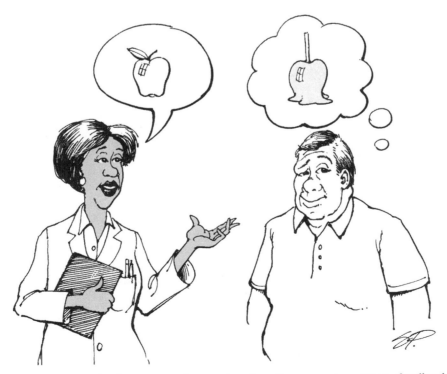

FIGURE 2.4. To determine whether or not the receiver has the correct message, feedback is necessary.

tients and clients is often due to fear of illness and its consequences (27). The job of senders is to generate in receivers those meanings for language that are closest to their own. Because meanings are not universal, they can be affected by external as well as internal influences. Communication environment, the distance between speakers, lighting, temperature, and colors are a few of the variables that can affect meanings ascribed to a message. These variables can be sources of interference and major factors in accounting for difficulty in generating in others the same meanings people intend. Toward the end of this chapter, under the heading "Barriers to Effective Communication," additional physical and psychological forms of interference are discussed.

VERBAL AND NONVERBAL COMMUNICATION

Verbal communication includes the actual words selected by the sender and the way in which these symbols are arranged into thought units. Nonverbal communication includes the communication environment, the manner and style in which the communication is delivered, and the internal qualities inherent in the sender and receiver that influence their interpretation of external stimuli. Although verbal and nonverbal communication occur simultaneously during interaction, each is discussed separately here in the context of their influence on the communication process. The salient point to remember here is that the lack of clear communication by the dietetics practitioner is the most common cause of poor employee performance. Conscious and clear communication is the key to every good relationship, with both clients and staff (28).

Employees are often hesitant to approach their supervisors, even if the superiors have explicit open-door policies. In order to open real lines of communication, certain companies have begun "Operation Speak-easy." This new form of meeting brings a group of employees together once a month with two or three top managers. The employees, who change monthly, serve as presenters from their departments, bringing forth suggestions, concerns, and questions (29). While this system is proving effective, it can only work in a supportive climate, which generally emanates from the management level.

To keep the communication channel open between the client or employee and the dietitian or dietetic technician, the professional needs to know how to create a supportive climate. A supportive climate is one where as one person speaks, the other listens, attending to the message rather than to her own internal thoughts and feelings.

Although maintaining a supportive climate is always a concern, it becomes especially crucial when the professional is attempting to discuss a topic the client or employee views differently, or attempting to resolve conflict and defuse anger. The behavioral sciences offer suggestions on what one can do verbally and nonverbally to create a supportive climate under conditions of hostility or stress (30).

Verbal Communication

When attempting to resolve conflict, sustaining a supportive climate is critical. Conflict can be positive and act as the catalyst to move a relationship forward. Contemporary organizational theory, in fact, states that conflict is essential for organizational development (31–33).

The verbal guidelines for creating a supportive communication climate are: *(a)* to discuss problems descriptively rather than evaluatively; *(b)* to describe situations with a problem orientation rather than in a manipulative way; *(c)* to offer alternatives provisionally rather than dogmatically; *(d)* to treat clients as equals rather than as persons of lower rank than oneself; and *(e)* to be empathic rather than neutral or self-centered.

Descriptive Rather than Evaluative. Ordinarily, when approaching topics that tend to provoke defensiveness in clients, professionals should think through the discussion prior to engaging the client, so that the problem area is exposed descriptively rather than evaluatively.

Whenever people hear others judging their attitudes, work, or behavior, they show an increased tendency to become defensive. Such comments as "You don't seem to be trying," "You don't care about cooperating," or "You are selfish" are based on inferences rather than facts. So when the other says, "I do care," "I am too trying," or "I am not selfish," the framework for an argument is set, with no way of proving objectively who is right or wrong. Instead of making judgments regarding another's attitudes, the safest and least offensive way of dealing with a touchy issue is to describe the facts as objectively as possible. For example, the professional tells a client that his continuing to eat four pork chops and a half pound of chocolates a day is frustrating to her as the client's diet counselor. The professional is confronting the problem honestly and objectively without being evaluative. The client can then address the topic of overeating rather than argue the professional's negative evaluation of poor attitude, lack of concern, or noncooperativeness.

Accusing an employee who has arrived late several mornings of being "irresponsible" and "uncaring" is likely to provoke a hostile refutation or cold silence. The employee may believe that being late does not warrant a reprimand. There may, in fact, be a reasonable explanation. Describing how being late is frustrating, causing problems to those who depend upon the employee, and causing work to back up, is honest, descriptive, and allows for nondefensive dialogue.

Problem-Oriented Rather than Manipulative. Orienting people to a problem rather than manipulating them promotes a supportive communication climate. Frequently, when people want others to appreciate their point of view, they lead them through a series of questions until the other reaches the "appropriate" insight. This is a form of manipulation and provokes defensiveness as soon as respondents realize they are being channeled to share the other's vision. It goes something like this:

"Three weeks ago I believe you told me you gained weight on the diet because your metabolism is slow, correct? Two weeks ago you told me that you gained weight because the diet itself was faulty, correct? We checked your metabolism, and it is normal, and I have assured you that someone of your size could not gain weight on 1200 calories a day. Today you tell me that you ate salty popcorn last night and that your weight gain for the third consecutive week is all water, correct? If you were dealing with a client like yourself, would you begin to get the feeling that this person is making a fool out of you?"

A discussion with the client would probably be more productive if the practitioner took a direct problem-oriented approach:

"In 3 weeks on a 1200-calorie diet you have gained 1 pound per week. After checking the results of your laboratory tests, I am certain that the diet should have caused a weight loss of 4 to 5 pounds. There seems to be a problem here. Let's discuss what the other possibilities might be."

Employees and clients respect professionals, even when they disagree with them, when they believe the professional is being straightforward and authentic. A slick, manipulative style ordinarily can be seen through immediately and causes others to become disdainful (28).

Although opening remarks should be planned descriptively rather than evaluatively, the practitioner, after making them, should allow for spontaneous problem solving without preplanned solutions. Creative, superior, and long-lasting solutions are more likely to occur when each person hears the other out fully and is heard in return. When one is intent on "selling" a solution, there is a natural disposition on the part of the other to block out conflicting opinions. The problem-solving process is discussed in detail in other chapters.

In the example of the previous paragraphs, the practitioner's subsequent remarks depend on how the client or employee responds to the directive to explain the underlying problem. The professional might need to wait several minutes for an answer. Providing excuses or putting words into the other's mouth is a mistake. The practitioner needs to learn the discipline of sitting supportively through the tension of silence until the client or employee responds. Frequently, the first explanations are those that people believe will not upset or shock the professional. The "real" reasons, however, may not be revealed until the client or staff member feels secure enough to risk shocking the professional without fear of being humiliated or embarrassed. After the first explanations are offered, dietitians or dietetic technicians would do best simply to repeat in their own words what was understood. Only when the clients or employees are comfortable enough, will they be able to express their authentic reactions, questions, or answers, these ordinarily being less logical, more emotional, and more risky to expose.

Provisional Rather than Dogmatic. When offering advice to clients or helping them to solve problems, the professional should give advice provisionally rather than dogmatically. "Provisionally" implies the possibility of the practitioner changing options, provided additional facts emerge. It keeps the door open for clients to add information. When advice is offered in a dogmatic way, it becomes threatening for clients or employees to challenge or to add their own information. A dogmatic prescription might be, "This is what you must do. I know this is the way to solve your problem." A provisional prescription might be, "Here is one thing you might consider," or "There may be other ways of handling this problem; perhaps you have some ideas too, but this is one thing you might consider."

Egalitarian Rather than Superior. In discussing problems, clients and professionals should regard each other as equals. Whenever the possibility of defensiveness exists, even between persons of equal rank, any verbal or nonverbal behavior that the other interprets as an attempt to emphasize superiority generates a defensive response. In the relationship between professionals and clients, or managers and employees, the dietitian's tendencies to emphasize status or rank may arise unconsciously from a desire to convince the other to accept their recommendations. Comments such as the following may cause the other to feel inferior, hurt, or angry: "As a lay person, you might not be able to grasp the theory, but it works," or "Just do what I ask; I've been doing this for 10 years." Certainly, there is nothing wrong with professionals letting clients know that they are trained and competent. In fact, clients often need and appreciate the reassurance. The manner in which it is done is crucial, however. A more effective and subtle way to solve problems with a client is to say, "I have studied this problem and dealt with other clients who have similar symptoms. I am interested, however, in incorporating your own insights and plans into our solution. You must be satisfied and will have to live with the diet, so please express your views too."

An employee making a recommendation to a manager that the manager had tried unsuccessfully many years ago might be told, "If I was in your shoes, I would think the same thing. Someday when you are more experienced, you'll know why it won't work." The subtle underscoring of the inferior relative status of the subordinate could be enough to cause a defensive battle. The professional would have done far better with a comment such as "I can understand why you say that. I have thought the same myself, but when I tried, it was not successful." Here the employee is left feeling reinforced and appreciated rather than humiliated. Showing respect for the clients' and employees' intelligence and life experiences and recognizing the human dignity in them facilitates receiving their cooperation.

In conflict resolution, problem solving, and the discussion of any issues that may be threatening to the client or employee, collaboration is far more effective than trying to persuade the individual to act according to the dictates of the professional. Collaboration has other virtues as well. People feel more obligation to uphold those solutions that they themselves have participated in designing. If individuals are trying the professional's solution, they may feel little satisfaction in proving the dietitian was right; however, if the solution is one that was arrived at through collaboration, there is genuine satisfaction in proving its validity. An additional reason for practitioners to involve others in problem solving is that often a valid solution that is superior to any the individual or professional would have discovered alone can be arrived at through collaboration. Two people sharing insights, knowledge, experience, and feelings can generate creative thought processes in each other, which in turn generate other ideas that would not otherwise have emerged.

Empathic Rather than "Neutral." Another verbal skill essential to maintaining a supportive climate is the ability to put oneself in the other's shoes. For a helping professional, however, that is not enough. To be effective in working with clients and employees, dietetics practitioners must be able to demonstrate in some way their desire to understand what it is those they are helping are feeling. This "demonstration" might be an empathic response to their comments. In an empathic response, the listener tells the other that he or she is attempting to understand not only the speaker's content, but also the underlying feelings. For example, a client might say, "For my entire life I have eaten spicy foods; they are a part of my culture. I don't know what my life will be like without them." The professional might then respond, "You feel worried that the quality of your life will change because of the severe dietary restrictions."

If the professional is accurate in her empathic remarks, the client will acknowledge it and probably go on talking, assured of being with a helper who listens. If the professional is wrong, however, the client will clarify the judgment and continue to talk, assured of being with a helper who cares. Thus, the dietetics practitioner need not be accurate in her inferences of the other's feelings as long as she is willing to try to understand them. In addition, empathic responses allow the professional to respond without giving advice, focusing instead on the individual's need to talk and to express feelings and concerns. Before clients or employees can listen to the professional,

they must express all of their concerns; otherwise, while the practitioner is talking, the clients or employees are thinking about what they will say when she stops.

An employee who has asked to be released from work on a busy weekend to attend a concert out of town might receive the following neutral response: "No offense, but a rule is a rule. If I make an exception for you, others will expect it." Alternatively, the employee would still feel sad about working but would feel less antagonistic toward the supervisor if he were to receive the following empathic response: "I realize how badly you feel about not being able to attend the concert, particularly because your girlfriend gave you the tickets as a birthday gift. I feel terrible myself having to refuse your request. I am truly sorry, but I can't afford to let you off." The supervisor, by letting the subordinate know that she has understood the employee's underlying feelings and that she is sympathetic, uses the most effective means of defusing the subordinate's anger or antagonism. There is additional discussion of empathy in other chapters of this text.

Paraphrasing, a Critical Skill for Dietetics Professionals. Most people have not incorporated the skill of paraphrasing into their communication repertoire. Even after a person realizes how vital this step is, and begins to practice it, he may feel uncomfortable. Often the person just beginning to use paraphrasing in his interactions feels self-conscious and fears others may be insulted or think he is "showing off" his professional communication skills. This fear itself, unfortunately, causes some people to alienate others, while trying to communicate with them. A hint for the professional feeling awkward about asking clients and staff to paraphrase would be to ask for the paraphrase by acknowledging the need to verify that what was heard is what the other intended. The dietetics practitioner might say, for example:

"I know that I don't always grasp everything immediately, and that frequently, I need to repeat what I think I have understood. My instructions today may be a bit complicated for someone who has never had to count food carbohydrates before. Just to be sure the instructions are understood as intended, would you mind explaining in your own words how you plan to manage this diet?"

Of course, it takes less time to ask, "Have you got it?" Asking this question is less effective, however. Because of the perceived status distinction between the helper and the person being helped, the latter may be ashamed to admit that he has not understood. Perhaps in the back of the client's mind is the thought that this can be read about later or that the patient in the next bed can be asked for an explanation after the professional leaves the room. When persons of perceived higher status ask others if they "understand," almost always the answer is,

"Yes." Another possibility is that the client or staff member honestly believes that he has understood, and for that reason has answered, "Yes." This understanding, however, may include some alteration of the original message, in the form of substitution, distortion, addition, or subtraction. The skill of paraphrasing needs to become "second nature" and automatic for the professional dietitian in verifying important instructions and significant client/staff disclosures.

Because of the anxiety attached to being in the presence of another of perceived higher status, the client or staff member may be less articulate than usual when describing symptoms or explaining a problem. The dietetics practitioner should paraphrase to verify that the message is being understood according to its intended meaning. The professional should avoid sounding too clinical with such comments as "What I hear you saying is . . ." or "Let me repeat what you just said"; rather, the language should be clear, simple, and natural. A comment such as "I want to make sure I am understanding this; let me repeat what you are saying in my own words" is more natural.

Two points need to be emphasized regarding paraphrasing: *(a)* Not everything the other says needs paraphrasing. It would become a distraction if, after every other sentence, the professional interrupted with a request to paraphrase. Paraphrasing is essential only when the discussion is centered on critical information that must be understood. *(b)* Paraphrasing often leads to additional disclosure and therefore tends to cause longer interaction sessions. People are so accustomed to being with others who do not really listen that when they are with someone who proves that attention has been paid by repeating the content of what has been said, they usually want to talk more. For the dietetics professional, this additional information can be valuable. Another benefit is that after the client or staff member has expressed all his questions and concerns and has cleared his mental agenda, he is psychologically ready to sit back and listen, or to solve problems. By talking too much or too soon, the professional may not be able to convey the entire message to the other, who may be using the difference in time between how fast the professional speaks and how fast his own mind processes information (the human mind operates five to eight times as fast as human speech) to rehearse what he is going to say next.

Nonverbal Communication

Of the two messages received simultaneously by receivers, verbal and nonverbal, ordinarily it is the nonverbal that is more influential. As receivers of messages, people learn to trust their interpretations of nonverbal behavior more than the verbal word choices consciously selected by the sender. Intuitively, they know that control of nonverbal behavior is generally unconscious, while control of verbal messages is usually deliberate.

Communication experts and social scientists feel that the image a person projects accounts for over half of the total message conveyed to another individual at a first meeting. Personal appearance, including clothing, hairstyle, and accessories, is one of the most important elements of the image. Personal space variables should be experimented with to determine where an individual feels most comfortable and how that distance makes others feel (34).

The chief nonverbal vehicles inherent in communicators are facial expression, tone of voice, eye contact, gesture, and touch. Receivers of communication perceive nonverbal behavior in clusters. Ordinarily one does not notice posture, eye contact, or facial expression isolated from the other nonverbal channels. For this reason, professionals need to monitor all of their nonverbal communication vehicles so that together the clusters are congruent with one another as well as with the verbal messages.

Facial expression is usually the first nonverbal trait noticed in interaction. A relaxed face with pleasant expression is congruent with a supportive climate. A supportive tone of voice is one that is calm, controlled, energetic, and enthusiastic. Supportive eye contact includes gazing at the other in a way that allows the communicator to encounter the other visually—to the extent of being able to notice the other's facial and bodily messages. Besides being an excellent vehicle for feedback, eye contact also assures the other of the dietetics professional's interest and desire to communicate. Attending to the other visually allows inferences of interest, concern, and respect. The professional's posture is best when leaning somewhat toward the person as opposed to away from him. Large expansive gestures may be interpreted as a show of power and, in general should be avoided.

Like eye contact, touch can work positively in two ways: *(a)* Through a gentle touch, a pat, or a squeeze of the hand, one can communicate instantly a desire to solve a problem without offending the other. Touch can communicate affection, concern, and interest faster than these messages can be generated verbally. *(b)* Like eye contact, touch is a vehicle for feedback. While an individual may look calm, controlled, and totally at ease, a touch can reveal nervousness and insecurity. These clues, when monitored by the dietetics practitioner, often provide insight. It is possible to react to them by spending more time putting the person at ease; by having the individual paraphrase to make sure information is being understood; and by making an effort to alter a communication style to be more overt in her support. People usually respond positively to touch, whether or not they are consciously aware of it.

Dietetics Professionals Must be Alert to Nonverbal Signals Emanating From the Other. Besides the professional's concerns with the environment and her own verbal and nonverbal behavior in her attempt to create a trusting climate between herself and others, she must also be sensitive to the nonverbal cues in other people. Even though the practitioner is being open, natural, caring, and attending to her own behavior and the environment, the internal anxiety, confusion, nervousness, or fear in people may be causing them to misunderstand or to react inappropriately. Two requirements for effective interpersonal communication, therefore, are that the professional observe the nonverbal cues in others and then respond to them in an affirming way.

If the client or employee is nodding to suggest understanding but looks puzzled, the professional needs to verify understanding by having the individual paraphrase important instructions or dietary recommendations. If the patient is flushed, has trembling hands, or tears rolling down his cheeks, the professional may need to deal directly with relieving anxiety before communicating instructions or explanations. Until the patient is relaxed enough to concentrate, optimal two-way communication is unlikely.

After talking with one another for only a few minutes, both the dietetics practitioner and the patient can sense the "warmness" or "coldness" of the other, as well as the degree of the other's "concern." Each person tends to generalize these impressions, while inferring additional traits in the other person. If the speaker has a gentle touch, pleasant expression, and looks directly into the eyes of the listener while talking, the listener may be inferring that this individual is a caring spouse, supportive community member, or loving parent. Once the initial positive impression has been created, the impression tends to spread into other areas not directly related to the originally observed behavior. The process can work in the reverse as well, negatively. If the professional does not look at the client while talking, or touches the client in a rough way and has an unpleasant facial expression, the inferences being created now may be arrogance, lack of concern, indifference, and "coldness." Even though these initial reactions, both positive and negative, may be inaccurate, faulty first impressions are common. The helping professional might not be given a second chance to win the client's trust and cooperation; the client's inferences regarding the professional's concern and positive regard need to be anticipated and begun at the initial encounter.

Positive Effect Must be Consistent. Seeing employees daily gives the practitioner (or manager) an opportunity to reinforce or alter the perceptions the other has. If one is cold, aloof, and uncaring on a daily basis, and suddenly, because it is time to conduct an appraisal or counseling session with an employee, acts differently, one will not be believed. The practitioner needs to be consistent in adding positive inferences to the impressions of staff and clients. Dietetics professionals must make a total commitment to the word-of-mouth process by listening and questioning effectively, taking appropriate action, focusing on a subordinate/client orientation,

delivering on promises, and teaching both employees and clients how to seek information efficiently (35).

Not only is it important to attempt to generate concern through one's own nonverbal behavior, manner, and disposition, it is also essential to control, whenever possible, the communication environment so that it too leads to positive inferences with a minimum of "interference." Attractive offices, rooms in pastel colors, soft lighting, intimate and private space for counseling, and comfortable furniture can all add to the client's or staff member's collective perception, promoting inferences that one is concerned. One recent empirical study, for example, reported that because so much of the dietitian's counseling takes place in a hospital setting, more attention must be given to creating an inviting educational atmosphere within the hospital environment (36).

Related indirectly to effective communication are the actual dress and physical appearance of the professional. Dress and appearance are usually consciously selected, and they are nonverbal communication vehicles. The female dietetics practitioner who is overly made up or too strongly scented, or the male practitioner who is wearing an earring or open shirt revealing a hairy chest, may be well meaning and competent; by their dress, however, they risk offending a more conservative person. Professionals communicate their image best when they are clean, and wearing clean and pressed clothing and only a mildly scented cologne. Because any ostentatious show of material wealth or status tends to provoke a defensive reaction in others, items such as expensive jewelry and other valuable possessions should not be worn.

Another aspect of effective communication is conflict management. In the workplace, the way to win an argument is to stop it as quickly as possible by settling the dispute rationally. This is not easy to do because generally people are programmed to respond to aggression in one of three ways: fighting back, running away, or becoming immobilized (37). Sometimes, when dealing with a hostile client or employee, the professional may want to remain calm and supportive, but her body may refuse to cooperate. Her face may turn red, her hands may begin to shake, and her voice may become loud and threatening. If this occurs, she should acknowledge that although she had wished to resolve the problem with the individual, she is feeling defensive and realizes that this might be upsetting the person. Because the individual sees the physical manifestations of the professional's defensiveness, the dietetics professional should acknowledge the reaction rather than attempt to feign control. Under these circumstances, further communication should be avoided and another appointment should be scheduled after regaining composure.

Among the requirements for effective interpersonal communication is the need for the dietetics practitioner to send verbal and nonverbal messages that are congruent with one another. If a client hears a practitioner say, "I want to help you; I'm concerned about your health and any possible recurrence of your heart problem as a result of improper diet," but at the same time sees the practitioner looking down at her notes rather than at him, making no attempt to connect physically through handshake or gentle touch, or looking frequently at her watch, the incongruous second message of impersonality or impatience will be more intense than the stated message of concern. Although the professional has said all the "right" words, she is, nevertheless, judged as insincere.

Helping professionals and managers who do not genuinely like working with people are destined ultimately to fail; often, however, professionals who do like people and care for their clients and employees fail as well. To be successful in working with others, the professional must develop congruent verbal and nonverbal communication skills. One can develop all the appropriate verbal skills and still be unsuccessful in calming a hostile employee or client or in securing an obstinate client's adherence to the dietary plan. Only when the professional treats others with respect, soliciting their opinions and responding to them, can an environment of trust and openness be created (38).

LISTENING SKILLS

Well-developed listening skills are an essential requirement for effective interpersonal communication between dietetics practitioners and their clients and staff (39). An individual with average intelligence can process information at speeds that are approximately five times that of human speech. The higher the intelligence, the faster the mind tends to process information. Some individuals can think at speeds of eight to ten times the rate of human speech. Thus, while practitioners are listening to their clients or staff members talk, they have time to be thinking about other things simultaneously. Everyone has had the experience of listening to a speaker and thinking about what the individual might be like at home or letting the mind wander to other topics. From the speaker's clothes, shoes, jewelry, diction, speech patterns, etc., people tend to fill in details and develop an elaborate scenario while they listen, more or less, to the presentation. The process of good listening involves learning to harness one's attention so that one is able to concentrate totally on the speaker's message, both verbal and nonverbal. Development of these skills is not difficult, but it does require a conscious effort and perseverance.

Listening is taught as an academic subject in the department of communication studies in most colleges and universities. Research projects conducted at the University of Minnesota, however, indicate that listening ability can be enriched only when the individual desires such enrichment and is willing to follow the training with practice (40). The following list of four of the most common issues related to poor listening is an excellent starting place for readers who desire to practice improving listening skills (25):

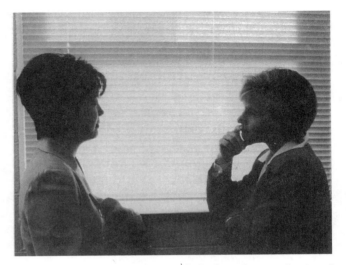

FIGURE 2.5. Listening is a skill that the professional needs to develop.

1. Most people have a limited and undeveloped attention span.

2. People tend to stop listening when they have decided that the material is uninteresting and tend to pay attention only to material they "like" or see an immediate benefit in knowing.

3. Listeners tend to trust their intuition regarding the speaker's credibility, basing their judgments more on the speaker's nonverbal behavior than on the content of the message.

4. Listeners tend to attach too much credibility to messages heard on electronic media—radio, television, movies, tapes, and so forth.

Listening can be improved with practice. The most important step in such improvement is resolving to listen more efficiently. Simply being motivated to listen causes one to be more alert and active as a receiver. The following are specific suggestions for improving listening (25):

1. Prior to engaging in the communication transaction, listeners should remind themselves of their intent to listen carefully.

2. The communication situation should be approached with the attitude of objectivity, with an open mind, and with a spirit of inquiry.

3. Listeners need to watch for clues. Just as one uses bold type and italics in writing, speakers use physical arrangement, program outlines, voice inflection, rate, emphasis, voice quality, and bodily actions as aids to help the listener determine the meaning of what is being said and what the speaker believes is most important.

4. Listeners need to make use of the thinking–speaking time difference and to remind themselves to concentrate on the speaker's message. They must use the

extra time to think critically about the message, to relate it to what they already know, to consider the logic of the arguments, and to notice the accompanying nonverbal behavior—all simultaneously.

5. Listeners need to look beyond the actual words to determine what the speaker means, and to determine whether the clusters of accompanying nonverbal behavior are congruent with the verbal message.

6. Listeners need to provide feedback to the speaker, either indirectly through nonverbal reactions or directly through paraphrasing, to verify that what is being understood by the listener is what the speaker intends.

Giving accurate feedback is the only way to prove that another person's message has been heard and understood (41). Ultimately, the most valuable listening skill is ongoing practice. Those who want to improve their listening must put themselves in difficult listening situations, must concentrate, and must practice good listening (42).

NEGOTIATION

Negotiation permeates human interaction; everyone on occasion needs to negotiate. Negotiation can be defined as a process in which two or more parties exchange goods or services and attempt to agree on the exchange rate for them (43). Negotiating with clients refers to the exchange of alternatives for dietary change between the dietetics professional and the client. Numerous books on the subject are available. The purpose of this section of the communication chapter is to introduce dietetics practitioners to the concept and to refer them to more detailed accounts (44–46).

Prior to actually engaging in the negotiating process, one needs to take time to assess one's own goals, consider the other party's goals and interests, and develop a strategy. Generally the process is considered to consist of five stages: preparation and planning, definition of ground rules, clarification and justification of one another's positions, the actual bargaining and problem-solving discussion, and finally closure and implementation. Negotiating with clients involves discussing several alternative dietary changes, involving the client in the selection of the alternative being considered, and modifying the options until they are acceptable.

The following suggestions can improve one's negotiating skills.

Begin with a positive overture. Concessions tend to be reciprocated and lead to agreements. Even a small concession is perceived as a positive overture and stimulates a reciprocal give-and-take climate.

Address problems, not personalities. There tends to be little value in focusing on the personal characteristics of the other. Negotiators understand that what is important is the other's ideas or position, and those can be disagreed with—not the individual personally. Separating the people from the problem and not personalizing differences is the mark of a seasoned negotiator.

Pay attention to initial discussions and offers. Everyone has to have an initial position, and it should be thought of as merely a point of departure. When initial offers are extreme and idealistic, the sophisticated negotiator remains calm and nonjudgmental and counters with a more realistic option.

Emphasize win–win solutions. Inexperienced negotiators often assume any gain must come at the expense of the other party. When one is patient and willing to tolerate the uncertainty and ambiguity that accompanies what seems like a deadlocked situation, creative thinking is most likely to occur with solutions that allow both people to be satisfied. This is called integrative bargaining and culminates with win–win solutions. When one enters into the process assuming a zero-sum game where one can only win if the other loses, missed opportunities for trade-offs that could benefit both sides occur. When conditions are supportive and options are framed in terms of the opponent's interests, synergetic solutions are most likely to surface in negotiations.

Create an open and trusting climate. To negotiate well, the negotiator needs well-honed communication skills, especially listening. Skilled negotiators ask more questions, focus their alternatives more directly, are less defensive, and know to avoid words and phrases that can irritate another. They have learned how to create an open and trusting climate, the kind of climate so critical for an integrative settlement (43).

There may be times in the professional life of dietetics practitioners when third-party negotiations are necessary, times when individuals or group representatives reach a stalemate and are unable to resolve differences through direct negotiations. There are four basic third-party roles: mediator, arbitrator, conciliator, and consultant. A mediator is a neutral third party who facilitates a negotiated solution by using reasoning, persuasion, and suggestions for alternatives. An arbitrator is a third party to a negotiation who has the authority to dictate an agreement. A conciliator is a trusted third party who provides an informal communication link between the negotiator and the opponent. Finally, a consultant used as a negotiator is an impartial third party, skilled in conflict management, who attempts to facilitate creative problem solving through communication and analysis.

Although there appears to be no significant direct relationship between an individual's personality and negotiation style, cultural background is relevant. The contemporary practitioner/negotiator will benefit from an understanding of the other's cultural context. Generally speaking, for example, the French tend to like conflict and tend to take a long time in negotiating agreement, not being particularly concerned about whether their opponents like or dislike them. The Chinese too tend to draw out negotiations, but they believe negotiations never end and are always willing to start over. Americans, however, are known for their impatience and desire to be liked. Many astute international negotiators often turn these characteristics to their advantage with Americans by dragging out negotiations and withholding friendship as conditional on the final settlement (47).

Negotiating skills improve with time and experience. One needs to understand the principles and look for opportunities to practice them. Dietetics practitioners need not wait for differences to begin learning. Practicing in one's private/personal life is often less threatening and can provide an excellent training field.

COMMUNICATING WITH LEGISLATORS

Knowledge of how to communicate with legislators has become another skill critical for health care professionals generally and dietetics professionals specifically. Thousands of voices compete for congressional attention as laws are written and money is provided for everything from health care to weapons (48).

Lobbying can be both effective and ethical. In a democratic society, in which government is designed to represent and protect the interests of all citizens and all parties, talking with legislators is exactly what people should do in order to ensure that decisions and legislation reflect a consensus and take into consideration the interests of all parties affected (49).

The word "lobbyist" was originally used in the 1830s to describe those who frequented the lobbies of U.S. public buildings and talked with legislators. Lobbying is protected by the U.S. Constitution, especially by the 1st Amendment's guarantees against interference with freedom of speech and the right to petition. Not only does it protect the public interests, lobbying is a respected, legitimate, and essential part of the democratic form of government (49).

Lobbyists range from teachers to homemakers, and organizations that maintain lobbyists in Washington, D.C. and state capitals include foreign governments, large business corporations, and citizens' groups ranging from the American Civil Liberties Union and Common Cause to the National Rifle Association of America.

Besides utilizing the services of professional lobbyists, organizations like The American Dietetic Association benefit from the networking and contacts made by the members of the profession. One of the most effective ways to make legislators aware of issues is at the grassroots level. It is naive to assume that government officials know everything they need to know about the professions related to nutrition. It becomes the members' responsibility to talk with elected representatives, get to know them, get on a first-name basis with them, and earn their trust and respect. The time to get networked with public officials, making sure they appreciate the point of view from the perspective of dietetics practitioners, is before they start considering legislation that might be harmful to the profession.

Some of the ways to get the message across include working with the profession's national association, writing letters, making phone calls, meeting with congressmen or senators in the home district, developing a relationship with the district administration assistant, and developing a relationship with health staffers who handle the issues relating to the dietetics profession.

Individuals, organizations, and professional associations can influence the way laws are made and enforced. The contemporary dietetics professional should consider the task of communicating with legislators as another professional responsibility. The professional, by the way, who learns how to communicate with legislators and develops a network of political connections becomes invaluable to the organization and develops increased power and prestige as a result (49).

BARRIERS TO EFFECTIVE COMMUNICATION

Thus far this chapter has dealt with what dietetics professionals can do verbally and nonverbally to ensure accurate communication with others. Most people tend to underestimate the forces and variables likely to impede the process. There are myriads of barriers that often alter perceptions, increasing the likelihood of inaccurate communication. Only after individuals are aware of these barriers can they begin to alter their communication to safeguard against them.

Meanings Are in People, Not Words

The major barrier to communication, which probably accounts for about 90% of the misunderstandings between people, is based on the communication principle that meanings are in people, not words. Communication scholars have been attempting to make people aware of the implications of this principle for more than 5 decades; however, it does not yet seem to be accepted and understood by most communicators. To comprehend the principle, one needs to understand the many ways in which humans differ one from another, and how these differences account for the variations in the way they understand and use language. With the possible exception of identical twins at birth, no two people have the exact same physiological makeup. Although a person may think that he is experiencing objective reality as he moves from one life experience to another, he is in fact interpreting objective reality subjectively through his body and mind.

To understand this point better, the reader can try to remember a time when he was not feeling like himself, a time perhaps when he was under strong medication or severe stress. If the medication or stress accelerated the processes of his nervous system, he noticed that he was more nervous, less tolerant, and perhaps more depressed than usual. If the medication slowed down these processes, he noticed that he was more lethargic, less enthusiastic, and less motivated than usual. In both cases, the objective reality would be interpreted differently than if he were in his normal state. The "normal" range, however, varies considerably. For some, being lethargic, moody, and slow-moving is normal. For others, being energetic, hyperactive, and tireless is normal. These two "normal" individuals might attend the same party, get married, or be involved in a helping relationship. Eventually, they will discover that each tends to interpret the same reality differently, with each assuming that his or her interpretation is the more "correct" one.

In addition to an understanding and appreciation of the uniqueness of each person's physiological profile, there is a need to consider that over time, even the same person experiences a range of sensation, which affects inferences about reality. As people grow older, their senses, moreover, change and begin to diminish. Two people sitting at a baseball game eating hot dogs might be having different sensual experiences. One is enjoying and savoring every mouthful, while the other is lamenting, "They just don't make them like they used to." The senses of sight, hearing, touch, smell, and taste all diminish over time. These internal changes add to the problem of inferring that because two people have heard the same message or shared the same experience, they, therefore, have the same "meanings" in their interpretation.

Two people of identical intelligence may interpret the same external stimuli differently. Some people are dispositionally oriented toward seeing details, are introverted, and are less emotional, while others with similar intelligence may tend to miss details, are more extroverted, and are more emotional. Although it is usually easier to communicate with someone who is cognitively similar to oneself, intelligence alone is not a predictor of ease of communication between individuals.

Culturally, people differ from one another, which causes them to have different interpretations of the same phenomenon. One of the authors (R.J.C.) is a second-generation Italian-American. When he traveled in Italy as a young student, he understood what it meant to be an Italian-American as opposed to a native Italian. He saw the world differently than his Italian-born cousins. Although he had never examined or challenged his values, he understood what it meant to be acculturated. The kind of home in which a person is brought up and the values he learns as a child continue to influence the way in which he interprets the world.

Many writers have pointed out the advantages of writing in English, the language with more extant words than any other. Theoretically, the extra number of words ought to allow writers and speakers of English to express "meanings" more precisely than communicators using other languages. When the language is examined carefully, however, other limiting variables emerge. No other language in the history of the world has had as many words to express extremes. There are dozens of synonyms in the English language for "bad," "terrible," "evil," and "horrible," as well as for "good," "beautiful,"

"wonderful," "terrific," and "fantastic." English has, however, only a scant representation of words that describe intermediate feelings and thoughts, middle-of-the-road positions, and other "gray" areas.

Philosophers have pointed out that thoughts are controlled to a great extent by vocabulary. One cannot think about something if one has no words for it. The inability to verbalize vague or intermediate areas of thought or feeling may distort one's perceptions of objective reality, increasing one's tendency to overreact and hindering the likelihood of easy collaboration.

Another idiosyncrasy of the English language involves its many words with multiple meanings. *The Oxford English Dictionary,* for example, includes some 15 definitions for the word "fast." A "fast" horse, for example, is one that runs with great speed, while a "fast" color is one that does not run at all.

Generating one's own meanings in others, which involves trying to arouse those meanings in the other that are closest to one's own, is an extremely difficult process. Because we are each unique physiologically, psychologically, socially, and culturally, and because we speak a language that is susceptible to many interpretations, the process of communicating accurately to one another is complicated.

In addition to the variables previously discussed, numerous other phenomena affect the accuracy of person-to-person transmission of messages. One such factor evolves from the predictable phenomena of substitution, addition, and simplification that occur as messages are passed from person to person. As messages are sent from sender to receiver, each receiver tends to alter the message unconsciously when she becomes a sender and passes it on to another.

While distortion of messages is predictable, additional complications arise from status distinctions between the interactants. When people who have the power to reward or punish others attempt to give instructions, teach a procedure, or merely relate a series of facts, their perceived higher status often makes understanding the message more difficult for receivers who perceive themselves to be of lower status.

Sensations similar to the tension, stress, and side effects of the adrenal secretions of prehistoric humans fighting for survival still exist in people today. When an employee is called before his boss, who wishes to explain the importance of the employee's task or a complicated procedure, the employee might become nervous, experience trembling hands, begin to perspire, feel his face become flushed, or develop the feeling of "butterflies" in his stomach. These "fight-or-flight" symptoms often make it even more difficult to think clearly. At the very time when one needs to be most alert, one may be subject to a physiological handicap.

The most salient implication for the dietetics practitioner engaged in helping clients or training staff is the need to compensate for this phenomenon by assisting her clients and employees in developing the appreciation and ability of paraphrasing. In the presence of health professionals, clients and staff members often experience tension and anxiety, which make it difficult for them to grasp messages. The dietitian and dietetic technician need to learn communication skills to compensate for this tendency. In addition to being natural, de-emphasizing status distinctions, using clear, concise language, and showing concern, the professional must consistently paraphrase the other, as well as have herself paraphrased, to verify that what was explained or taught was understood.

Selective Perception is Rampant, Although "Selectors" are Unconscious of It

A final barrier to communication is the human tendency to perceive information selectively, and to be intolerant of others who interpret the information differently. General Motors, for example, did a study several years ago to determine who reads Pontiac advertisements. The corporation learned that the major consumers of information about Pontiac automobiles are Pontiac owners. Each person tends to tune in to information that supports their already existing attitude and tends either to distort or not to hear information that refutes their existing attitudes. The exercise below will help to demonstrate the point: Count the "F's" in the following statement:

FASCINATING FAIRYTALES ARE THE
RESULT OF YEARS OF SCIENTIFIC STUDY
COMBINED WITH THE EXPERIENCE
OF CREATIVE MINDS

Most people looking at the message above for the first time, and told to count the number of "F's" see three. Even after being told that there are actually six, some people continue to see only three. How many do you see? Although many people believe themselves to be open-minded, unprejudiced, and able to see all sides of an issue, this simple test provides some evidence that there is the tendency in each of us to lock onto an expected view of reality and miss the objective truth.

This tendency to perceive reality selectively is unconscious. In general, people are unaware of which stimuli their minds are selecting to attend to and which stimuli are being ignored. For this reason, stereotypes, biases, and prejudices are likely to emerge and distort interpretations of messages. Such distortions carry implications for professionals. The increase in foreign-born and minority employees and clients in the United States will further challenge the management and client skills that had been effective with "traditional" Americans.

In dealing with clients or staff members, practitioners must consciously attempt to verify perceptions as a safeguard against selective distortion. One of the best ways to accomplish this is to listen actively, paraphrasing and making empathic responses. If the empathic response or paraphrasing is inaccurate and represents selective per-

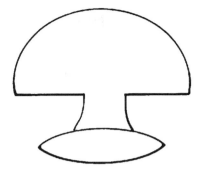

FIGURE 2.6. What do *you* see? Compare your perception with that of another person.

ception, the other person has the opportunity to clarify. To maintain organizational cohesiveness and effectiveness, dietetics professionals must become conscious of their own biases and stereotypes and must develop, stretch, and risk in the process of developing appropriate techniques for dealing with the actual differences among foreign-born, minority, and nonminority employees and clients (50).

This chapter has presented numerous suggestions for improving the dietitian's and dietetic technician's communication competence with clients and staff. One can, however, read and reread this chapter, pass a quiz on the material with a grade of A + , and still be ineffective in practicing communication skills. To develop communication skills, readers must begin immediately to put into practice what has been read. They should not be discouraged if they cannot employ all skills immediately. Months of conscious attention to these skills are needed before they become a part of one's natural approach to clients and staff.

Nothing is as frightening to humans as the fear of uncertainty and ambiguity. When people have the opportunity to try out new communication behavior, forces within them tend to pull them toward their past behavior. Even when the old strategies are unsuccessful, they generally tend to be repeated because the probable outcomes are predictable.

The professional who is serious about increasing her communication competence needs to swallow hard and stretch, forcing herself to attempt the new behavior. The time to begin is now. One need not have access to clients or staff. People can exercise these skills just as effectively in their personal as in their professional lives. Despite all the problems, improved communication is possible, and the professional who is aware of the problems and the recommended safeguards to minimize them is going to be more effective.

REVIEW AND DISCUSSION QUESTIONS

1. In the helping professions, what conveys the professionals' effectiveness with their clients and staff?

2. What are the common elements of the definition of communication?

3. What are the components of the communication model?

4. What are the verbal guidelines for creating a supportive communication climate?

5. Of the two messages received simultaneously by receivers, which is more influential, verbal or nonverbal?

6. What are the four most common poor listening habits?

7. What are some specific suggestions for improving listening?

8. What is selective perception and why is it a barrier to communication?

SUGGESTED ACTIVITIES

1. After filling out the questions below, join with classmates in groups of three to share and discuss your responses with one another.

    A. What types of nonverbal signals from your instructor or supervisor indicate to you that he or she is getting angry?
        a.
        b.
        c.

    B. What nonverbal cues indicate that you are getting angry?
        a.
        b.
        c.

    C. List some of the nonverbal signals that you send when you are talking and someone interrupts you.
        a.
        b.
        c.

    D. List some of the nonverbal signals you send when you want to signal confidence or approval of the other person.
        a.
        b.
        c.

    E. List changes you might make in the room where you are reading to alter its climate positively.
        a.
        b.
        c.

2. Write a two-paragraph description of a current interpersonal conflict you are experiencing. Be sure to indicate: *(a)* the behavior on the part of the other individual that has caused you a problem, and *(b)* what "feelings" you are experiencing as a result of that behavior. Do not sign your name unless you want to be acknowledged. After the instructor has collected the descriptions, he or she may read them and either invite students to participate in role-playing of the situations, using the guidelines for supportive verbal and nonverbal behavior, or engage the class in a case study discussion of how the communication skills might be employed to resolve the conflict.

3. One can increase his or her knowledge of nonverbal behavior by viewing others talking but not hearing what they are saying. Turn the television to a soap opera or talk show, turn off the volume, and watch the nonverbal behavior, trying to interpret it. After 3–5 minutes, turn the volume up. Then again, turn off the volume. Do this several times and attempt to grasp the verbal messages without the sound by merely interpreting the nonverbal behavior. Take notes and be prepared to share your experience in class.

4. As an in-class exercise, silently jot down your general "meanings" for the nonverbal behaviors listed below. Compare answers with classmates. Is there general agreement on all or is there a range of answers? Where answers vary, discuss the possible reasons why.
    a. Lack of sustained eye contact
    b. Lowers eyes/looks away
    c. Furrow on brow
    d. Lips are tight
    e. Bites lip or lower lip quivers
    f. Nods head up and down
    g. Hangs head down
    h. Shakes head right to left
    i. Folds arms across chest
    j. Arms unfolded
    k. Leans forward
    l. Slouches, leans back
    m. Hands tremble
    n. Face is flushed
    o. Holds hands tightly
    p. Taps foot continuously
    q. Sits behind a desk
    r. Sits nearby without any intervening objects

5. The following is an exercise that the reader might try with friends. The first person expresses the message to the second, who in turn expresses it to the third, and so on until six people have heard it. Ordinarily, the message is audiotaped and played back. This allows the participants to see the many ways in which messages are altered as they pass from person to person.
    Message:

    There has been an accident, and I must report it to the police. It is necessary, however, for me to get to the hospital as soon as possible.
    The cement truck, heading east, was turning left at

CASE STUDY

Joan Stivers, RD, noted on the medical record that her patient, John Jones, aged 63 years, was 5'11" tall and weighed 250 lbs. A retiree, he was recently diagnosed with Type II diabetes mellitus. Joan stopped by his hospital room to see him, introduced herself, and told him that the purpose of her visit was to discuss his current food intake. During the conversation, Mr. Jones and his roommate were watching a baseball game on television and periodically commented briefly on the plays and players. Finally, Mr. Jones said, "You need to talk to my wife, not me. She does the cooking." Just then, the physician came by to make rounds.

1. Identify the barriers to communication.

2. What should the dietetics professional do to overcome the barriers?

the intersection when the sports car, heading west, attempted to turn right. When they saw that they were turning into the same lane, both honked their horns, but each continued to turn without slowing down. Actually, the truck appeared to be speeding up just before the crash.

REFERENCES

1. Contento I. (senior author). The effectiveness of nutrition education and implications for nutrition education policy, programs, and research. J Nutr Educ 1995;27(special issue):6.

2. Anderson E. Getting through to the elderly patients. Geriatrics 1991;46:5.

3. Greene M, Adelman R, Friedmann E, et al. Older patient satisfaction with communication during an initial medical encounter. Soc Sci Med 1994;38:9.

4. Sandwith P. Building quality into communications. Training Dev J 1994;48:1.

5. Bebbington P. The content and context of compliance. Int Clin Psychopharmacol 1955;9:5.

6. Morris L, Schulz R. Medication compliance. Clin Ther 1993;15:3.

7. Booth T. The use of depth interviewing with vulnerable subjects. Soc Sci Med 1994;39:3.

8. Khayat K, Salter B. Patient satisfaction surveys as a market research tool for general practices. Br J Gen Pract 1994;44:382.

9. Carter H. Confronting patriarchal attitudes in the fight for professional recognition. J Adv Nurs 1994;19:2.

10. Levinson W, Stiles W, Inui T, et al. Physician frustration in communicating with patients. Med Care 1993;31:4.

11. Charles S. The doctor–patient relationship and medical malpractice litigation. Bull Menninger Clin 1993;57:2.

12. Berglund S. Why patients sue physicians. J Ark Med Soc 1991;87:11.

13. Kushell E, Ruh S. Dealing with conflict. J Nurs Adm 1996;26:2.

14. Murphy C, Sweeney M. Conflict resolution with end of life decisions in critical care settings. Medinfo 1995;8:2.

15. Hanna B. Improving communication . . . "over the sink". Nurs Manage 1994;25:7.

16. Deckard G, Meterko M, Field D. Physician burnout. Med Care 1994;32:7.

17. Piscopo B. Organizational climate, communication, and role strain in clinical nursing faculty. J Prof Nurs 1994; 10:2.

18. Newton J, Hutchinson A, Hayes V, et al. Do clinicians tell each other enough?. Fam Pract 1994;11:1.

19. Kirk D, Shanklin C, Gorman MA. Attributes and qualifications that employers seek when hiring dietitians in business and industry. J Am Diet Assoc 1989;89:494.

20. Owen A. Challenges for dietitians in a high tech/high touch society. J Am Diet Assoc 1984;84:285.

21. Eckerling L, Kohrs M. Research on compliance with diabetic regimens—applications to practice. J Am Diet Assoc 1984;84:805.

22. Carnevale AP, Gainer L, Meltzer A, et al. Workplace basics: the skills employers want. Training Dev J 1988; 42:22.

23. Smith S. Dealing with the difficult patient. Postgrad Med J 1995;71:841.

24. Baker K. Improving staff nurse conflict resolution skills. Nurs Econ 1995;13:5.

25. Samovar L, Mills J. Oral communication, message and response. Dubuque, IA: William C Brown, 1986.

26. Fielden JS. Why can't managers communicate? Business 1989;39:41.

27. Tindall W, Beardsley R, Kimberlin C. Communication in pharmacy practice. Philadelphia: Lea & Febiger, 1994.

28. Matejka JK. Opening doors: good relationships as good management. Personnel J 1988;67:74.

29. Anderson JS. Blueprint for real open-door communication. Personnel J 1989;68:32.

30. Gibb J. Defensive communication. J Commun 1961;11: 141.

31. Valentine P. Management of conflict. J Adv Nurs 1995; 22:1.

32. Fritchie R. Conflict and its management. Br J Hosp Med 1995;53:9.

33. Littlefield V. Conflict resolution. J Prof Nurs 1995;11:1.

34. Davidson J. Shaping an image that boosts your career. Market Commun 1988;13:55.

35. Haywood KM. Managing word of mouth communication. J Serv Market 1989;3:55.

36. Picus SS. Evaluation of the nutrition counseling environment of hospitalized patients. J Am Diet Assoc 1989;89:403.

37. Bernstein AJ, Rozen SC. How to cool it when things heat up. Sales Market Manage 1989;141:66.

38. Field L, Knowles L. Can we talk? The key to a productive management pattern. Can Manager 1989;14:21.

39. Wachs J. Listening. AAOHN J (Official J Am Assoc Occup Health Nurses) 1995;43:11.

40. Nicholas R, Stevens L. Are you listening? New York: McGraw-Hill Book Co, 1957.

41. Lewis DV. The art of active listening. Training Dev J 1989;43:21.

42. Buher P. What attributes does the better manager possess? Supervision 1989;50:8.

43. Robbins S. Essentials of organizational behavior. Englewood Cliffs, NJ: Prentice Hall, 1997.

44. Fuller G. Negotiators handbook. Englewood Cliffs, NJ: Prentice Hall, 1991.

45. Breslin J, Rubin J. Negotiation theory and practice. Cambridge, MA: Harvard Law School Press, 1993.

46. Kennedy G. Field guide to negotiation. Boston, MA: Harvard Business School Press, 1994.

47. Robbins S. Organizational behavior. Englewood Cliffs, NJ: Prentice Hall, 1996.

48. Congress A to Z. CQ's ready reference encyclopedia. Washington, DC: Congress Q Inc, 1988.

49. Klemp R. Lobbying. Vital Speeches 1993;59:19.

50. Ballard L, Kleiner B. Understanding and managing foreign-born and minority employees. Leadership Organiz Dev J 1988;9:22.

three

INTERVIEWING

Most people have engaged in the interviewing process at one time or another. A person applying for a new position interviews the employer concerning the job opening and in turn, is interviewed by the employer. When one seeks medical care, the physician takes a medical history using interviewing techniques. The client or hospitalized patient may be interviewed at great length and by more than one person. A considerable amount of time is spent in gaining information from an individual in order to advise, counsel, or assist him. Dietetics professionals apply interviewing skills with their patients, clients, and employees.

Interviewing may be defined as a guided communication process between two people with a predetermined purpose and an exchanging or obtaining of specific information. The interview is more than a question-and-answer session, although questions are the means of determining the subject matter of the interview. The goal of the interview is to collect valid and accurate data from the respondent while maintaining an interpersonal environment conducive to disclosure. These data include both rational and emotional reactions of the individual.

Development of interviewing skills requires practice and repetition over time. Anyone conducting an interview for the first time may expect to feel quite uncomfortable. While some advance planning concerning the content and process of interviews is helpful and important, the warm human relationship that develops between two people differs each time, and no two interviews are exactly alike. Knowing the principles and process of interviewing, using them, and frequently evaluating the results can help students and practitioners to improve their skills.

Developing listening skills is also important, as an effective interviewer must be a good listener. Skillful listening requires concentration on the verbal and nonverbal behavior and perception of what is important in the respondent's behavior. One listens not only for facts, but also for attitudes, feelings, and values.

This chapter examines the principles and process of interviews, the conditions that facilitate interviews, the three parts of an interview, the use of different types of questions, and the types of interviewer responses.

TYPES OF INTERVIEWS

For the purpose of illustrating the interviewing principles and process, two examples of interviews are referred to in this chapter—the diet history and the pre-employment interview. Although a full delineation of the content of these types of interviews is beyond the scope of this book, a brief explanation of each follows. For more detailed information on content, other sources should be examined (1-7).

A diet history, obtained by interview, is an account of a person's food habits, preferences, eating behaviors, and other factors influencing food intake. It may be used in medical nutrition therapy to assess the nutritional status of the individual, to establish a nutrition care plan, to prioritize nutrition intervention, or to check for appropriate and inappropriate eating habits prior to nutrition counseling. While there currently is no gold standard method for estimating one's usual dietary intake, approaches utilized frequently are the 24-hour recall, the record of usual daily food intake, and the food frequency checklist.

In the 24-hour recall, the interviewer asks the client to recount, qualitatively and quantitatively, all foods and beverages consumed in the previous 24-hour period. The second method, the usual daily food intake, elicits a record of what the client usually consumes during one day. In both approaches, the portion sizes, the methods of food preparation, the between-meal snacks, the times of day food is consumed, the use of vitamin and mineral supplements, and any alcoholic beverages consumed require consideration.

Neither method is considered to have a high degree of accuracy in assessing the nutritional status of the individual, and each suffers certain deficiencies. For example, the previous 24-hour period may not have been typical of what the person normally eats, and the usual daily intake this week may differ considerably from previous weeks and may undergo seasonal variations. An additional point is that the food intake Mondays through Fridays often differs from that of weekends.

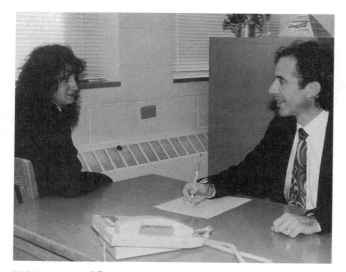

FIGURE 3.1.   The manager interviews a job applicant.

One method to increase the accuracy of the diet history is to use a food frequency checklist with it. A food frequency checklist determines the daily or weekly frequency of consuming basic foods, such as meats, milk, breads, cereals, fruits, vegetables, fats and oils, sweets and desserts, beverages, and snack foods. Portion sizes may be included on the list. With the previously mentioned methods, a skillful interviewer obtains more accurate and usable information than an unskilled one.

In the management of personnel, the dietetics professional uses interviewing skills with prospective employees. Several applicants for the same position may be interviewed to obtain information on which to base the hiring decision. The same basic interviewing principles are used, but for a different purpose. Federal legislation outlaws discrimination in hiring based on race, color, religion, national origin, sex, age, and disability. "Pre-Employment Interview Questions" (see below) give examples of some interview questions that are permissible and others that are not recommended. Those responsible for pre-employment interviews should consult additional resources to determine the content of questions that may be considered discriminatory (1–4).

Pre-Employment Interview Questions

Permissible Questions and Their Significance

In general, questions asked in pre-employment interviews should be job-related or predictive of success on the job. They should elicit information to compare the individual's qualifications and interests with those of the job description for the vacant position. The following are examples with their significance:

1. "Tell me about yourself." Gives general impressions.

2. "Why do you want to work for our company?" Tells what the person knows and whether or not there is a fit with the company's needs.

3. "Tell me about your previous work experience. What did you do on your job?" Gives knowledge, skills, and abilities.

4. "What are your greatest strengths and weaknesses as a worker?" Gives skills and abilities.

5. "What kind of work interests you?" Tells interest and motivation.

6. "What subjects in school did you like most? Least?" Shows interests.

7. "What was your grade point average? Class rank?" Shows mental ability.

8. "While in school, what extracurricular activities did you participate in that have a bearing on this job?" Shows diversity of interests, interpersonal skills, and teamwork.

9. "What organizations do you belong to that are relevant to the job you are applying for?" Shows interest and interpersonal skills.

10. "What offices have you held?" Shows leadership ability and acceptance of responsibility.

11. "What are your career goals? Where do you see yourself in five years?" Shows any short- or long-range plans and whether or not they are congruent with those of the company.

12. "What hours do you prefer to work?" Tells availability various hours of the day and days of the week.

Questions That Should Not Be Asked

Certain subjects can be the basis for complaints of discrimination on the basis of race, color, sex, marital status, national origin, religion, age, and disability. For this reason, the following questions are examples of ones that should be avoided in pre-employment interviews:

1. "Are you a citizen of another country?"

2. "What is your religious faith?"

3. "Are you married? Single? Divorced? Expecting?"

4. "What is your maiden name?"

5. "Where does your spouse work?"

6. "Who will baby-sit for you?"

7. "Do you have plans to start a family?"

8. "What is your date of birth? Date of graduation from school?"

PURPOSE OF THE INTERVIEW

Prior to the interview, the purpose should be clearly identified and communicated. A diet history may serve one of several purposes. The interviewer may use it as a basis for calculating the individual's daily nutrient intake, comparing it with anthropometric and laboratory data in nutritional assessment. It may be initiated prior to establishing a nutrition care plan because a patient is at high risk for nutritional deficiencies. The history may be used prior to initiating nutrition counseling and education to identify what nutritional problems the client has and to provide a baseline for gauging change. A history can also help to determine a person's current food habits and the necessary changes when instituting counseling on a modified diet, such as a sodium-restricted diet.

In the case of a job opening, the purpose of the interview is to determine which applicant best meets the qualifications for the vacant position as described in the job description, and whether the opening is suited to the person's talents. The decision of which applicant to hire is based on the interview and other sources of information, such as the application form and references. A secondary purpose is to "sell" the company and to give applicants information about the position and the organization on which to base their own decisions regarding possible employment with the company. The interviewer both gives and gathers information.

The interviewer should communicate the purpose of the interview to the interviewee. With clients and patients, one can also stress that the interview is necessary to provide better advice, service, or health care to the individual. With job applicants, one may note that it is important to find an employee who will be satisfied with the company and the position. If the purpose is clear and understood, better cooperation from the interviewee may be anticipated.

CONDITIONS FACILITATING INTERVIEWS

For effective interviewing, a number of conditions should be considered. They include the following (8, 9):

1. Attentiveness, including attending to nonverbal behavior

2. Rapport

3. Freedom from interruption

4. Psychological privacy

5. Physical surroundings

6. Emotional objectivity

7. Personal context of the respondent

8. Note taking

Attentiveness

Attentive listening helps to create a climate in which the interviewee can communicate more easily. The professional needs to develop listening skills and to listen with empathy rather than to talk extensively. Listening is an active, not a passive, skill. The professional assists interviewees in gathering and communicating their thoughts and feelings. To understand the complete message, the interviewer must listen to the verbal message while observing the nonverbal behavior, such as, facial expressions and tone of voice. At the same time, the interviewee is observing the nonverbal behavior of the professional. Frequent looking at one's watch, failure to maintain eye contact, sitting back in too relaxed a posture, frowning, yawning, and tone of voice all may convey a negative message and inhibit effective interviews.

Rapport

Rapport should be established early in the interview. Rapport is the personal relationship established between the interviewer and the respondent and is a key to a good interview. It deals with emotional aspects, the building of a warm and supportive climate, the release of stress, and the smooth flow of conversation in a nonjudgmental atmosphere.

The interviewee should be put at ease and relieved of anxiety and uncertainty of what is planned, since people react more favorably in situations that they understand and accept. Examples of positive nonverbal behaviors include smiling when appropriate, having an approving facial expression, nodding approval, giving undivided attention, speaking confidently, and making people feel that one is interested in what they are saying. When the individual has been seen previously, less time is needed to develop rapport; a comment on something from a previous visit may be sufficient.

Excessive deference, although it may be flattering to the professional, may actually inhibit the development of rapport with patients. Patients, overwhelmed by the professional's expertise, may give information they think is being sought instead of medically useful information. Building trust in the relationship is the key to rapport.

If the person has been kept waiting for a long time, negative feelings may occur, and the person may appear angry, belligerent, or unfriendly. Recognizing that these emotions interfere with establishing a good relationship, the dietetics professional should apologize and attempt to reduce these feelings by saying, for example, "I'm

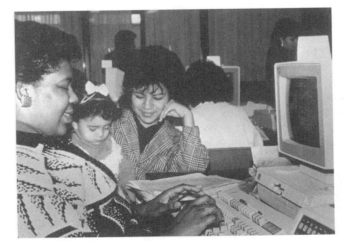

FIGURE 3.2. After completing a nutrition history, nutrient analysis may be completed on a computer.

sorry you had to wait so long. I was busy with another patient, and it took longer than I expected. I can understand if you are annoyed.''

Rapport may be inhibited by addressing people by their first names, a practice usually restricted to close friends and family. This may be interpreted as lack of respect by some people, especially those who like the tradition of formal address or who are older. When in doubt, use both names, such as ''Mary Smith'' or ''Mrs. Smith.'' A first name should be used only with permission of the interviewee, after an inquiry, such as ''Do you prefer to be addressed as 'Mary' or 'Mrs. Smith?''' Using the person's preferred name does not show excessive concern with tradition, but is simply another tool for promoting rapport.

Freedom from Interruptions

Freedom from interruption furthers the impression that one is genuinely concerned about the person being interviewed. The professional should arrange to have phone calls held, and if a phone call should come despite such an arrangement, one should explain to the caller that a conference is in progress, and should ask to return the call later. Upon hanging up, the professional should apologize for the interruption, and then resume the interview.

Psychological Privacy

Psychological privacy is enhanced by geographical privacy, but is not absolutely necessary for psychological privacy to exist. Since they may discuss private matters, the interviewer and interviewee should be alone. A quiet office without interruption is preferable. At the patient's bedside in a hospital setting, however, others may be present in the room. Whenever possible, arrange the setting so that the interview cannot be overheard, is not interrupted, and promotes the giving of undivided attention.

The interviewee should understand that the conversation will not be repeated later. In a professional relationship, the confidentiality of patient, client, and applicant information must be respected. Anecdotes and stories should not be shared with others over coffee breaks, lunch, or at social gatherings.

Physical Surroundings

Other variables related to the location of interviews include comfort, distance between parties, and seating arrangements. These may either help or hinder an interview, and may or may not make the other person feel more like communicating. Comfort concerns proper furniture, lighting, temperature, ventilation, and pleasant surroundings. A comfortable setting where eye contact can be maintained should be arranged. Preferably the parties should be at the same head level, since standing over a patient lying in bed may trigger deferential behavior. The optimum distance between people involved in

an interview is 3 or 4 feet, or about an arm's length (10). The most formal seating arrangement is for one person to sit across the desk from another, while a chair along the side of the desk is less formal and makes people feel more equal in status. Two parties seated without a table is informal, but when it is necessary to view materials, a round table is less formal since it avoids the head-of-the-table position. In general, the fewer the furniture barriers, the better. A clean desk top also removes distractions.

Emotional Objectivity

Emotional objectivity is another essential for effective interviewing. Personal feelings and preferences should be controlled and not revealed to the interviewee. The client should feel free to express all feelings and attitudes and in the process, may express some that are contrary to those of the professional. An attitude of acceptance, self-control, and concern for the interviewee should be maintained, with a desire to understand behavior, rather than judge it.

Interviewers should be aware that a professional relationship is most easily established with persons of similar socioeconomic status, ethnic group, and age, while barriers to the relationship may arise when these factors differ. The professional needs to learn about, understand, and accept the cultural differences, value systems, and lifestyles of other groups. Exploration of one's own attitudes towards those who are different may be necessary.

The interviewee should feel free to discuss all matters without fear of condemnation, since any such expression will block the progress of the interview. A raised eyebrow, a look of shock or surprise, or an incredulous follow-up question (e.g., ''You had three pieces of pie and two milkshakes for lunch?'') may cause an obese woman to change or end her story. The professional should seek to understand the circumstances, not to pass judgment on them. The respondent who does not find the professional an understanding person is unlikely to converse freely.

Interviewers should develop an awareness of their own conscious and unconscious prejudices. These include not only racial or religious preferences, but also exaggerated dislikes of people and their characteristics, such as, obese, poorly dressed, or uneducated people, aggressive women, meek men, highly pitched voices, redheads, and weak handshakes. Interviewers who identify their areas of intolerance may be better able to control their expression and avoid nonverbal behaviors revealing prejudices.

Personal Context

Interviewees bring to the interview their own personal contexts or systems of beliefs, attitudes, feelings, and values that must be recognized. Concerns about perceived threats to health can be so frightening, for example, that they preoccupy and block conversation. The professional would do well to recognize that the respondent's situation may have both subjective and objective aspects. That a man has had a heart attack is a medical fact, but his subjective feelings about his illness may be equally important. Fear, resentment, anger, anxiety, dependence, or regression may be underlying emotions that interfere with cooperation. An understanding of the psychological reactions to illness and ways of dealing with them may be necessary, and a sense of caring and concern is helpful.

One may need to facilitate the venting and feelings and to acknowledge them before going on to the interview. A job applicant may have been laid off recently from a position held for 10 years, which is a fact. The subjective way the individual feels about the situation, however, is as important as the situation itself. Anxiety, nervousness, and depression may be evident. The professional should be alert for nonverbal and verbal clues about the person which give a frame of reference for understanding.

Usually, the interviewer has some information about the person in advance, which may prove helpful in understanding the personal context of the interviewee. In the hospital setting, the medical record is a source of information on the social and economic circumstances that may influence the treatment—marital status, number in household, age, occupation, economic status, religion, level of education, physical health, level of activity, medications, weight, height, and medical history. In pre-employment interviews the application form should be examined in advance, since it contains information on education and previous work experience. The job description for the vacant position describes job duties and qualifications.

The professional should keep in mind that people may be suffering from problems of which they are not consciously aware or problems that they are unable to express. Job applicants may be nervous or apprehensive about the impression they are making. Patients may be worried about their medical problems and how these will affect their jobs or lifestyle. While the interviewer may be focusing on obtaining a diet history and giving counseling, the patient may be thinking about adjusting to a new disease or completing arrangements for hospital discharge by 1:00 PM. By putting people at ease, by encouraging them to talk freely, and by assisting them to organize their thoughts and feelings, the empathetic, skilled listener may ease or eliminate these problems.

Cognitive approaches conceptualize four distinct stages that an individual goes through in response to another's questions, each of which may lead to errors in responses. Comprehension is the first stage in which the interviewee interprets the meaning of the questions. In the second stage, retrieval, the respondent searches short- and long-term memory for an appropriate answer. Third, in estimation/judgment, the interviewee evaluates the relevance of the information from memory, decides whether or not it is appropriate, and possibly combines various bits of information. In the fourth and final stage.

response, other factors may be weighed, such as how sensitive the information is, whether or not the answer is socially expected or desirable, the amount of accuracy to provide, and so forth. The individual then provides a response to the question (11).

Note Taking

Another factor to consider is the impact of note taking. The inexperienced interviewer may find it necessary to take notes, which may raise suspicion on the part of the interviewee and hamper the flow of communication. To avoid such concern, the dietetics professional should ask for the interviewee's permission to jot down a few notes, and should explain why they are necessary and how they will be used. The practitioner may ask, for example: "Is it all right if I take a few notes so that later I can review what we said?"

Writing constantly throughout an interview interferes with both parties. The interviewee may be distracted or apprehensive, and the professional has less time for listening carefully and developing continued rapport with the person. Attention should be concentrated on what is said, not on writing.

Notes should be as brief as possible, and eye contact with the interviewee should be maintained while writing. Interviewers should train themselves to remember conversations from a limited number of key words, phrases, or abbreviations. A breakfast of orange juice, cereal, toast, and coffee with cream and sugar, for example, may be abbreviated, "OJ, cer, tst, C-C-S," while a pineapple-cottage cheese salad may be noted as "P/A-CC sld." Taking brief notes during an interview may be difficult initially for students who are accustomed to taking notes during classroom lectures, sitting passively and filling notebooks with what is said; however, this skill can be developed with time.

Comprehensive notes should be dictated or written immediately after the person has departed. Waiting 15 minutes or longer, seeing another client or job applicant, or accepting phone calls may cause the interviewer to forget essential information. Notes are necessary for comparing and ranking job candidates who may be seen on different days. Only relevant job-related comments should be written since unsuccessful candidates may sue for discrimination later.

PARTS OF THE INTERVIEW

Each interview can be divided into three parts. They include the following:

1. Opening
2. Exploration
3. Closing

The initial phase, or opening, involves introductions and establishing rapport, a process of creating trust and good will between the parties (10). The exploration phase includes the use of questions to obtain information

TABLE 3.1.

The Interview Process

PHASES	TASKS
Opening	Introductions
	Establish rapport
	Discuss purpose
Exploration	Gather information
	Explore problems
	Explore both thoughts and feelings
	Continue rapport
Closing	Express appreciation
	Review purpose
	Ask for comments/questions
	Plan future contacts

while maintaining the personal relationship, as the interviewer guides and directs the interview with responses. In the final phase, the interview is closed and any future contacts are planned. Table 3.1 summarizes the interview process.

Opening

The opening sets the tone of the interview—friendly or unfriendly, professional or informal, relaxed or tense, leisurely or rushed. Introductions may establish several conditions. Interviewers should greet the client, and state their name and job title, e.g., "Good morning. I'm Judy Jones, a registered dietitian." A smile, eye contact, a handshake or placing a hand on the other's hand or arm, and friendly face and tone of voice are supporting nonverbal behaviors. It is possible to be professional without being cold, distant, and formal.

In the hospital setting, it may be necessary to verify who the patient is. The individual may ask, "Are you Mary Johnson?" If answered affirmatively, one may respond, "I'm glad to meet you, Mrs. Johnson. How do you prefer to be addressed?" The professional may add how she prefers to be addressed.

If the person's physician has requested the contact, the professional may mention this. "Did Dr. Smith tell you that he asked me to visit you?" If the client answers, "No," one should explain the fact that the physician requested the contact. A discussion of the nature and purpose of the interview may follow, along with how the interviewee will benefit from the interview. Stating one's name and immediately unleashing a barrage of questions should be avoided.

Discussion may center initially on known information from the medical record or from the application form of job applicants. Alternatively, the weather, sporting events, holidays, a national or international event, or any topic of joint interest may be appropriate for opening the discussion. Small talk is important in developing and building the relationship between two people. When the conversation appears to be artificial, however, the interviewee may become uncomfortable.

When interviewees initiate the appointment, it is preferable to let them state in their own words their problem or purpose for coming. The dietetics professional may ask, "What brought you to the Friendly Company to seek employment, Mrs. Johnson?" or "How have things been going since we last talked?" or "When we talked on the phone, Mrs. Smith, you mentioned that your doctor told you that you have borderline diabetes." When interviewees are given the chance to express themselves first, the interview begins with their agenda, which is preferable.

Although it may be time-consuming for the busy professional, the opening exchange of either information or pleasantries is important and should not be omitted. Rapport, a degree of warmth, a supportive atmosphere, and a sense of mutual involvement are critical components in the interview (10). Willingness to disclose information about oneself is influenced by the level of trust established in the relationship, and cooperation and disclosure are crucial to the success of interviews. Interviewees quickly develop perceptions of the situation and make decisions about the amount and kind of information they will share. Mrs. Johnson and Mrs. Smith form impressions of the interviewer just as the professional does of them. The purpose should be clearly stated prior to directing the conversation to the second stage.

Exploration Phase

In the second stage the interviewee is asked a series of questions. A good interviewer has preplanned and prepared an "interview guide," an outline of information desired or topics to be covered. The guide should not only tell what questions will be asked, but also how questions will be phrased in order to elicit the most information in the least amount of time.

Topics should be arranged in a definite sequence. In a diet history, for example, the interviewer may desire information about beverages consumed, eating in restaurants, portion sizes, meals, methods of food preparation, and snacks. Put in sequence that list includes meals, portion sizes, methods of food preparation, snacks, beverages, and eating in restaurants. See "Questions and Directives for Diet Histories." In a pre-employment interview the sequence may be previous work experience, career goals, education, present activities and interests that are job-related, and personal qualifications. Specific questions intended to gain information about the applicant's qualifications, as compared with those on the job description, should be planned in advance. Refer to "Pre-Employment Interview Questions."

Questions and Directives for Diet Histories

1. "Tell me about any diet you have followed previously or are currently following."
2. "Can you tell me about any problems you have had with your diet and what caused them?"
3. "Tell me about the people in your family who eat together and any dietary problems they have."
4. "Who is responsible for grocery shopping, meal planning, and meal preparation?"
5. "I need to get an idea of what you are eating now. Please start with when you arise and tell me about the first thing you have to eat or drink with the amount."
6. "Tell me about what you eat or drink next including the amount."
7. "What about later in the day?"
8. "How are your meats and vegetables usually prepared?"
9. "We haven't talked about snacks between meals. What do you have between each of your meals and during the evening or before bed?"
10. "What time of day are your meals?"
11. "What about alcoholic beverages?"
12. "What about meals in restaurants? How often do you eat out and what would you eat?"
13. "What about vitamin and mineral supplements?"
14. "To summarize what you have told me, can you tell me how many servings you eat daily or weekly of these foods? Milk? Cheese and other dairy products?" (Continue with food frequency checklist.)

While it ensures that information is gathered in a systematic manner, the interview guide does not have to be followed strictly. The interviewer should be thoroughly familiar with the questions and not have to refer to them constantly. Knowing the purpose and significance of each question is important so that questions are not asked in a perfunctory manner and so the interviewer does not accept superficial or inadequate answers. Asking a job applicant about offices held in organizations, for example, is an attempt to seek information about leadership ability and the acceptance of responsibility, while inquiring about plans over the next 5 years is an attempt to learn about short- and long-range goals. Refer to the "Pre-Employment Interview Questions." To answer fully, interviewees must see how the questions are relevant to their needs. With patients or clients, the dietetics professional can explain that the answers to questions are a basis for nutrition counseling or education. Appendix A contains supplementary information on questions to ask and to avoid in nutrition interviews.

USING QUESTIONS

Questions play a major role in interviews. The wording of questions in interviews is as important as one's manner and tone of voice. A friendly approach in asking the questions communicates the desire to understand and be of assistance. The kind of questions asked should require the other person to talk 60 to 70% of the time. Questions that are highly specific or may be answered with one word or with "Yes" or "No" should be avoided initially, but may be necessary later to follow up on specific information.

Knowledge of the kinds of questions to use and skill in using them are important to successful interviewing as well as to counseling. Questions may be classified in three ways: open or closed, primary or secondary, and neutral or leading (10). Table 3.2 summarizes the advantages and disadvantages of different kinds of questions.

Open and Closed Questions. Open questions are broad and give the interviewee great freedom in respond-

TABLE 3.2.

Advantages and Disadvantages of Questions

KIND OF QUESTION	ADVANTAGES	DISADVANTAGES
Open	Gives interviewee control Communicates trust/interest Less threatening Tells what the person thinks is important	Time-consuming May get unneeded information
Closed	Gives interviewer control Provides quick answers	May get incomplete answers Short answers force more questions
Primary	Introduces new topics	
Secondary	Elicits further information	
Leading		Reveals bias of interviewer Directs person to one answer
Neutral	More accurate answers	

ing while giving the professional an opportunity to listen and observe. Two examples of open questions are:

"Can you tell me a little about yourself?"

"Can you tell me about your eating habits?"

At the beginning of the interview, open questions are less threatening, communicate more interest and trust, and reveal what the interviewee thinks is most important. Disadvantages are that they may involve a greater amount of time, the collection of unnecessary information, and lengthy, disorganized answers.

Additional examples of open questions, but with moderate restrictions, are:

"What about your meals?"

"What diet have you been following?"

"What did the doctor tell you about your diet?"

"Can you tell me about your job responsibilities in your previous position?"

"How did you become interested in this position?"

Closed questions are more restrictive, that is, they limit answers. Some closed questions are more limiting than others, as for example:

"Who cooks the food at home?"

"Can you tell me about any snacks you eat?"

"What skills do you have that are important for the job?"

Closed questions give the interviewer more control, require less effort from the interviewee, and are less time-consuming. Disadvantages include the inhibition of communication, which might result if the interviewer shows little interest in the answers, taking more questions to obtain the same information, and getting answers that may not reveal why the respondent feels as he does.

Primary and Secondary Questions. Questions may also be classified as primary or secondary. Primary questions are used to introduce topics or new areas. The following are examples:

"Now that we have discussed your most recent position, can you tell me about your former job with Smith & Co.?"

"Now that we have discussed the food you eat at home, tell me about what you eat in restaurants."

Note that mentioning what was just said shows that one has been listening.

Secondary questions attempt to obtain further information or explanation which primary questions have failed to elicit; they may be referred to as "follow-up" questions. Interviewees may have given an inadequate response for many reasons, including poor memory, misunderstanding of the question or amount of detail desired, and the feeling that the question is too personal or irrelevant, or that the professional would not understand the response. Specific follow-up questions, such as the following, may be asked:

"How much orange juice do you drink?"

"What do you use in your coffee?"

"In your previous position, how many people did you supervise?"

Neutral and Leading Questions. Neutral questions are preferred to leading questions. Leading questions direct the respondent to one answer in preference to others, an effect that may be unintentional on the part of the interviewer. Leading questions reveal the bias of interviewers, which they themselves may not realize. Listed below are examples:

"You eat breakfast, don't you?" "Yes, of course."

"You aren't going to eat desserts anymore, are you?" "No."

"What do you eat for breakfast?" "An egg and toast."

Two of these questions assume the client consumes breakfast, and in these instances, people will probably answer as they feel they are expected to, even if they usually omit the meal. Clients may change their answers on the basis of a nonverbal appearance of the dietetics professional of surprise, disgust, dislike, or disagreement with what clients are saying. To receive uninhibited responses from clients, the interviewer should try to avoid these appearances.

The practitioner's language and wording must be understood by the client if successful communication is to take place. One does not need to impress people with medical and dietetic vocabulary. Complex terminology should be avoided, or used sparingly, and only when one is sure that the client understands. The following may be misunderstood:

"People with the type of hyperlipidemia you have should avoid eating foods containing saturated fatty acids and emphasize monounsaturates and polyunsaturates instead."

When the interviewer senses that too many questions are being asked and the respondent may be developing a "feeling of interrogation," one may introduce some questions as a statement or directive (1). For example: "How has your diet been going?" may be changed to "I'd be interested in hearing how your diet has been going." "How did you become interested in this position?" may be changed to "I'd be interested in some of the reasons you decided to apply for this position." This makes the interview more conversational.

Questions should be asked one at a time and the interviewer should concentrate on listening carefully to the answers rather than thinking ahead to the next question to be asked. Further discussion of questions is found in Chapter 4 on "Counseling."

Sequencing Questions. Questions are often arranged in a "funnel" sequence (10). A funnel sequence begins with broad, open questions and proceeds to more restrictive ones. For example:

"Tell me about the food you eat during a day."

"What do you have for snacks between meals?"

"We haven't discussed alcoholic beverages—what about them?"

Beginning with open-ended questions poses the least threat to the client and induces a response. The person then volunteers much information, making it unnecessary to ask additional questions. At times, an inverted funnel sequence may be preferable. In pre-employment interviews, for example, applicants may feel more comfortable dealing with a specific question than with a broad, open one, such as, "Tell me about yourself," when they are apprehensive and unsure of what to say or what the interviewer expects.

In taking a diet history, questions or statements starting with "What" or "Tell me about" elicit better responses than "Do you. . .?" Examples include the following:

"I'd like to get some background about your daily food intake starting with when you arise in the morning. Tell me about the first meal or food you eat during the day—what you eat, and in what amounts."

"Tell me about the next meal or food you eat. What would it be like?"

"Now that we have discussed your meals, can you tell me about coffee breaks or the types of snacks you eat between meals and the times of day you eat them."

"We haven't talked about beverages. What about beer, wine, and alcohol?"

These questions or statements allow people to tell their stories in their own way.

Questions that do not require a sufficient answer or may be answered with one word or "Yes" or "No" are less productive, such as the following:

"Do you eat breakfast?" "Yes."

"Do you drink orange juice?" "Yes."

"Do you eat cereal for breakfast?" "No."

"Do you like milk?" "No."

"How often do you eat meat?" "Once a day."

A series of short, sequential, dead-end questions from the professional's list of information to be gathered prevents people from telling their stories their way, and information may be omitted as a result.

In the follow-up visits, open questions should be broad to allow the client to determine the focus of the interview. Examples are, "Tell me how the diet is going," and "What progress have you made since we last talked?" The professional should begin discussion with whatever is of current concern to the patient. For opening questions, the interviewer should also refer to the records regarding the client's background and problems.

Some recommend avoiding questions beginning with "Why" (9, 10, 12). While asking "why" may seek information, it may also indicate disapproval, displeasure, or mistrust, and it appears to ask for justification or explanation, for example:

"Why don't you follow your diet?"

"Why don't you eat breakfast?"

"Why did you resign from your job?"

"Why were you late for your appointment?"

Clients may react defensively or explain their behavior in a manner they believe is acceptable to the dietitian.

"Because I don't understand my diet."

"I'll start eating breakfast tomorrow if you think I should."

"Because there was no chance for advancement."

"Because the traffic was heavy."

If threatened by a "why" question and unwilling to reveal the answer, the individual may answer in an evasive manner, in which case nothing is gained.

RESPONSES

In the verbal interaction of medical interviews, interviewer responses may be divided into six categories (8):

1. Evaluative
2. Hostile
3. Reassuring
4. Probing
5. Understanding
6. Confrontation

In the discussion of each type, responses to the following statement by Mrs. Jones, an obese woman, are compared: "I haven't lost any weight this week. I ate just a few cookies. The diet doesn't work."

Evaluative Response. In the evaluative response, the interviewer makes a judgment about the person's feelings or responses or implies how the person ought to feel. The evaluative response leads to the offering of advice by the professional for the solution to the client's problem. An example is, "I suggest that you stop buying those cookies, Mrs. Jones." Note that the evaluative response leads to giving advice, not information. Little attempt is made to understand the psychological needs of the patient or the reasons that the cookies were eaten. The recipient of the advice has the choice of following it or not. At times, some people ignore advice as a means of maintaining their independence.

Hostile Response. In the hostile response, the professional's anger is uncontrolled, and the response may lead to antagonism or humiliation of the client. The following response is an example: "You're not acting very mature, Mrs. Jones. I've told you before to avoid all sweets and desserts if you want to lose weight." The hostile response may lead the client to a reply that retaliates: "How would you know about dieting? Look how thin you are." A vicious cycle of angry, hostile responses results, destroying the professional-to-client relationship. The fact that the client is anxious about the inability to follow the diet has been ignored by the professional. The interviewer who is frustrated by the client who is not following the diet should avoid responding with anger.

Reassuring Response. With a reassuring response, the client is prevented from working through her feelings since the interviewer suggests that there is nothing to worry about. Frequently, a client's expressions of anxiety are followed by the dietetics professional's reassuring response that things will improve and that the person should not worry, as illustrated by the following: "Don't worry about it, Mrs. Jones. It takes time to adjust to new eating patterns. You'll do better next week." This response suggests that the problem does not exist, or that the professional does not want to discuss it. Such responses make it difficult to solve the client's problem or to discuss it further. Admission of failure with the diet may have been difficult for the client, but it indicated a desire to discuss the problem.

Probing Response. The probing response is an attempt to clarify or to gain additional information in helping respondents recall details. In dietary interviews, for example, details on food quantities, added ingredients, preparation methods, and snacks are probed frequently.

Probing implies that the person should give more information so that the professional can assist in solving the problem. "So you think the diet doesn't work, Mrs. Jones. I wonder if you could tell me a little more about that." This helps the person to tell her story, and further information can be obtained.

There are a number of probing techniques, which may be used to facilitate better interviewee responses in addition to secondary or follow-up questions. They should be nondirective, so as to avoid leading people to specific answers, nonthreatening, and nonjudgmental. A brief silence may be effective, as may repetition of the last phrase spoken by the client or a summary sentence. Closing probes may elicit important additional information. Probing further in the case of superficial and vague responses, as well as probing for feelings about events, is suggested in the following paragraphs.

When a more detailed response is desired in the case of superficial answers, the following may be asked:

"Can you tell me more about that?"

"What do you do next?"

"Please explain a little more about. . ."

"Anything else?"

To obtain clarification if the answer is vague one may respond:

"Could you clarify for me what did you mean by. . .?"

"I don't think I quite understand. . ."

Paraphrasing is another technique to ensure that the information is clear and correct. By repeating, summarizing, or rewording what was said, interviewers show that they are trying to understand.

When the person seems hesitant to go on, the interviewer may remain silent, pausing for the respondent to gather her thoughts and continue. The professional should appear attentive, with perhaps a thoughtful or expectant look, but should avoid eye contact for the moment. While the inexperienced interviewer may find silence uncomfortable and embarrassing and push on too quickly, a more experienced interviewer realizes that too hasty a response may cause part of the story to remain untold or change what is disclosed. If the interviewee does not go on within 30 to 60 seconds, however, she may perceive the silence as disinterest or disapproval; the interviewer should commence before that impression can occur.

A technique useful in breaking a silence is to repeat or echo the last phrase or sentence the person has said, raising the tone of voice to a question. For example:

"I follow my diet except when I eat out." "Except when you eat out?"

"I especially enjoy doing special projects with coworkers." "Special projects with your coworkers?"

Repetition, however, should not be overdone, or it has a parrotlike effect. If this is noticed by the respondent, it will inhibit conversation.

A summary sentence stated as a question also elicits further elaboration. For example:

"You say you already know how to plan a diabetic diet?"

"You think this company is the one you want to work for?"

Other probes are:

"Go on."

"I see."

"I understand, Mrs. Jones. Please continue."

"Uh huh."

"Hmmmmm."

"And next."

"Oh?" or "Oh!"

"Really?"

"Very good!"

"That's interesting!"

"I see," "I understand," and "that's interesting" may give a feeling of acceptance and encourage conversation or elaboration of a point of view. "Very good" gives the person a pat on the back, and is another kind of acceptance comment. Nonverbal probes include giving a quizzical look, leaning forward in the chair, and nodding of the head.

Understanding Responses. In the understanding response interviewers try to understand the person's message and re-create it within their own frame of reference. People have more rapport with those who try to understand them, and this may lead to more cooperation on the part of the client. "You are feeling concerned because you haven't lost any weight, Mrs. Jones, and you are wondering if it was something you ate, or a problem with the diet." The understanding response assists the person to clarify what was stated. The person also feels accepted even if her behavior has not been perfect. The client will feel safe in expressing her sentiments, and exploring them further. The client who believes that the professional is an understanding person may cooperate more fully in the interview.

Note that the professional should focus on the client's feelings and attitudes, rather than only on the content of what is said. In the example given, the client may be expressing her feelings of disappointment with the diet, her dissatisfaction with lack of progress in weight loss, her frustration in changing eating habits, or her fear of the dietetics professional's response to the fact that no weight has been lost.

The understanding response should be most helpful in assisting the client to recognize problems and to devise her own solutions. She may progress from initial negative feelings to more neutral ones and finally to more positive attitudes and solutions. Expressions of sincere sympathy may assist in building bridges in personal relationships, especially in response to information about death, prolonged illness, discomfort, or other problems. A quick response may be "Oh, my!" or "I'm very sorry to hear that."

It is necessary to differentiate and understand both the content of a message and the feelings. To determine the content, one may ask oneself, "What is this person telling me or thinking?" Feelings may be classified as positive, negative, or ambivalent, and these may change as the interview progresses (8). In identifying feelings, ask, "What is this person feeling, and why is he feeling that way?"

One may use the following sentence in paraphrasing the person's statement to verify one's understanding. The answer may be inserted into a format, such as "You feel. . .because. . ." Although one may have an incorrect impression, such as a feeling that a person is bored when the person actually is fatigued, the interviewee will usually provide the correct interpretation, thereby furthering the interviewer's understanding; this process demonstrates that one is trying to understand.

To avoid overuse of the same phrase and sounding mechanistic, the phrase can be varied, as for example: "Do I understand correctly that you feel. . .?" "You seem to be saying that you are feeling . . .," "I gather that . . .," "You sound . . .," or "In other words, you are feeling . . . ."

Interviewee responses that suggest feelings about an event may provide an important key to the person's behavior. How patients or clients feel about their lifestyles,

their diets, or their health is critical to dietary adherence. Food behaviors may be influenced by psychological, cultural, and environmental variables that are important to understand.

Job applicants may also express feelings about previous work experience, relationships with superiors and subordinates, and activities and interests. Preceding a statement with "I think," "I feel," or "I believe" gives a signal that the statement expresses opinions, beliefs, attitudes, and values. Follow-up probes may be the following:

"Can you explain more about your feelings?"

"What do YOU think about that?"

"What do you think causes that?"

Confrontation. Confrontation is an authority-laden response in which the interviewer tactfully and tentatively calls to the person's attention some inconsistency in the person's story or words and actions, pointing out the discrepancy to the individual (12). For example:

"I'm a bit concerned. You say you have no problem with the diet and yet you have not lost any weight for a month. What do you think is the problem?"

"You say that you liked your previous supervisor, but you didn't get along well with him?"

This response challenges and encourages the person to recognize and cope psychologically with some aspect of behavior that is self-defeating or to examine the consequences of some behavior. It should be used nonjudgmentally as discussion centers on resolution.

Confrontation is an advanced level skill that should not be used by an inexperienced interviewer or when good rapport and a supportive atmosphere are missing. Otherwise such responses can become threatening or appear punitive, and will inhibit conversation.

During the interview, one can examine not only what the person says, but also what is not said. Are there gaps in the information that the interviewer should try to fill? One should also note nonverbal behaviors, such as, tension, inability to maintain eye contact, hand movements, fidgeting, and facial expressions of discomfort, nervousness, anger, or lack of understanding. The nonverbal behaviors may be inconsistent with the verbal message, or may add to it.

While interviewers should adjust the pace of the interview to that of the respondent, they are also responsible for the direction of the interview. When the topics for discussion are inappropriate, the skilled interviewer brings the conversation back to appropriate areas. The patient talking about his wife or his children, for example, must be brought gently back to the diet history. A job applicant discussing a recent visit to Spain must be brought back to relevant topics. People who are especially talkative may ramble frequently, requiring more direction and leadership on the part of the interviewer. In these cases, restating or emphasizing the last thing said

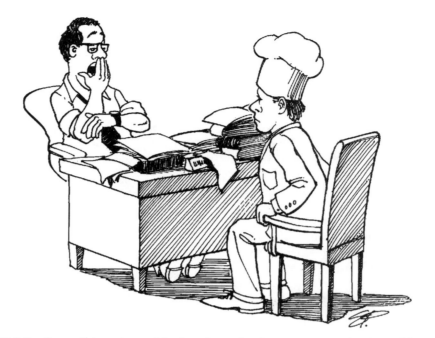

FIGURE 3.3. Some things to avoid when interviewing or communicating with another.

that was pertinent to the interview and asking a related question may be helpful.

Closing

The third part or closing of the interview takes the shortest amount of time but should not be rushed or taken lightly. A word of appreciation sincerely expressed, such as thanking the person for his or her time and cooperation, is a common closing. Another suggestion is to review the purpose of the interview and declare its completion. One may ask if there are any questions they would like to ask or any other comments they want to make, which may elicit important new information for which adequate time should be available. For example, "What else would you like to ask or tell me about?" The time, place, and purpose of future contacts should be mentioned. To a hospitalized patient, the professional may say, "I'll stop by to see you tomorrow to discuss your diet with you." With a client, arrangements for a future appointment may be made. To make sure that each has understood the other, plans may be paraphrased.

As a courtesy to job applicants, they should be told approximately when the employment decision will be made and how they will be notified if selected, for example, "We are interviewing additional candidates, but if selected, you'll hear from us in about a week by telephone." For those not selected, a letter may be sent thanking them for their applications and interest in the company and telling them the position has been filled. This letter is a public relations effort, which may be handled by the human resources department. The applicant who hears nothing after an interview may react negatively or telephone again for information. One may signal

the close of the interview by breaking eye contact, placing hands on the arms of the chair, standing up, offering to shake hands, smiling, and walking the interviewee to the door.

Interviewing is a skill, and as with other skills, it takes practice to develop. The inexperienced interviewer needs to plan in writing what topics need to be covered and in what sequence. Various types of questions can be prepared in advance in an appropriate sequence for the three parts of the interview. Physical surroundings and freedom from interruption should be planned. These conditions put the professional in a better position to concentrate on the interviewee and on the process of developing rapport, noting the verbal and nonverbal responses, and providing understanding responses with empathy. The interview session should be followed by a self-evaluation to determine areas that went well, as well as those that could be improved for the next interview.

REVIEW AND DISCUSSION QUESTIONS

1. What are the possible purposes of a diet history or nutrition interview? Of a pre-employment interview?
2. What conditions facilitate an interview?
3. Explain the three parts of an interview. What occurs in each part?
4. Differentiate between the following types of questions: open and closed; primary and secondary; and neutral and leading.
5. Explain the six types of responses.

SUGGESTED ACTIVITIES

1. Watch an interview on television noting the parts of the interview, techniques used, and verbal and

nonverbal responses. Write up your reactions and analysis.

2. Observe a television interview show. What types of questions are asked? What kinds of responses does the interviewer obtain?

3. Plan an interview guide specifying content and sequence. Write examples of various kinds of questions, such as, open and closed, primary and secondary, neutral and leading. Which kinds of questions do you prefer to answer?

4. Divide into groups of two for role-playing with each person interviewing the other in turn. Use various types of responses, such as probing, paraphrasing, and understanding. If three people are available, the third may serve as evaluator.

5. Make an audiotape of a simulated or actual interview, if participant's permission is granted. Complete an evaluation.

6. Make a videotape of a simulated or actual interview, if participant's permission is granted. This will show both the verbal and nonverbal behaviors as well as any personal idiosyncrasies. Complete an evaluation.

7. Turn on the television set without the sound. Try to interpret the nonverbal behavior you are seeing.

8. Arrange the furniture in a room or office for an optimum interviewing setting.

9. Change the following technical words that are used by professionals into terms that will help a client to understand their meanings:

Fiber

Nutrients

Sodium

Lipids

Protein

Serum glucose

Carbohydrates

Low density lipoproteins

Polyunsaturated fatty acids

Saturated fatty acids

Colitis

Gastric ulcer

Hypertension

Fluid intake

Osteoporosis

10. Directions: Read the lettered statements below. Identify both the thought the person is expressing and the feelings the person may be experiencing. Write a paraphrased statement reflecting the content or thought.

A. "I've had diabetes for 6 years. They put me on a diet and insulin injections when I first found out about it, and I check my blood sugar sometimes. The diet isn't too bad."

B. "I'm expecting my second baby. I never paid any attention to what I ate during my first pregnancy and my baby was healthy."

C. "The doctor told me that I can go home tomorrow, but I live alone so I have no one to help me with a diet, and I'm in no hurry to leave."

D. "Joan talks to people all day long and doesn't get her work done. The rest of us have to finish for her or we get yelled at."

E. "I've been working here for 10 years. Now you come in as a new supervisor and want to change everything around. What's wrong with keeping things the way they are?"

CASE STUDY

Delores Maynard is a 55-year-old woman who made an appointment with Joan Stivers, a registered dietitian in private practice, because of her interest in losing weight.

D.M. is 5′2″ tall and weighs 190 pounds. She says that she has no health problems. She is married with two grown children. She is unemployed at present.

Joan: "What brings you to our appointment?"

Delores: "Well, I need to lose a lot of weight."

Joan: "Tell me about any other times you tried to lose weight."

Delores: "I wasn't overweight until after I was married and bringing up two kids. Then I've gradually gained weight. Over the years, I've tried many different diets. I lose weight. But I gain it all back, and sometimes more. My husband thinks I should lose 50 pounds.

1. What questions would you ask in obtaining her nutrition history? Put them in sequence. Discuss the reason that each question is important in assisting the client.

2. What related questions would you like to ask, such as questions about meal preparation, food shopping, vitamin-mineral supplements, family meal practices, snacks, eating in restaurants, and weekend meals?

3. What other questions would you explore related to her family or lifestyle?

F. "How do you expect me to get all this work done? First you tell me to do one thing, and then you tell me to do another."

Directions: Write a second paraphrased statement reflecting the feelings in the above examples, such as:

"You seem to be *feeling* (angry, depressed, lonely etc.) *because* . . . ."

"It sounds like you *feel* . . . ."

"I hear you saying that you *feel* . . . . Tell me if I'm understanding you accurately."

Example: Client: "My friend and I are both dieting. She has lost weight, but I haven't even though I have been trying."

Counselor: "You seem to be *feeling* upset *because* your friend has lost weight and you haven't."

After writing your own paraphrase, discuss your paraphrase with others.

REFERENCES

1. Drake Beam Morin, Inc.: Selection interviewing for the 1990's. New York: Drake Beam Morin, 1993.
2. Sherman AW, Bohlander G, Snell S. Managing human resources, 10th ed., Cincinnati: South-Western, 1996.
3. Mathis RL, Jackson JH. Human resource management, 8th ed., St. Paul: West, 1997.
4. Umiker W. Selection interviews of health care workers. Health Care Superv 1988;6:58.
5. Thompson FE, Byers T. Dietary assessment resource manual. J Nutr 1994;124:2245S.
6. Dikovics A. Nutritional assessment: case study methods. Philadelphia: George F. Stickley, 1987.
7. Hankin JH. Dietary intake methodology. In: Monsen ER, ed. Research: successful approaches. Chicago: American Dietetic Assoc, 1992;173–186.
8. Bernstein L, Bernstein RS. Interviewing: a guide for health professionals. 4th ed. Norwalk, CT: Appleton-Century-Crofts, 1985.
9. Benjamin A. The helping interview with case illustrations. Boston: Houghton Mifflin, 1987.
10. Stewart CJ, Cash WB. Interviewing: principles and practices. 7th ed. Madison, WI: Brown & Benchmark, 1994.
11. Jobe JB, Mingay DJ. Cognitive research improves questionnaires. Am J Public Health 1989;79:1053.
12. Evans DR, Hearn MT, Uhlemann MR, et al. Essential interviewing: a programmed approach to effective communication. 4th ed. Pacific Grove, CA: Brooks/Cole, 1993.

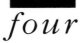

four

COUNSELING

Counseling may be defined as a process that assists people in learning about themselves, their environment, and methods of handling their roles and relationships. It involves problem solving, identifying goals, and change. Counselors assist individuals with the decision-making process, resolving interpersonal concerns and helping them to learn new ways of dealing with and adjusting to life situations.

In recent years, the profession of dietetics has experienced profound changes as the scope of practice has broadened. As the roles and responsibilities of dietetics practitioners have changed, so too has the need for knowledge and skills in different subjects. According to the 1995 Commission on Dietetic Registration Dietetics Practice Audit, one area of educational preparation of dietetics professionals that needs greater emphasis is communication. Role delineation studies conducted by the American Dietetic Association in the areas of clinical dietetics, community dietetics, and food-service systems management confirmed the need for dietetics practitioners to be knowledgeable of the process of communication in general, and the techniques of counseling in particular (1-6).

One's own needs for being a counselor affect the helping interactions. It is essential that counselors become aware of their own motivations in choosing to help others. Generally these include doing good, having contact with people, earning a living, and fulfilling a personal commitment. Often, however, there may be deeper motivations as well. Helping satisfies basic needs; it may provide a salary, but it also satisfies psychological needs. For example, counselors may become involved in helping others to resolve problems or to satisfy personal needs for power, prestige, and the dependency of others.

A counselor's needs do affect the process of helping others. For example, a counselor with a strong need to be needed might extend a helping relationship unnecessarily to gratify the need. Counselors with a need for power may take too much control over their counselees' situation or give too much advice. Counselors who have a need to be seen as competent can also interfere with the process of helping. If they tend to take personal responsibility for their counselees' successes and failures, they will become upset when counselees do not change. Counseling is influenced by the counselors' personal needs and motivations; therefore, it is crucial that counselors understand these needs prior to engaging in counseling to ensure that their personal needs do not interfere with their efforts to help (7).

There is no one correct way to counsel. Just as different clients will have different personalities, therapists will differ in personality and disposition. Adherence to a single therapy may limit the scope of the counselor-client relationship. A variety of theories and strategies are available and may be incorporated in a style that allows the counselor to adapt them on a contingency basis, depending on the needs of the counselee. There is an appropriate sequence: assess, plan, implement, evaluate, readjust as needed, and follow up. One plan of action, however, ordinarily will neither suffice nor always be appropriate for a particular client.

This chapter presents an overview of the counseling process as it applies to dietetics practitioners. There are currently approximately 40 different therapy models, approaches, or theories with only a few being most commonly used (8). These numerous theories and approaches exist to facilitate understanding, growth, and/or change on the part of the client seeking assistance, and each approach has its validity and its proponents. The chapter provides a brief overview of a few of the most popular counseling theories and approaches, followed by a more detailed description of the existential-humanistic client-centered approach, the one currently used most by dietetics practitioners.

Counseling is explored as a four-stage process, with the first stage concentrating on the development of a trusting, helping relationship between the counselor and counselee. The next three stages center on problem solving. The second half of the chapter focuses on two specific approaches to counseling, classified as nondirective and directive and concludes with a discussion of a specific type of work-related counseling, performance appraisal. Detailed discussions of other appropriate and relevant theories of dietetics counseling are presented in the chapters on behavior modification, counseling and cognitions, nutrition counseling, and multicultural communication.

It is not within the scope of this chapter to convert the reader into a practitioner of any one of the counseling theories presented. Dietetics practitioners can, however, learn to use components of a variety of counseling theories and integrate them effectively into their own counseling style. There are currently available several advanced books devoted entirely to discussions of counseling for dietary management (8, 9).

In addition to reading about various theories applicable to dietary management, the dietetics practitioner can take advantage of the many workshops and seminars conducted in different sections of the country. Attending such workshops affords the opportunity to learn more about the various theories from those who use them. Many colleges offer master's degrees in counseling and are likely to include courses that examine a variety of counseling theories.

PREVALENT THEORIES AND APPROACHES

Reality Therapy

Reality therapy was developed in the 1960s by William Glasser, MD, a board-certified psychiatrist (10). Reality therapists view human nature in terms of behavior, believing that human behavior is motivated by two basic needs common to all: the need to love and be loved, and the need to feel worthwhile to ourselves and others. People are responsible for their behavior, and behaving in a responsible manner helps people fulfill their needs. Clients are helped and encouraged to make value judgments about their own behavior, and once the chosen behavior is viewed as responsible, clients' feelings about their behavior tend to become positive. Adapting the concepts of this theory and the steps for implementation into dietary management affords the dietetics practitioner a structured, effective approach for assisting the client to change inappropriate eating behaviors (9).

Behavioral Counseling

Behavioral counseling has evolved from the early theories of behaviorism. The focus of behavioral counseling is on examining current behaviors and learning new ones. Counseling applications of this theory are discussed in the chapters on behavior modification and cognitions. In the chapter on cognitions, the point is made, however, that feelings and thoughts may come before the behavior, not after. For example, a person feels upset, so he eats.

Cognitive-Behavioral Approaches

Cognitive-behavioral approaches, which include psychoeducational and rational-emotive therapy, generally take less time in comparison to other contemporary theories and deal both with what a person does and what a person thinks. The goal in this therapy is to identify problem behavior and irrational beliefs, then to design strategies for immediate action plans. Psychoeducational therapy more specifically involves a process of learning about oneself and gaining self-understanding and self-knowledge. Once the patient has grown in the understanding, she is ready to learn to regulate her behavior in accordance with some standard. This therapy is intended to teach one to "manage" physical and mental impulses. The rational-emotive therapy, developed by Albert Ellis, is based on the premise that negative self-talk and irrational ideas are a major cause of emotion-related difficulties (11, 12). The therapy is intended to provide the client with insight to stimulate both logic and emotion simultaneously in the direction of the planned change. For the nutrition therapist the goal might be to help the client think, for example, that her serum cholesterol is too high and that foods lower in fat are preferred and also to "feel" emotions, like concern or fear, in order to sustain the effort toward change.

The Family Nutrition Approach to Counseling

The family nutrition approach to counseling involves relatives or significant others who live in the client's household in assisting clients to make necessary dietary changes to prevent or to control diet-responsive diseases and to maintain client adherence to nutrition advice over the long run. Family counseling is regularly practiced among dietetics practitioners in cases involving children and adolescents (8). Recent articles also discuss the need to educate the child or adolescent with diabetes in developmentally appropriate ways and to include the family in this process (13). Family therapy is appropriate where the client's problems are related to his relationship or function in the family. For such clients working with his or her family and in the family context promotes more rapid improvement and fewer relapses than when treated individually.

The Nondirective Approach to Counseling — Rogerian

The nondirective approach to counseling is often called "client-centered" and is best represented by the writing of its originator, Carl Ransom Rogers. Dr. Rogers' theory was first presented in his book *Counseling and Psychotherapy* (1942), and was further refined in subsequent publications (14, 15). Although the theory is constantly developing, changing with experience and research, there seems to have been no basic change in its assumptions. The theory is one of the more detailed, integrated, and consistent theories currently existing and has led to, and is supported by, a greater amount of research than any other approach to counseling (16). Rather than providing a complete description of the theory, the following discussion is intended to acquaint the reader with some of its more salient assumptions, particularly those related to the counseling techniques described later in this chapter.

Contrary to the common concept that people are by nature irrational, unsocialized, and destructive of themselves and others, a basic assumption in the client-centered point of view is that humans are basically rational, socialized, and realistic. All people, if their needs for positive regard from others and for positive self-regard are satisfied, possess an inherent tendency toward realizing their potential for growth and self-actualization. Counseling releases the potentials and capacities of the individual.

One of the most important characteristics of this theory is the relationship it suggests between the counselor and the client. The underlying assumption is that the client cannot be helped simply by listening to the knowledge the counselor possesses or to the counselor's explanation of the client's personality or behavior. Prescribing "cures" and corrective behavior are seen as being of little lasting value. The relationship that is most helpful to clients, that enables them to discover within themselves the capacity to use the relationship to change and grow, is not a cognitive, intellectual one. Rogers states, "I believe the quality of my encounter is more important in the long run than is my scholarly knowledge, my professional training, my counseling orientation, the techniques I use in the interview" (17). There are four specific characteristics that Rogers suggests the counselor possess for the therapy relationship: acceptance, congruence, understanding, and the ability to communicate these to the client.

The counselor needs to be accepting of clients as individuals, as they are, with their good and bad points, their conflicts and inconsistencies. Only after clients are convinced that they are accepted unconditionally and nonjudgmentally can they begin to trust the counselor. Recent research, moreover, has indicated that trust is not a nebulous feeling that people have about other individuals; instead, it is focused on predictability, genuine concern, and faithfulness (18).

Ideal counselors are characterized by congruence within the counseling relationship. They are unified, integrated, and consistent, with no contradictions between what they are and what they say. These counselors are able to express outwardly to their clients what they are feeling within themselves. Their verbal and nonverbal behaviors are consistent.

The counselor must experience an accurate, empathic understanding of the client's world as seen from the inside, sensing the client's world as if it were his or her own, but without losing the "as if" quality. This empathy is essential to nondirective therapy. The understanding enables clients to explore freely and deeply, and develop a better comprehension of themselves.

It is of no value for the counselor to be accepting, congruent, and understanding if the client does not perceive or experience this. The acceptance, congruence, and understanding need to be communicated to the client verbally and nonverbally. Rogers is definite in his belief that these not be "techniques," but a genuine and spontaneous expression of the counselor's inner attitudes (16).

If the counselor has these characteristics and is able to communicate them to the client, then a relationship develops that is experienced by the client as safe, secure, free from threat, and supportive. The counselor is perceived as dependable, trustworthy, and consistent. This is a relationship in which change can occur.

The administrative practitioner, moreover, working with staff, must be able to make the transition from technical professional to helping professional with a priority-oriented, tightly focused coach/counselor approach. This requires being a good listener, having intuition, providing feedback both on data and feelings, and providing inspiration (19).

COUNSELING AS A FOUR-STAGE PROCESS

In accordance with the theoretical assumptions of nondirective counseling, many counselors, trainers, educators, and theoreticians consider counseling to be a four-stage process. The first stage, "involving," includes the development of rapport, empathy, and a trusting relationship. The three subsequent stages are referred to as stage II, "exploring"; stage III, "resolving"; and stage IV, "concluding." They deal with the implementation of specific behavioral change strategies and techniques directed at the client's problem. Counseling deals simultaneously with both content and feelings. Trained counselors realize that only after the client's underlying feelings have been exposed and talked about can the content behind those feelings be discussed. Each stage requires special counseling skills that may have a particular utility and relevance at that stage (20).

The first stage, involving, may be initiated by either the client or the counselor, but the goals of this stage remain the same—to give clients clear expectations of the counseling process and a level of comfort and trust enabling them to interact authentically and effectively with the counselor. The counselor's sincere concern and caring must be established during this stage or the remainder of the counseling process is likely to be ineffective. Concern and caring are often expressed in ways other than words. The old adage is valid: actions speak louder than words. If the counselor seems uninterested, the counselee is likely to feel uncomfortable and confused. Attentive nonverbal behavior allows one to infer caring and concern and creates the impression that the counselor is capable and effective. Counselors need to be conscious of eye contact, body posture, hand and arm movements, facial expressions, and vocal quality because these are the signals by which clients infer the degree of attentiveness, caring, and concern. A counselor's words can make a difference, however. They can encourage the counselee to discuss a concern with greater openness or they can limit the counselee's disclosures. One must learn a new set of verbal responses, each of which is useful for a specific purpose.

Stages II, III, and IV relate more specifically to the recognition and initiation of specific behavior-change strate-

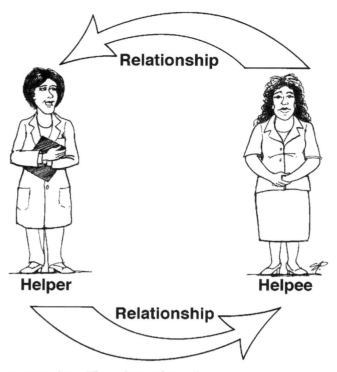

FIGURE 4.1. The relationship is key to successful counseling.

gies. Stage II, exploring, can begin once trust has been established. The goal is to discuss the nature of the specific problem in concrete rather than vague terms. The counselor's role is to encourage the counselee to enlarge on all issues and provide details related to the problem.

In stage III, resolving, the counselee's goal is to begin planning some actions to resolve the problem. The counselor, mostly through the use of questions, attempts to collaborate, suggest alternatives, and serve as a resource to the counselee.

The final stage, concluding, is intended to verify for the counselee the plan for subsequent actions. The counselor may reinforce the proposed actions of the counselee, but the primary task is to make certain that both counselor and counselee agree on what has occurred during the session and on all subsequent actions that are to take place. In the remainder of the chapter, nondirective counseling, directive counseling, and a specific category of directive counseling, "performance appraisal," are examined, using the four stages described above as the framework for discussion.

DIRECTIVE AND NONDIRECTIVE COUNSELING

Counselees perceive the two counseling strategies of directive and nondirective differently, and their responses to each style differ as well. Directive counseling tends to be most appropriate when the counselor is aware of the problem and/or is concerned about the behavior of the

counselee but the counselee is unaware of the problem or is avoiding acknowledging it. Nondirective counseling tends to be most appropriate when the counselee has insight and calls on the counselor to assist in the problem solving.

In the first instance, directive counseling, the counselor initiates discussion or summons the counselee. In the second instance, nondirective counseling, the counselee is aware of the problem and seeks help from the counselor. Counselees tend to be far more likely to become defensive and resist problem solving under the conditions of directive counseling. For this reason, counselors employing the method need to be especially sensitive to all verbal and nonverbal behavior, being supportive while attempting to explore the problem areas.

Unresolved employee complaints and concerns, for example, can result in formal grievances, serious performance difficulties, or legal disputes. Staff complaints fall into two categories: verbal and nonverbal. The latter may be expressed through careless or late-to-work habits, absenteeism, sleeping on duty, and horseplay. The manager needs to be receptive and alert to complaints and concerns and defuse them before they become more serious. Feedback from and to employees can be obtained through regularly scheduled staff or work unit meetings, the company's performance appraisal system, or counseling sessions (21). Directive counseling tends to occur most often in the manager-subordinate relationship rather than in the dietitian-client relationship. In general, directive counseling techniques are used to expose poor employee performance when employees are unaware or unwilling to expose it themselves.

When working with employees, dietetics professionals will generally have occasion to use both the directive and nondirective approaches to counseling; when working with clients, however, the nondirective approach tends to be used almost exclusively. It is the preferred counseling method when dealing with clients who need to plan and set wellness goals or with employees who have sought out the help of their manager or supervisor. Frequently, counselors employ a combination of both methods, but for discussion purposes, each is described separately, with the nondirective method described first.

Application of Nondirective Counseling

INVOLVING STAGE

When a client seeks out a professional directly, or when a client or patient has been referred by a physician, the dietetics practitioner should first allow clients to expose their concerns fully before giving any suggestions. The dietetics practitioner may be rushed and anxious to prescribe a diet regimen, but the regimen is likely to be ignored unless the patient has participated in the plan and has developed trust and a sense of confidence in the professional. An earlier chapter has elaborated on the necessity for clients to vent all of their concerns so that they are mentally receptive to listening. It is the nondirec-

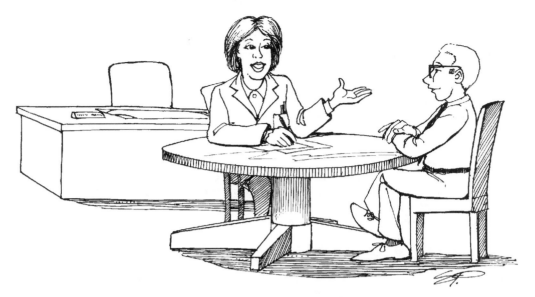

FIGURE 4.2. A casual setting creates a better rapport.

tive counselor's responsibility to encourage "venting." Sometimes patients are ill-at-ease with professional helpers and hesitate to talk. Practitioners may need to learn to tolerate some silence and to be reassuring and supportive when they attempt to induce clients to reveal underlying concerns.

Because underlying problems are frequently emotional rather than logical and are not likely to be revealed until the counselee trusts the counselor, the counselor's learning to respond without giving advice or passing judgment is essential. A client's excessive overeating or apparent lack of motivation in adhering to a diet may be due to some illogical and emotional stimulus rather than to a lack of discipline. He may be aware of the problem and may want to correct it, but before he reveals his underlying rationale and/or emotional conflict, he is likely to be seeking assurance that he will not be humiliated or embarrassed for doing so.

EXPLORING STAGE

There is little value in counselors making recommendations until they have first fully understood the client's perspective and gained the client's trust. Clients become far more receptive to hearing their counselor's advice when they are certain that they have said all they want to say and that their words have been understood. During the exploring stage, the dietetics practitioner attempts to provide insight for the counselee by clarifying perceptions and attempting to discuss the problems in concrete terms.

Several techniques can be used to motivate clients to contribute to the counseling session during the exploring stage. Small talk at the beginning of the interview can help relax the interviewee. The location of the interview, as well as the physical surroundings, can create different

moods and should, therefore, be carefully selected. All interruptions should be eliminated during the entire interview period, and note taking should not interfere with the client-interviewer relationship. If there are forms to be filled out, they too should be personalized as much as possible (22).

Not all clients are articulate and able to express themselves. Although they may want to express themselves, they may have a difficult time exposing their concerns. The counselor can offer assistance by asking questions that stimulate full explanations. Two kinds of questions used in counseling are "open-ended questions" and "closed-ended questions." Understanding the distinction between the two is important because each tends to elicit a different response from the counselee. The use of directives or "encouragers" and active listening are helpful.

Closed-Ended Questions. Closed-ended questions are designed to be answered by brief responses (often by one or two words, or by "yes" or "no"). They are good for eliciting specific data quickly. Examples include questions, such as, "When did you notice you were gaining excess weight?" or "Where do you tend to do most of your eating?" and "When do you find yourself craving sweets most?"

Open-Ended Questions. Open-ended questions are designed to encourage longer answers. They are good for eliciting responses in the other's own words, and for encouraging the other to enlarge on an idea and to reveal all concerns. The major difficulty with open-ended questions is that they take longer to answer and can be frustrating when specific data are needed and time pressures are present. They tend to be characterized by the words "how," "what," and "why." "How did you initially try to lose weight on your own?"; "What sorts of treatments have you tried in the past?''; and ''Why do you want to be a size three?'' are examples of open-ended questions.

The skill of asking specific closed-ended questions when a short and concise direct answer is desired and open-ended questions when a fuller and more subjective answer is desired is not natural for most people. The explanation and examples given previously may make it seem simple. It is not! Developing this ability takes practice, and both students and professionals wishing to increase their competence in question formation should make a conscious effort to practice it whenever possible. Over time, the skills become automatic and one begins to frame questions easily, either to elicit specific answers or to allow the counselee to move the discussion subjectively into other areas.

Use of Directives. There will be times when even open-ended questions fail to lead the client to expand on an idea or give additional information. The response may be a simple shrug of the shoulders, or ''I don't know'' or ''I don't remember.'' When this occurs, there is an additional verbal response possible from the counselor that is often effective. It is called a ''directive.'' A directive involves the use of a command rather than a question. It should not, of course, sound like a command and put the client on the defensive, but when delivered in a gentle, supportive manner, directives often do what open-ended questions cannot do with hesitant clients—get them to talk more. Examples of directives include comments such as ''Talk more about . . .''; ''I want to know what you think of . . .''; ''Tell me your ideas on . . .''; ''Expand on your thoughts regarding . . . .''

Use of Encouragers. In addition to the use of open-ended questions, closed-ended questions, and directives, counselors need to develop their ability to use nonverbal ''encouragers.'' Encouragers are sometimes verbal utterances such as ''Yes, yes,'' ''Ah, ha,'' or ''Hmmmm,'' or some other sound that indicates to the client that the counselor is listening and comprehending. These utterances should be accompanied by such nonverbal signs as nodding the head, leaning forward toward the client, and making other facial expressions that suggest interest, understanding, and the desire for the client to go on speaking. Frequently, the best way to get the client to talk more is for the counselor to remain silent when the client stops talking. After a few moments of silence without the counselor filling in the awkward moments, the clients are apt to go on talking if they have more to add.

Active Listening. It has been mentioned that prior to the counselors' acts of asking questions, probing into specific areas, giving advice, or disclosing their own experiences, they must first be certain that they have understood the problems as the client intends. This is done through the use of active listening—paraphrasing and responding empathically. After the counselor has understood the original problem to the counselee's satisfaction, and at each subsequent stage in the counseling process, the counselor needs to repeat the verification process through paraphrase and empathic responses. Communicators need to remember that they don't know what they don't know. Everyone is subject unconsciously to selective perception and communication distortion. For that reason, a summary paraphrase and an empathic reaction are appropriate at each stage in the counseling process. Besides verifying that she is understanding the counselee as intended, the paraphrase summary often provides real insight for the counselee. Just hearing the same comments in another person's words can help the counselee to see new possibilities and to provoke new insight.

The underlying principle governing the use of nondirective counseling is that when clients seek help, they are often the people in the best position to solve their own problems and to suggest corrective behavior. The job of the counselor is to help counselees to understand their problems more clearly and, in nutrition counseling, to make them aware of alternatives available for solving the problem. In nondirective counseling, the technique for doing this is called ''mirroring.'' The counselor ''mirrors'' or reflects back to the counselee what has been said. When this is done in a supportive manner, without the subjective values and judgments of the counselor added, the process tends to stimulate creative thinking and understanding in the counselee. Part of the ''supportive manner'' for counselors includes the ability to make responses without sounding clinical. A comment such as ''What I hear you saying is . . .'' may be interpreted as sounding clinical and officious. It is more supportive to say, ''I just want to be sure I'm understanding. Is this what you are saying . . . ?''

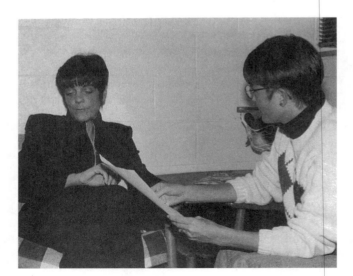

FIGURE 4.3. The person's nonverbal behavior gives clues to her reaction.

RESOLVING STAGE

Once the total problem has been explored and understood, the counselor and counselee can move on to examine the criteria for solving the problem, which form the framework for any solution. The specific purpose of this stage is to assist the counselee in setting goals and identifying resources for resolving the problem. As mentioned earlier, all stages of the process are primarily interrogative for the counselor. The practitioner moves through the stages by asking questions, not by judging. The counselor might say to someone with high blood pressure and a problem of eating too many high-sodium foods, for example, "What are some low-sodium snacks that could be substituted for potato chips?" To someone whose problem is eating too many high-calorie desserts and whose goal is to lose weight, she might ask about the possibility of selecting fruit for dessert for the next 7 days or the possibility of purchasing lower-fat meats for the next week.

Throughout the process, discipline is required of counselors. Often, they will be tempted to say, "Can't you see, this is what you need to do!" or "This is what you must do." The problem in being prescriptive, that is, telling the counselee what he or she must do to solve the problem, is that the solutions arrived at in that manner are not really the counselee's; they are the counselor's. Solutions that people have struggled to form themselves are more likely to work than ones "given" them by another person. If the solution prescribed by the counselor does not work, the counselee can always say, "I told you so," or "You didn't really understand what I meant." Also, when counselors dictate solutions to counselees, they are likely to receive the response, "Yes, but . . ." from the counselee. The counselee tends to rationalize a reason for rejecting whatever the counselor prescribes. Although the alternative method takes longer and requires more discipline, counselors will be more effective in the nondirective process if they coach the counselee to make all decisions whenever possible.

After the criteria for a solution are made clear, the counselor needs to help the counselee formulate several alternative solutions. This process may take time, discipline, and patience. Frequently, one solution is obvious, while other possible solutions remain in the client's unconscious. Counselors with discipline and patience can bring other potential solutions to the consciousness of their clients by helping them to focus on other possibilities and not allowing them to rush off on refining the single first alternative. Some open-ended questions useful at this stage are "What solutions have you tried already?" "What are some things that might help?" "Are there other possibilities you haven't yet thought of?" Allowing time for silent reflection on the part of the counselee during this process is critical.

After several alternatives have been listed, the counselor may add other possibilities. As the nutrition expert, the professional has knowledge and insight to suggest alternatives unknown to the client. It is important, however, to add additional suggestions in a way that leaves the counselee free to reject any and all. The difference between "Here is one thing you might consider" and "Here is what you need to do" is that if the former is accepted as the solution, the counselee considers it his or her own idea and will be committed to making it work; if the latter is selected, the counselee considers it the counselor's idea and is less committed to making it work.

There will also be times when the alternative selected by the counselee is obviously a poor choice. Here the counselor may be tempted to say, "Can't you see what a poor solution that is?" or even worse, "That is a terrible idea." Rather than pass negative judgments, the counselor would do better to assist the counselee in understanding the weaknesses in the solution. This can be done through the use of open-ended questions that will foster the counselee's involvement in evaluating the solution. The counselor might ask, for example, "What would happen if you tried that? Would the situation get better or worse?" In this way, the counselee, not the counselor, is rejecting the solution.

CONCLUDING STAGE

It is possible for a client to go through the entire process previously described and not internalize the agreed upon solution and action plan. Because most people are not accustomed to being counseled, and because of the status distinction between the counselor and counselee, the counselee may feel a heightened anxiety, which causes him or her to distort meanings and block clear understanding. The client may be agreeing and nodding understanding when, in fact, nervousness is hindering clear perception. Another possibility is that while the counselee is nodding and agreeing, and the counselor is nodding and agreeing, each thinks he or she is in consensus with the other; however, as pointed out in Chapter 2, meanings are in people, not in words. It is possible that each person has interpreted the agreed upon solution differently. For those reasons, closure of the counseling session needs to include a final paraphrase by the counselee that includes action plans. As a result of the session, the counselee should have plans to do something to correct the problem, and both the client and the counselor need to be in agreement on what that action is to be. The chapter that deals specifically with nutrition counseling expands on the concepts presented here.

Applications of Directive Counseling

Employee counseling can be defined as the discussion of a work-related problem to eliminate or reduce it. Problems might include such things as performance and discipline on the job as well as the need for professional and/or skill development. Unless managers have advanced degrees with appropriate clinical counseling experience, counseling their staff should be limited to the job-related concerns mentioned previously and should not include probing into personal problems such as depression, drug abuse, alcoholism, and midlife crisis. For such personal problems, the manager should provide referrals, recommending professional therapists, psychologists, or psychiatrists. When employee counseling loses its problem-performance orientation, it runs the risk of being interpreted as meddling or an invasion of privacy.

Directive counseling is the method used for discussing job-related problems with subordinates when the employee is unaware of the problem, has already been warned about the problem and has not corrected it, or is aware of the problem but hopes that the manager is not. Often, managers tolerate abusive and inappropriate behavior from subordinates, rather than confronting and counseling them directly to improve. Among the reasons this inaction often occurs are the following: managers may be afraid of handling the counseling poorly and making matters worse; they may be afraid of losing an otherwise good employee if the employee objects to being called in for counseling; they may be afraid of being confronted in return and becoming defensive themselves; they may be afraid of retaliation from the employee, either by his spreading stories to the other staff members or by his engaging in some kind of subversive activity on the job; or they may be worried about losing the friendship and respect of the employee. Because directive counseling has the potential to make matters worse, these fears are legitimate, especially for managers who have not had training in directive counseling or in conflict resolution.

Training in directive counseling is essential for managers. Often, individuals who are extraordinary in their professional expertise or ability to perform a professional task are selected to manage others. Promoting technical professionals into management without first providing them with adequate training for the job is like sending individuals to bat with two strikes against them. Directive counseling, like nondirective counseling, can bring two people closer interpersonally, but only when the counselor understands the underlying principles and is sensitive to the need to preserve the self-concept of the counselee.

Managers who fear confronting employees directly and who tolerate poor work behavior may be creating additional morale problems among the rest of the staff. Resentment swells in those who are cooperating and attending to their occupational obligations. When they see others of equal rank and salary doing less or doing poorly and getting away with it, their own morale sags.

Directive counseling of employees is a form of discipline, and those administering it need to understand the concept. The root of the word "discipline" comes from Latin and means "to train" or "to teach." The attitude of the counselor needs to be that of a caring teacher who wishes to assist the other in improving. The objective of employee counseling is to change workers' behavior and develop productive members of the organization (23).

The best way to address and improve poor performance involves a three-step process. Step one is to be ready to face the facts and recognize that waiting for things to change simply will not work. It is essential to make sure that the employee understands that management is seriously dissatisfied with work performance, that the need for change is urgent, and what specific changes in performance are needed. If the employee has objections, the objections should be carefully considered, and modifications in the requirements should be made if merited. Step two is to establish clear objectives and a timetable to meet them. Step three and a last resort is to terminate the employee in an honest and straightforward manner (24, 25).

INVOLVING STAGE

In opening the discussion with the counselee, the counselor must be explicit in the desire to solve a problem rather than to punish. The manager's aim is to improve the subordinate, not to get an apology. One way of keeping the conversation from becoming threatening is to keep remarks performance-centered rather than to make judgments about the staff member. It is more supportive and factual to say, "You have been late six times in the past 2 weeks," for example, than to say, "Lately you don't seem to care about your job; your attitude is poor." Inferences are not facts. The manager could not possibly know the quality of the employee's "caring" for his job or the condition of his "attitude," but she does know the objective facts—that the employee has been late six times in 2 weeks.

EXPLORING STAGE

Throughout the interview, the counselor focuses on objective facts, being specific about what she has seen, what she wants in terms of improved behavior, and what action she will take if she does not get it. If others have been complaining, and if the manager is unable to document the examples from personal observation, it would be best to postpone the session until she has direct observation to illustrate to the employee. Saying such things as, "Some of the staff members have been complaining about your behavior," or "Word has gotten to me," will make the employee suspicious of coworkers and hinder the possibilities for future trusting relationships among the staff.

RESOLVING STAGE

As in nondirective counseling, the counselor should provide adequate opportunity for employees to tell their side of the story, and their remarks should be paraphrased as well. As pointed out in the "Count the 'F's'" exercise in Chapter 2, not only do people not know what they do not know, but they easily fall into traps of seeing, hearing, and selectively perceiving what they expect to see and hear. Giving employees an opportunity to tell their side of the story and then paraphrasing it, and empathizing with what the employee is feeling, usually leads to collaboration in the conflict-resolution process. There may be extenuating circumstances that no one on the staff is aware of that account for the dysfunctional behavior of the employee. Having employees explain the problem from their own perspective may add significant insight and understanding.

When attempts at collaboration do not work, managers can shift to another mode of solving the problem. They can use a win-lose mode, insisting that it be their way "or else." They may win the battle but lose the war if they use this mode too often. They can back down when they see the employee becoming defensive and allow the employee to continue the poor performance. They can attempt to compromise with the employee and agree to some exceptions if the employee agrees to improve soon. Too often, however, managers rush to compromise and negotiate behavior change with employees because this approach is less stressful than collaboration. The problem with compromise is that neither party leaves fully satisfied. Employees resent being called about a problem and being asked to change, and the managers resent that they have been unable to bring about the optimal behavior they had originally hoped for. In "real life," there may be times when the best approach is any one of the four discussed previously. Collaboration is not always possible, and so it may be necessary on occasion to use one of the others. Managers, however, need to understand that their first approach should be to try to collaborate on solutions with employees as a first and preferred mode of problem solving.

CONCLUDING STAGE

After an agreement on a solution has been reached, the counselor should describe as specifically as possible what the consequences will be if the agreed upon changes in the employee's behavior are not actualized. At the moment, less tension and a shorter discussion might result from simply saying, "You had better straighten up or else"; however, in the long run, it is far more effective to be exact. One might say, for example, "If you are absent without notice again, I am going to file a warning notice with human resources." The manager needs to remember at this point not to exaggerate the consequences or to mention consequences she has neither the authority nor the intention to carry out. If the employee does continue the dysfunctional behavior and the manager fails to implement the consequences, the manager is implicitly fostering a norm that others will expect to be applied to them. She is giving one extra chance beyond the final warning. Also, she risks developing the reputation of being "all bark and no bite," and of being an ineffective manager.

If managers have been too lenient in the past, tolerating poor work behavior from the staff and avoiding con-

frontation in the form of directive counseling, they will encounter resistance if they suddenly insist that everyone must perform optimally. Staff members tend to assume that supervisors are partially to blame because they did not object to their behavior in the past. In such cases, counselors need to admit their share of the blame for lax supervision in the past. They need to acknowledge their own responsibility for not attending to the problem sooner, and then to work with the staff on ways of correcting the poor performance. Professional confrontation is an effective and equitable management tool and should not be avoided.

While verifying understanding is important in nondirective counseling, it is even more important in directive counseling. The tendency for employees to experience physiological stress symptoms from the threat of being called in by the manager heightens the possibility of their misunderstanding some of the communication. Both the manager and the staff members need to paraphrase one another to verify that each has understood the other and that they agree on the final solution.

A final step that is appropriate for directive counseling of subordinates is for managers to assure subordinates that they really do want them to succeed. An expression of confidence and support can help ensure successful implementation of an action plan that both parties have agreed upon. Rather than saying, "Well, let's see what will happen," the manager provides more motivation by saying, "I think these are the kinds of ideas that can make a difference." Employees should be reminded that they are an important part of the unit, that the manager does indeed care for them personally, and that their contributions to the staff are valued. If the action plan includes a multistep process for improvement, it would be wise to set follow-up dates for meeting with subordinates. Doing so not only confirms commitment, but also adds incentive to begin changes.

The processes of counseling are far more effective if a trusting relationship exists between the counselor and counselee. In the case of directive counseling between a manager and a subordinate, there is an ongoing and consistent relationship before the counseling as well as after it. The manager cannot vacillate between being unfeeling, bureaucratic, officious, and cold toward subordinates most of the time and being suddenly supportive, caring, and trustworthy during the counseling session. Subordinates begin inferring the degree of trustworthiness and caring on the part of managers from the time of their first encounter with them, with each subsequent encounter adding to their perceptions. Being a manager of other people is actually a "helping profession" in itself. The manager needs to lay the foundation for that trust early and continuously. Directive counseling is characterized by both a caring and a determined effort to correct dysfunctional behavior affecting work performance.

Managers must attend to the supporting nonverbal behavior throughout the directive counseling interview. They should select a private place free of interruptions. The spatial dynamics of the location should allow the two people to feel at ease as feelings are being shared and help is being given to solve the problem. The manager needs to act, talk, look, and gesture in a manner that allows the subordinate to infer that the purpose of the counseling session is to change dysfunctional behavior, not to reject or punish him. Finally, the manager has to remember to allow adequate time for full expression of thoughts, scheduling multiple sessions when appropriate.

PERFORMANCE APPRAISAL: A SPECIFIC APPLICATION OF DIRECTIVE COUNSELING

The manager has an obligation to conduct work-related counseling sessions with employees. These should be held as often as necessary, assisting the staff in their professional development as well as dealing with career problems as they occur. Counseling employees can be considered a form of staff development and training.

Above all, the manager should not postpone employee counseling until the annual or semiannual performance appraisal interviews. Allowing problems to accumulate and handling them all at one time may seem more time-efficient, but in the long run this strategy is generally ineffective, for problems may accumulate beyond easy resolutions. Dealing with issues one at a time as they occur is highly advisable.

Performance appraisals are a specific type of counseling in which professionals engage. Unfortunately, too often most organizations assume that no special training is required to conduct such an interview and that all one needs to do with staff is to observe, take notes, perhaps fill out an evaluative form or checklist provided by the organization, and attempt to "motivate" the employee to improve according to the counselor's prescriptions. This portion of the counseling chapter describes what the counselee/employee and the manager each need to do to prepare for the appraisal counseling session.

Employees need to be very clear on the criteria used in their performance evaluations and the kinds of work-related behavior that are likely to reflect positively or negatively. Both the supervisor and the employee share the obligation to clarify one another's expectations of the standards long before the actual appraisal occurs.

The tone of a performance review should reflect the desire of the organization not to punish but to isolate skills and competencies that are currently deemed appropriate and others that need improvement, so that remedies could be considered and developed as needed. As discussed in Chapter 9, "Motivation," behavior that is reinforced is repeated and behavior that is punished, unless perceived as warranted, will meet with resentment, if not with hostility. Perceived punishment is the least effective way to alter human behavior.

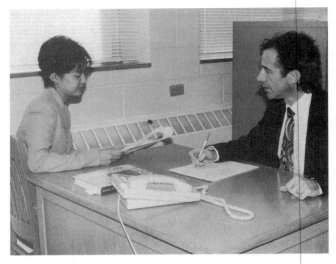

FIGURE 4.4. A quiet setting is important for performance appraisal.

The manager's ability to exercise optimal communication skills throughout the performance appraisal counseling sessions is critical. Appraising another person's performance is one of the most emotionally charged of all management activities. The impression subordinates receive about their assessment has a strong impact on their self-esteem and subsequent performance. Positive affect toward the employee needs to be demonstrated daily and routinely; it must become part of the manager's "style." One's sense of belonging, competence, and worthiness in the workplace are the three most critical ingredients of one's sense of professional self-esteem, and the appraisal session can either heighten or diminish them.

Statistically speaking, the performance of half of all employees is below the median, yet evidence suggests that the average employee's estimate of his or her own performance level generally falls around the 75th percentile. A survey of more than 800,000 people found that most individuals see themselves as better than average. Seventy percent rated themselves above average on leadership, and when asked to rate themselves on "ability to get along with others," none rated himself or herself below average. Sixty percent rated themselves in the top 10%, and 25% saw themselves among the top 1%! Similarly, a survey of 500 clerical and technical employees found that 58% rated their own performance as falling in the top 10% among their peers doing comparable jobs and a total of 81% placed themselves in the top 20%. The point of sharing these statistics is that unless the manager reinforces the appraisal with quantitative data and/or specific examples, any negative constructive criticism may come as a surprise to the employee, who may well have an inflated perception of his or her skills and competencies. Even good news may not be as good as the employee had anticipated (26).

Appraisal approaches vary. They include behavioral approaches such as rating scales, peer rating or ranking, and outcome approaches, such as, management by objectives and goal setting (27–30).

Listed below are specific suggestions for conducting performance appraisal interviews. Although there is frequently crossover and dovetailing among the stages of counseling, the suggestions have been grouped according to the stages in which they would ordinarily occur.

Involving Stage

Employees themselves should be trained to engage in self-evaluation. Prior to the interview they should be taught how to evaluate themselves, and, more importantly, to consider what the organization generally, and the appraising manager specifically, can do to help them perform better. The manager at this time must exercise one communication skill particularly well—listening. If there is anything the employee requests that can be granted, she should be accommodated.

The "upward communication" from the employee to manager that occurs during the appraisal allows the employee to experience the organization's desire to develop him or her, acknowledging the individual's needs, strengths, and proclivities. Rapport is more easily maintained when the counseling session occurs at an appropriate time, when all parties are prepared to talk at length, and in an appropriate place, one that is private without being intimidating and where there will be no interruptions.

The appraiser needs to define herself in the role of coach or mentor during the counseling session. By the conclusion of a carefully planned performance appraisal the interpersonal relationship between mentor and mentee is enhanced. The appraiser should verbally acknowledge the performance appraisal counseling session as a development tool. This gives appraisees who want additional training, knowledge, and expanded visibility the opportunity to identify themselves.

Exploring Stage

The appraiser should spend time acknowledging the subordinate's strengths, letting the subordinate know how aware the appraiser is of his contributions. Specific "chapter and verse" examples go a long way here. It is extremely affirming to hear someone in a position of influence acknowledge one's gifts, strengths, efforts, and dedication.

Although there are generally numerous opportunities in performance appraisal counseling to use techniques ordinarily associated with nondirective counseling, it is, nevertheless, considered a form of directive counseling. The counselor is advised to be directive, specific, and exact—giving dates, times, circumstances, and examples of problems to be solved, so that the employee/counselee

understands what needs to be altered and what will happen if appropriate improvements do not occur. For this reason the pre-preparation by the appraiser is time-consuming but tends to be far more worthwhile for the counselee.

Time needs to be provided for the subordinate to make recommendations to the appraiser. Prior to the session, the appraisee should be invited to prepare suggestions, requesting that any suggestions for improvement be given with specific examples, so that they can be understood. The appraiser/counselor has an opportunity during this "turning of the tables" activity to model behavior by not becoming defensive or contradicting the other's reality. The appraiser should attempt to listen carefully, verifying the understanding of what could be done differently to be more effective in working with this particular subordinate. If several subordinates make the same constructive comments, appraisers should very seriously consider altering their behavior and acknowledge their efforts to accommodate subordinates.

The focus throughout the counseling session should be on the future rather than the past. The appraiser may bring up examples from the past, but the emphasis is best kept on what can be learned from the past so that work-related tasks and interactions will be more effective.

Resolving Stage

Performance appraisal counseling is an opportunity for new and improved ideas to emerge. When both the supervisor and the subordinate remain nondefensive and talk about how work could be done more effectively, synergy often occurs. Without being accusatory, appraisers need to train themselves to make comments, such as, "There seems to be a problem here," and "What might we consider doing to improve the situation?"

The counselor needs to plan so that the social climate during the session remains supportive and facilitates a healthy rapport. If things get out of hand, however, and the communication breaks down during the appraisal, it should be terminated and rescheduled for another time. Confrontations and arguments rarely lead to collaboration. Remember, the purpose of appraisal counseling is to agree on steps for improvement; in a confrontation the more powerful "boss" may "win," but at the expense of destroying rapport and the spirit of collaboration.

For a performance review to have long-term effectiveness, the counselees/subordinates need to feel some "ownership" and commitment to whatever is agreed upon; therefore, they should be encouraged to participate actively. Some individuals will be anxious to share their views, while others will be reluctant, shy, or fearful. The most powerful way to get the other to participate is silence. Wait and listen; once others are convinced the appraiser is genuinely interested in their perspectives, they will provide it. Although it has been stated elsewhere in this text, it bears repeating: people don't know what they don't know. In listening and paraphrasing and not interrupting, the appraisers may discover new data that alters their perceptions of the original appraisal.

Concluding Stage

The leading cause of stress among American workers is the absence of feedback. The performance appraisal counseling session is an opportunity to reduce stress by making sure the subordinate has all her questions answered regarding her performance. Before concluding not only should the appraiser clear her own agenda of discussion topics, but she should also provide time for the appraisee to ask questions and paraphrase her understanding of what needs to occur prior to the next appraisal.

The session should conclude on a positive note. The subordinate should paraphrase any action plans or future goals agreed upon. Even though one may look like one is in agreement and understands, the tension of the experience sometimes clouds clear communication. The session, therefore, should conclude with the subordinate and appraiser both reassuring one another that they have been understood and that the appraiser does intend to work with the subordinate in areas in which improvement is necessary.

The model described above works best when quarterly appraisals are the protocol. When each session concludes with short-term goals for improvement and a time schedule that permits brief meetings to accommodate and fine-tune or amend goals, subsequent sessions then become opportunities to review goals from previous meetings while formulating additional ones.

In summary, performance appraisal counseling is a two-way process, with each party providing feedback to the other. The skills required to optimize the counseling session do not come naturally to most people. Training in the appraisal counseling process is essential. For managers the training should occur during their education or mentoring process; for subordinates, however, it generally is up to the manager to teach communication skills that enable each to experience growth through discussion of performance.

REVIEW AND DISCUSSION QUESTIONS

1. What are the four stages of counseling?

2. Explain the difference between directive and nondirective counseling.

3. What should the attitude be of a counselor who is administering directive counseling?

4. What is the three-step process involved in directive counseling?

5. What is a closed-ended question?

6. What is an open-ended question?

7. What is a directive?

8. What is active listening and how is it used in the counseling process?

9. In the concluding stage, what should a counselee do at the close of the counseling session?

SUGGESTED ACTIVITIES

1. During the next week, make arrangements to view a practitioner's counseling session, noting particularly what occurs during stage I, "Involving." What behavior on the part of the dietetics practitioner facilitates the building of rapport and trust?

2. During the following week, make three efforts to express caring for another, using nonverbal behavior. What do you do, and how does the other respond?

3. Using a videotape recorder, meet with another individual and record 10 minutes of interaction and conversation. Comment on the quality of your verbal and nonverbal behavior. What kind of messages might one infer from your demeanor?

4. In groups of three, develop a conversation around the topics presented in this chapter. Before one person can respond to what another has said, however, he will need to paraphrase to the other's satisfaction what the other has just said.

5. During the next week, practice paraphrasing after others talk. What reactions do you get? Does your paraphrasing tend to cause the other to go on talking?

6. In round-robin groups of five, each person expresses a statement, and the person to the right should attempt to identify a feeling expressed in the statement. After three rounds, discuss the reactions of the group to the attempts at empathizing.

7. Write both a paraphrase and empathic comment to the following comments made by a counselee:
   A. I feel awkward discussing my eating habits. I feel I must be disgusting to you.
   B. People tend to think I'm jolly, but I don't believe they take me seriously.
   C. I am at a point now where I don't believe I will ever lose the weight.

8. Form triads consisting of a counselor, counselee, and observer. Each individual should take a turn in each of the roles for 7 minutes. The counselee should play the role of an obese client, and the counselor should use paraphrasing and empathizing, along with open-ended and closed-ended questions, to facilitate disclosure and problem solving. After each round, the observer should share his reactions to the counselor's approach and encourage

CASE STUDY

Connie, a Clinical Dietitian, has worked at Sun Valley Hospital, a 300-bed community hospital, for 3 years. Her immediate supervisor, Jill, a Chief Clinical Dietitian, is preparing her performance evaluation. While preparing Connie's evaluation, Jill noted that more than 50% of the goals for Connie's performance had not been met. During Connie's evaluation, she asked Jill why her merit increase was smaller than the year before. Jill indicated that since 50% of her goals were not met, she would not be entitled to a full merit increase, but only a percentage based on the goals that were met. Connie left the evaluation session angrily, stating "I don't think this is fair."

1. What can Jill do to avoid such confrontations in the future?
2. Who should prepare the goals? The employee, the manager, or both?
3. Should time frames have been set for each of the goals? Why?
4. Should a professional's goals be checked for progress made and appropriateness of direction?
5. What are the communication steps that Jill should take to avoid a future misunderstanding?

feedback from the counselee to the counselor. From the counselee's perspective, what did the counselor do that helped their interaction; what did he do that hindered it?

9. Write an open-ended question for each of the statements below:
   A. I never have any fun at a family gathering anymore. Being on this diet has taken the fun out of my life.
   B. I dislike my supervisor at work. No matter what I do, he criticizes me.
   C. Since I developed these health problems, it seems that all I do is think about my diet.

10. After each of the statements below, write responses in the form of a closed-ended question, an open-ended question, or a directive.
    A. My work situation is impossible. It seems that I'm the scapegoat for everybody. I'm beginning to wonder if I should consider looking for another job.
    B. It doesn't seem fair to me that I should have to work weekends when the staff members who have been here only 2 years longer don't have to.
    C. It seems easy every morning to promise myself that today I will stick to the program you designed for me. By noon, however, I begin thinking that I'll never be able to comply with the diet for the rest of my life, so why bother?

REFERENCES

1. Kane MT, Cohen AS, Smith ER, et al. 1995 Commission on dietetic registration dietetics practice audit. J Am Diet Assoc 1996;96:1.
2. Baird S, Armstrong R. Role delineation for entry-level clinical dietetics. Chicago: American Dietetic Assoc, 1981.
3. Baird S, Sylvester J. Role delineation and verification for entry-level positions in community dietetics. Chicago: American Dietetic Assoc, 1983.
4. Baird S, Sylvester J. Role delineation and verification for entry-level positions in food service systems management. Chicago: American Dietetic Assoc, 1983.
5. Kane MT, Estes CA, Colton DA, et al. Role delineation for dietetic practitioners: empirical results. J Am Diet Assoc 1990;90:1124.
6. Kane MT, Estes CA, Colton DA, et al. Role delineation study for entry-level registered dietitians, entry-level dietetic technicians, and beyond-entry-level registered dietitians. Chicago: American Dietetic Assoc, 1989; Vols. 1-3.
7. Danish S, D'Augelli A, Hauer A. Helping skills: a basic training program. Trainee's workbook. 2nd ed. New York: Human Sciences Press, 1989.
8. Helm KK. Nutrition therapy: advanced counseling skills. Lake Dallas, TX: Helm Seminars, 1995.
9. Hodges P, Vickery C. Effective counseling: strategies for dietary management. Rockville, MD: Aspen Publications, 1989.
10. Glasser W. Control theory. New York: Harper Row, 1984.
11. Ellis A, Dryden W. Rational-emotive therapy. Nurse Pract 1987;12:16.
12. Ellis A, Harper R. New guide to rational living. North Hollywood, CA: Wilshire Book Co, 1975.
13. McKelvey J, Borgersen M. Family development and the use of diabetes groups. Pat Educ Counsel 1990;16:61.
14. Rogers C. Client-centered therapy. Boston: Houghton Mifflin, 1951.
15. Rogers C. On becoming a person. Boston: Houghton Mifflin, 1961.
16. Patterson CH. Theories of counseling and psychotherapy. New York: Harper Row, 1966.
17. Rogers C. The interpersonal relationship: the core of guidance. Harv Educ Rev 1962;32:416.
18. Johnson K. How to create trust. Broker World 1989;9:100.
19. Luzaszewski J. How to coach executives. Commun World 1989;6:38.
20. Kinlaw D. Helping skills for human resource

development: a facilitator's package. San Diego: University Assoc, 1981.

21. Pratt H. Employee complaints: act early and be concerned. ARMA Rec Manage Q 1989;23:26.

22. Kaplan A. How to fire without fear. Personnel Adm 1989;34:74.

23. Pizzano J, Pizzano R. The key to an effective client interview. Legal Assist Today 1988;5:61.

24. McClenahen J. Training Americans for work: industry's monumental challenge. Indust Week 1988;237:52.

25. Herman S. Ready, aim or fire? Personnel Adm 1989;34: 132.

26. Robbins S. Essentials of organizational behavior. 5th ed. Englewood Cliffs. NJ: Prentice Hall, 1997.

27. Queen V. Performance evaluation. Nurs Manage 1995;26: 52.

28. Sheridan D. Staff development through performance appraisal. Nurs Staff Dev Insider 1995;4:4.

29. Davidhizar R, Giger J, Poole V. Taking the dread out of annual performance evaluations. Health Care Superv 1995;13:33.

30. Buckley J. Evolution of peer review. Crit Care Nurs Q 1995;18:48.

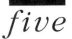

five

NUTRITION COUNSELING

Nutrition counseling is a major responsibility in the practice of many dietetics professionals. Since medical problems, such as diabetes mellitus, cardiovascular disease, renal disease, hypertension, and obesity, have a nutrition component, practitioners are frequently involved in counseling individuals with these problems for the improvement of their health. Many patients and clients are referred by a physician as part of either treatment or prevention. Some are self-referred, such as in corporate wellness programs, in sports nutrition, and in weight control. Counseling clients about normal nutrition for children or during pregnancy are other examples.

The importance of shaping food choices to enhance health and to reduce the risk of chronic diseases is well established. Medical nutrition therapies have been used in the treatment of diseases for many years. Medical nutrition therapy has been defined as "the use of specific nutrition services to treat an illness, injury, or condition" (1). It involves two phases: *(a)* "assessment of the nutritional status of the patient or client," and *(b)* "treatment, which includes diet therapy, counseling, or use of specialized nutrition supplements" (1). The assessment may include a nutrition history, lifestyle data, results of laboratory tests, exercise, medications, and other medical problems. The individualized intervention or counseling, derived from the assessment, includes setting goals for clinical outcomes, problem solving, alternatives for the client to consider, negotiating dietary goals for change, and enhancing self-management. Evaluation and follow-up should be included.

These services, provided by dietetic technicians registered and registered dietitians, may be provided in many settings, including inpatient and outpatient facilities, such as hospitals and medical centers, long-term care facilities, schools, and in private practice, public health agencies, home-care agencies, media, industry, and corporate wellness centers.

Nutrition counseling is a collaborative process that assists individuals in learning about themselves, about their eating habits as a part of their total environment, and about methods of coping with their dietary problems. The overall process may be divided into two separate functions: interviewing and counseling. Interviewing, discussed in Chapter 3, involves the gathering of information and requires considerable training and practice to elicit accurately the selective information vital to the counseling process. Counseling, per se, is a process involving listening, accepting, clarifying, and helping clients to form their own conclusions and develop their own plans of action as outlined in the counseling chapter. The professional interprets and evaluates information, guides the client's thinking toward focusing on goals, and translates for the patient the regimen prescribed by the physician. This chapter examines nutrition counseling specifically.

The purpose of nutrition counseling is to change behavior for the improvement of health. The following model depicts this relationship (2):

Nutrition counseling & education → Changes in food intake (Compliance) → Altered risk factors → Desirable health outcomes → Economic benefits

Nutrition counseling should lead to changes in food intake that alter the risk factors for disease and produce better health outcomes. Although conclusive evidence is not available to prove the first link that nutrition counseling always results in changes in food intake, counseling is the most reliable means of bringing about patient adherence to recommendations. Examples of economic benefits for patients, providers, and payers are the cost savings that result from a reduction in the incidence of or severity of a disease, such as reduced hospitalization expenses or increased job productivity.

In the person with diabetes, for example, the purpose of nutrition counseling would be to change from current eating patterns to nutrition self-management of diabetes. For the pregnant woman, the purpose might be to add to her diet those foods that meet the nutrient needs of pregnancy while maintaining appropriate caloric levels.

Nutrition counseling involves deliberation and collaboration between two parties (the dietetics professional or counselor and the client or counselee), during which values may be examined, knowledge imparted and acquired, new ways of dealing with life situations learned,

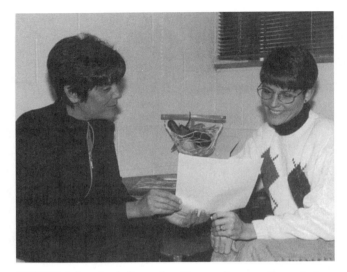

FIGURE 5.1.   An informal setting enhances the relationship and is appropriate for counseling.

goals set, and decisions made. The counselee is assisted in setting goals and planning new and different actions.

Since the purpose of counseling is to promote change in eating behaviors, the counselor should remember that choosing to change one's food intake is affected by complex psychological factors and is never easy for people. Continuing with one's current, comfortable lifestyle and avoiding change represent the path of least resistance. The client's resistance to change may occur at an unrecognized, subconscious level and should be expected and probed by the counselor. Models trying to predict change, as discussed in Chapter 1, include the Health Belief Model and Stages of Change. The client's stage of change should be explored since better results may be expected when the intervention is tailored to the individual's stage of change. Other chapters explore behavior modification, cognitive restructuring, self-efficacy, and relapse prevention. The goal-setting process is discussed in this chapter. Since there is no one unifying theory, the professional must be prepared to use several strategies to promote dietary change.

Changing one's eating patterns is probably one of the most difficult lifestyle changes an individual has to make owing to the fact that dietary habits are long-standing and have been associated with pleasure from the time mother offered the bottle or the breast; in addition, dietary habits may provide psychological relief for emotions, such as boredom, frustration, and stress. At the same time, food is associated with status, comfort, security, and celebration.

The ideal situation for nutrition counseling consists of a process over a period of time in which the client develops a growing awareness of his food intake and dietary practices, and of how these factors influence his health. The process of assisting people in establishing and maintaining good nutrition habits is a complex task, as it re-

quires people to make permanent changes in their eating habits.

Eventual client self-management is the goal of all counseling. Counseling must provide the knowledge, skills, attitudes, and behaviors that are needed by the client for living independently. The client should take increasing responsibility over time for the dietary change process. Nutrition counseling cannot be a one-time service. Follow-up counseling is necessary until the individual is self-sufficient. As an old adage states: Give a man a fish and you feed him for a day. Teach a man to fish and you feed him for a lifetime.

The amount of time required to perform nutrition services has been reported to range from 45 minutes to 12 hours or more. A consulting nutritionist employed in a corporate health office reported, for example, that initial visits lasted 45 to 60 minutes, with follow-up appointments of 15 to 30 minutes (3).

California dietitians spent an average of 53 minutes at an initial session of cholesterol-related counseling (4). Participants in the Modification of Diet in Renal Disease (MDRD) study met with a dietitian monthly. The mean time spent by a dietitian counseling participants was 183 ± 70 minutes during months 1–4, and declined to 116 ± 41 minutes per visit during the third year of the study (5). Guidelines for persons with non-insulin-dependent diabetes mellitus suggest a first visit of 1–1.5 hours (6). If the hospital clinical dietitian has insufficient time for counseling, patients can be referred to consultant dietitians in private practice, and to community resources for out-patient follow-up.

A number of models of the nutrition counseling process may be found in the literature (7–10). Models help one to examine and understand the steps in a complex process. A model for medical nutrition therapy includes the following four parts (9):

1. Assessment of the person's metabolic and lifestyle parameters including dietary, behavioral, physical, social, and cognitive environments.

2. Goal setting.

3. Intervention and treatment to achieve the goals.

4. Evaluation of outcomes and follow-up.

ASSESSMENT

Nutrition assessment uses a comprehensive approach to defining nutritional status by using a number of sources of information: dietary intake, medical history including medications taken, laboratory data, anthropometric data, and lifestyle and other influences. The assessment assists in identifying the nutrition goals for change, the type of nutrition intervention designed to achieve the goals, and the evaluation of the outcomes.

The first step is to gather in advance data or information about the client that may have an impact on treatment. In a hospital or clinic setting the medical record is the source of data about the patient. Height, weight,

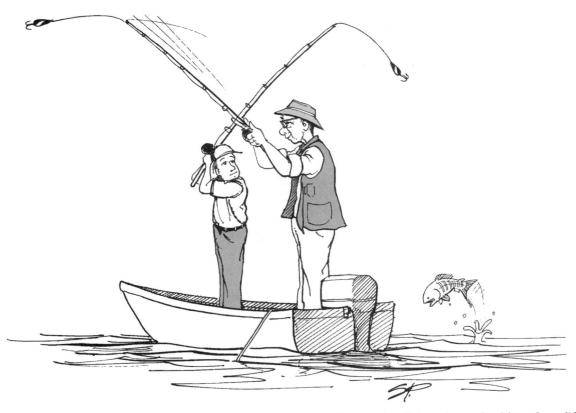

FIGURE 5.2. Give a man a fish and you feed him for a day. Teach a man to fish and you feed him for a lifetime.

pertinent laboratory values, medications, and medical history should be noted. A number of factors may impact upon eating patterns, including family status, occupation, income, educational level, ethnicity, religion, physical activity, physical disabilities or impairments (seeing, hearing), and place of residence (10).

Information that is unavailable from the medical record may be obtained during the interview, by use of a self-administered questionnaire, or by collecting anthropometric and dietary data. Nutrition counselors are expected to know their clients physiologically, psychologically, socially, and economically, i.e., they should know what factors influence their clients' eating and lifestyle behaviors. Counselors must view their clients as individuals living and interacting in an environment that influences their motivation and capabilities for change.

A second source of data is one's own records kept from previous counseling sessions or previous contact with the client. These records should be reviewed prior to follow-up counseling. Since the purpose of counseling is to promote change, the dietetics professional needs to collect and assess data that indicate what changes need to be made, what the client wants to discuss, and what personal and lifestyle factors may promote or interfere with changes in eating patterns. After informing the client of the purpose of the interview and after having established good rapport with the client, the counselor

may take a nutrition history from the client by using the interviewing skills discussed in Chapter 3.

The assessment may have a number of important functions. These include making both parties aware of the current nutrition patterns, problems, and misinformation, as well as health history. The stage of change, as discussed in Chapter 1, can be determined so that the intervention is planned appropriately. The assessment also provides baseline information from which to gauge progress, alerts both parties to the demands placed on the patient so that realistic goals can be identified, provides both parties with ideas for developing the nutrition intervention, provides an opportunity to continue rapport, and enables the counselor and client to work together on a plan for gradual changes that is a congruent with the client's lifestyle (9). Screening for the risk of malnutrition, for example, may require a full nutrition assessment in some illnesses, such as cancer and AIDS (11). This will assist in determining and prioritizing appropriate nutrition interventions.

The dietetics professional may collect data on current eating habits, on the physical, social, and cognitive environments, and on previous attempts to make dietary changes (10). Behavioral assessment and cognitive assessment are discussed in later chapters. The physical environment includes where meals are eaten (at home or in restaurants and in which rooms of the home), and events that occur while eating (watching television or reading).

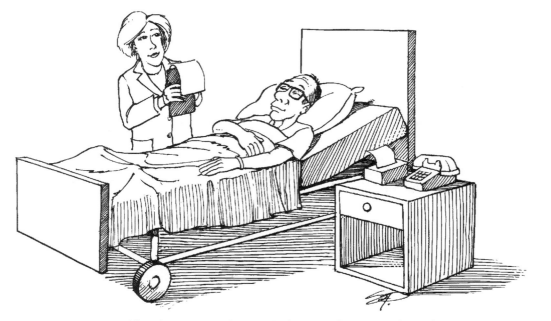

FIGURE 5.3. The dietetics professional obtains information from the patient.

The social environment, which may or may not be supportive, includes family members, friends, social norms, and trends involved with eating behaviors (e.g., popular food customs of a bridge club, drinking buddies).

The cognitive or mental environment involves the client's thoughts and feelings about food, self-image, and self-confidence. It concerns what clients say to themselves about their food habits and life, since personal thoughts may or may not promote successful change. Some thoughts may be positive, such as "I love a steak and baked potato," or "My favorite snacks are potato chips and beer." There may be negative and self-defeating thoughts, or thoughts of failure, boredom, stress, and hunger. Examples include "It's too difficult," "It's not worth it," "I can't do it," "I've been on diets before, always failed, and regained all of the weight I lost," or "I'm happy the way I am and don't want to change." Further information on cognitions is found in a later chapter. Since behavior is influenced by beliefs and attitudes, one needs to explore these in relation to the medical condition, nutrition, diets, and health. The client's educational level and any language barriers should be noted. Further information is found in Chapter 7, "Modifying Cognitions."

After the data are gathered, they should be analyzed and interpreted. Influences on eating patterns should be identified, and alternative food choices noted. Changes may be thought of as problems to be solved by setting goals with the client. This information is baseline data on the client prior to counseling and is recorded later and referred to in future counseling sessions.

GOAL SETTING
The counseling relationship was described in the previous chapter. Counselors should clarify that the responsibility for change rests with the client, but that they are willing to be of assistance in solving problems and making new plans. It is recommended that nutrition interventions be based on the self-management approach (9, 12, 13). This involves clients in their own health care and has them take an active part in their treatment.

Before problems are explored in the exploring stage of the counseling process, it is advisable to discuss with the client, show approval for, and reinforce those current food choices that do not need changing, i.e., what the individual is already doing right according to the diet prescription. Problems—foods that should be omitted or foods or cooking practices that should be changed—may be discussed next, perhaps starting with the counselor's estimation of what is most important. The conditions and circumstances surrounding food behaviors need to be explored. This stage of counseling requires the skills of the helping-process model discussed in an earlier chapter: listening, questioning, accepting, clarifying, and helping clients find solutions to their problems and develop their own plan of action. Counseling should not be directed solely at the client's knowledge, but also at feelings, attitudes, beliefs, and values, which have strong and powerful influences on dietary behaviors. Reasonable and appropriate alternatives may be suggested by the counselor, leaving the final decision on which alternative is preferred to the client. Knowledge is a tool only if and when an individual is ready to change and motivated to change. One may ask any of the following questions:

"Which of these alternatives or changes do you think you could try?"

"What would be the easiest?" "The hardest?"

"Is this the right time to make changes?"

"Do you think you can succeed?"

"What foods could you substitute?"

"How will things be better or worse after you make the change?"

"How do you feel about making that change?"

The client weighs the pros and cons of the options.

At the resolving stage, one or two priorities for change should be selected by the client, not the counselor, for the next week or so. Clients who are enthusiastic about making total changes immediately are setting themselves up for frustration and possible failure that may lead to abandoning the dietary changes altogether. The counselor should guard against this. Slow, steady changes that will persist over time are preferable.

The session with a client needing a sodium-restricted diet, for example, may uncover the following problems:

1. Uses salt in cooking and at the table.
2. Snacks include crackers and potato chips.
3. Uses some high-sodium spices and flavorings.
4. Likes bacon, ham, and salami.
5. Eats lunch in a restaurant.
6. No one else in the family is on a sodium-restricted diet.
7. Wife does the grocery shopping and does not read labels.

The problems can be reinterpreted into positive goals for change. A four-step process may be followed in using goal setting with clients: *(a)* goal identification, *(b)* goal importance assessment, *(c)* goal roadblock analysis, and *(d)* goal attainment (14–16).

Goal Identification

The first step is goal identification. Because clients will be more committed to changes they select, the counselor may inquire which one or two of the problems the individual wants to address first, by saying "Which one or two changes do you think that you can make this week?" When people play a significant role in selecting goals, they hold themselves responsible for progress and engage in self-evaluative mechanisms in the process. If goals are imposed by the counselor, individuals do not accept them or feel personally responsible for fulfilling them. If these goals impose severe constraints and burdens, they can render the pursuit aversive and breed dislike rather than nurture interest (17).

Goals selected by the client should be positively stated as concrete behaviors. Goals should be specific, measurable, reasonable, attainable, and timely. A goal should specify what the individual will do or what one is trying to achieve. The following are examples of goals:

"I will eat fruit instead of baked desserts today."

"I will purchase salt-free pretzels for a snack."

"I will walk for 20 minutes on Monday, Wednesday, and Friday this week."

The degree to which goals create incentives and guides for action is partly determined by their specificity (17). Clear, attainable goals produce higher levels of performance than general intentions to do the best one can, which may have little or no effect, such as "I'll look for low-sodium foods the next time I am at the grocery store." When goals are set unrealistically high, performance may prove disappointing. If the client selects problems numbered one and two from the earlier list, for example, these can be reinterpreted into goals for change as follows:

"I will use low-sodium seasonings in cooking and pepper at the table."

"I will eat fruits and low-sodium crackers for snacks."

Note that the positive statement of using low-sodium seasonings is preferable to the negative goal of avoiding salt. It is easier to do something positive than to avoid doing something.

Goals should provide a degree of challenge, and are standards against which performance attainments are compared (17). To be realistic and reasonable, goals should be based on one's past and current behavior. The first challenge should be only a small step away from the current behavior, not a major change, and be matched with the client's perceived capabilities for achieving it. The counselor should guide individuals toward those goals that clients believe they can realistically accomplish. Goal setting may also be an important part of disease management. Outcomes of interventions may include clinical parameters, such as blood pressure, body weight, lipid levels, and blood glucose levels (7). However, they may be influenced by factors unrelated to the desired dietary changes.

Hopefully, the client will have a successful change experience, not failure, if first assignments are not difficult, before returning for follow-up counseling. This is especially important when the individual has negative thoughts or a previous failure at dietary change. Each succeeding subgoal should present new challenges in the mastery of a new subset of skills. Small steps lead to major gains.

A distinction must be made between short-term goals and distant or end goals. The relationship between attaining goals and expenditure of effort to do so differs for each (17). Short-term subgoals that are challenging, but attainable with effort, are likely to be more motivating and self-satisfying. Self-motivation can be increased by progressively raising subgoals even though the long-range goals are difficult to realize. For example, individuals need to commit themselves to the goal of following the dietary regimen or goal today, rather than a long-term goal of never eating high-fat foods again. When the distant future is the focus, it is easy to put off the goal and decide to start tomorrow.

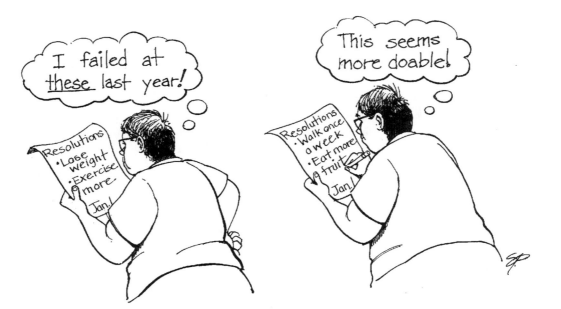

FIGURE 5.4.   Goals should be specific, measurable, and short-term.

Persistence that leads to eventual mastery of an activity is thus ensured through a progression of subgoals, each with a high probability of success. When self-satisfaction is contingent upon attaining challenging goals, more effort is expended than if easy goals are adopted as sufficient.

Goal Importance Assessment

In the second step, after identifying goals, the counselor assesses the goal importance by asking, for example, "On a scale of 1 to 10 with 10 being the highest, how important is that goal to you?" What the counselor thinks is important does not matter. Goals that are not perceived as important by the client are unlikely to be achieved. Other goals should be set instead.

Most of the activities that we now enjoy at one time held little or no interest for us because we were not exposed to them. Certain sports, kinds of music, hobbies, and our career choices are examples of activities we learn about and enjoy over time. Subgoals for dietary change, if valued, can cultivate people's intrinsic interest, enlist sustained involvement in activities that will build new skills and competencies, and increase motivation and self-perceptions of efficacy (17). Those who do not set any goals achieve little change in performance.

The strength of one's goal commitment is affected by several factors. The value the person places on the activity, the perceived attainability of the goals, and binding pledges people make to others concerning their future performance all make a difference (17). The practitioner needs to inquire about these. "Do you think you can do it?" "How important is it to you?" "Is there someone else with whom you can share your plans?"

In a clinical trial, for example, intense dietary counseling lowered low-density lipoprotein cholesterol (18).

Goal setting involving a focus on two or three goals was used in the initial counseling session. The second session provided positive feedback on dietary and serum cholesterol changes and continued the goal-setting process. A team approach and counseling for 3 to 4 months enhanced dietary compliance.

Using goal setting, a second intervention with women set 20% of calories from fat as the goal. Twenty dietary behavior change sessions were held. Results showed that 77% met the goal in 6 months and more than two-thirds were maintaining it 2 years later (19).

Goal Roadblock Analysis

In the third step, obstacles to achieving the goals are examined. "What problems do you see in achieving this goal?" "What might interfere?" "How do you feel about this change?" may be asked. It is important to discuss the problems thoroughly along with the impact of physical, social, and cognitive environments on the goals selected for change. Roadblocks may be lack of knowledge, such as about the fat content of foods, lack of skills, such as cooking skills or skill in reading food labels, inability to take risks, and lack of social support at home (14–16).

It is advisable to tell the client to expect some problems since some things may come up that were not thought of during the counseling session. If aware of the possibility of problems, the client may avoid abandoning the diet with the first lapse or obstacle. After all, Michael Jordan does not make a basket every time he shoots the ball. But he keeps on trying. Supplying a phone number for questions may resolve unexpected problems.

Goal Attainment

In the final step in the goal-setting process, if the obstacles are overcome, clients can discuss what specific steps they plan to take in achieving the goals. For example, the goal of using low-sodium seasonings may require their identification and purchase, the acquisition of new recipes for using them, and the modification of favorite recipes to use them.

By selecting a level of performance, individuals create their own incentives to persist in their efforts until their efforts match the standards of the goals. Clients compare results against the goals continuously so that they know when they are succeeding. The personal standards against which performance attainments are compared affect how much self-satisfaction is derived from the subgoal. Feedback on progress of how one is doing is provided by cognitive comparison and self-evaluation. By making self-satisfaction conditional on a selected level of performance, individuals create their own incentives to persist in their efforts until their performances match their internal standards (17, 20).

The attainment of subgoals builds motivation, competencies, interest, and self-perceptions of efficacy. Motivational effects do not derive from the goals themselves, but from the fact that people respond evaluatively to their own behavior (17). They note how well they are doing. When individuals commit themselves to goals, perceived negative discrepancies between what they are doing and what they seek to achieve create self-dissatisfactions that can serve as incentives motivating enhanced effort.

Without standards against which to measure performance, people have little basis for judging how well they are doing nor do they have a basis for judging their capabilities. Subgoal attainments increase self-perceptions of efficacy, and self-satisfaction sustains one's efforts. Attainments falling short of the goals lower perceived self-efficacy and the way one feels about oneself.

INTERVENTION AND TREATMENT

The information from the assessment and goal setting is the basis for the nutrition care plan and nutrition intervention (9, 11). They suggest the information, knowledge, and skills the client needs in order to make dietary changes. The counselor judges what information to provide, how much information can be absorbed at each session, at what educational or literacy level, and what handouts and media to use as supplements. The amount of information to provide and the best method of doing so must be individualized.

The intervention may include information, for example, on the following: reading food labels, adapting recipes, menu planning, restaurant eating, principles of healthful eating, food safety, nutrients in selected foods, nutrition supplements, nutrition misinformation, fat, carbohydrate, sodium or calorie counting, nutrient-drug interactions, managing appetite, and the relationship of nutrition to the medical problem. In addition, the client needs to know about exercise, self-monitoring, and self-

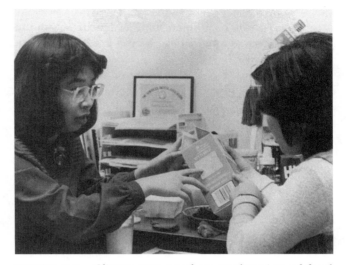

FIGURE 5.5. Clients may need an explanation of food labels.

management. Problem-solving skills for meal planning and preparation and food purchasing may be needed. Culturally sensitive interventions are important in meeting the needs, desires, and lifestyles of ethnic clients.

The client's commitment to specific action behaviors and at specific times may be obtained. The counselor may wish to know if there are others with whom the client can discuss the goals since a public commitment may make it more likely for goals to be accomplished. Practitioners frequently ask their clients to keep self-monitoring records of food intakes and environments, which they should bring to the next appointment as a way for them and the counselor to learn about factors affecting eating behaviors, and as a demonstration of their commitment to change. Clients' personal records, observations, and analysis of their environments will contribute to their personal understanding. Chapter 6 on ''Behavior Modification'' discusses this matter in more detail.

By the end of the counseling session, the client should not only know what to do and how to do it, but also be committed to doing it. Clients should be asked to summarize their plans to check for understanding and commitment. The client has to perceive and accept the need for change. Motivation for change should be explored as well as the dangers in continuing the current dietary patterns. Solely providing information about a dietary regimen is frequently not enough to interest or enable people to improve their eating habits. Counseling involves much more than distributing printed diet materials to clients.

In one study, the intervention consisted of eight weekly sessions, followed by six biweekly sessions, and then monthly sessions for the rest of the year (21). The goal was to decrease total fat intake to 20% of baseline calories and increase complex carbohydrate consumption to reduce cancer risk. Individual counseling sessions were offered twice. Women were taught fat counting, self-monitoring, reading labels, recipe modification, and other strategies.

In the Modification of Diet in Renal Disease (MDRD) study, the intervention emphasized long-term adherence (22). Dietitians counseled participants about protein intake, weight loss, sodium restriction, and fat modification for managing hypertension and hypercholesterolemia, meeting with patients monthly. Dietary and anthropometric data were collected during the nutrition intervention. Instruction included self-monitoring of protein intake, goal setting, and problem solving for meal planning and preparation, food purchasing, and eating out. After 24 months, maintaining motivation, promoting self-efficacy, preventing relapse, and sustaining adherence were emphasized.

EVALUATION OF OUTCOMES AND FOLLOW-UP

An outcome is the measured result of the counseling process. Outcome data identify the benefits of medical nutrition therapy in patient and client care. As systems of quality control, nutrition counselors may wish to evaluate several things: *(a)* the success of the client in following the goals set and in implementing new dietary behaviors; *(b)* the degree of success of the nutrition intervention including its strengths and weaknesses; and *(c)* their own personal skills as counselors. Records of the problems and goals, of the factors influencing them, and of the intervention should be kept by the counselor for future measurement of client change. Examples of outcomes are changes in weight; glycemic, lipid and other laboratory values; blood pressure control; patient acceptance and progress at self-management; improvements in knowledge, skills, and dietary changes; and lifestyle changes. These indicate the impact of the intervention and can be used to evaluate the effectiveness of the treatment. The counselor and client can engage in evaluation jointly.

A measure of success, such as eating differently in an overweight person, is obvious. Other outcome measures may be indicators of quality of care. The blood pressure and lipid levels of cardiovascular patients can be monitored, although they are more difficult to evaluate since they depend on factors beyond dietary adherence. Despite the client's commitment to dietary change, results may not reflect his adherence to the regimen. Monitoring of both glycemic and lipid levels helps to assess results in clients with diabetes mellitus (23). These outcomes can be used by the medical team working together to adjust the treatment to achieve and maintain treatment goals. Therefore, medical nutrition therapy is an ongoing process. Further information on

evaluation is found in Chapter 12, "Implementing and Evaluating Learning."

Frequent follow-up for reassessment, further intervention, coaching, and support is essential until the client is self-sufficient. Discussion at subsequent sessions should focus first on what went well, i.e., the successful experiences and subgoals reached, no matter how small. Such positive focus helps clients feel that they can have some control over their eating, health, and life, and builds a sense of personal mastery and coping ability. Self-monitoring records kept by the client should be examined jointly and discussed, and problems should be resolved. Overlooking the records indicates to the client that they were not considered important. If things are going well, new subgoals for change may be established jointly. Support and reinforcement to strengthen desirable habits along with gradual, planned changes should continue as long as necessary until the client is successful at self-management.

Enthusiasm for change may decline the first week and even more in the second week, as problems develop. Therefore, frequent follow-up appointments should be scheduled. For long-term follow-up with clients with diabetes mellitus, for example, appointments every 3 to 6 months for children and every 6 to 12 months for adults are recommended. Dietitians in tertiary care settings who do not have the opportunity for follow-up may need to refer patients to dietitians in outpatient clinics or in private practice since one session with a client is insufficient to promote long-term change in health counseling. The minimal requirements for a successful nutrition counseling program and long-term change are active patient participation in the planning, execution, and evaluation of various nutrition change strategies, continuity of care for an extended period, and treatment strategies tailored to the individual's needs (10).

DOCUMENTATION

The Joint Commission on Accrediting Healthcare Organizations (JCAHO) sets standards that are required to address quality of care issues in the health care environment. Documentation is essential to quality patient care and reimbursement, and health care professionals need to meet the provision in the JCAHO standards. A summary of the medical nutrition therapy should be communicated to the medical team and/or other referral source in the medical record. The total assessment, the measurable goals set and plans to achieve them, the nutrition intervention, and the evaluation should be documented clearly and concisely in the permanent medical record. All discharge instructions must be documented and provided to the organization or individual responsible for the patient's continuing care (24).

As the client returns for follow-up appointments, re-

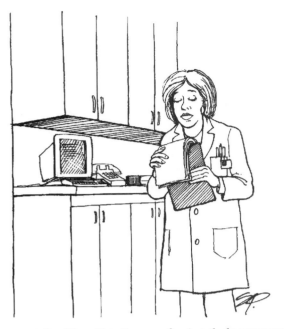

FIGURE 5.6. The dietetics professional documents in the medical record.

sults of health outcomes and goals achieved should be noted. Changes in weight, meal intake, tolerance problems, results of new laboratory values, medications and their nutritional significance, and skills in self-management may be assessed. Follow-up reassessment with new goals and interventions should be recorded. Appropriate referrals should be included.

EXPANDING ROLES FOR DIETITIANS

The concept of expanded roles and of the medical intervention specialist is a challenge to dietitians who want to expand their counseling in matters other than diet. An intervention specialist is defined as a clinician "who promotes adherence to a variety of prescribed medical and life-style interventions through the health behavior counseling process" (25). Articles in the literature suggest that the dietitian can prepare to counsel clients in other areas.

The concept originated in clinical trials, in which dietitians effectively counseled study participants on adherence to taking drugs as well as on adherence to diet. Many clients, for example, those with diabetes mellitus and hypercholesterolemia, are treated with both medication and diet. Counseling in areas of stress management, exercise, and smoking cessation are other examples. Sedentary obese clients may be counseled about exercise principles, such as the speed, frequency, and duration of walking.

Requirements of education and experience for intervention specialists are essentially the same as those for registered dietitians with added knowledge of the topic area and additional training in interviewing and behavior counseling (25). Intervention specialists do require, of course, more time with the patient than the usual one or two counseling sessions afforded to some clinical dietitians. The dietitian needs extra time in this counseling approach to achieve long-term health behavior change in cases of adherence problems.

Dietitians need to train for this role and to promote it as being of significant benefit to physicians and their patients. The intervention specialist can coordinate several different prescribed treatments that require behavior changes by the patient. Currently, drug, diet, exercise, stress management, smoking cessation, and physical therapy treatments are often prescribed with no provision for monitoring success of their incorporation into a client's lifestyle. Close cooperation and coordination between the patient, the intervention specialist, and other members of the medical team can help improve the quality of health care.

Some dietitians have expanded into career paths as study coordinators. The individual is responsible for the day-to-day operations of a clinical study (26). The registered dietitian can also assume the prominent role of case manager (27). The Diabetes Control and Complications Trial (DCCT) showed, for example, that the registered dietitian was an important contributor to health care delivery, research, and case management (28). In the DCCT, the dietitian's role expanded as the team recognized the relationship between adherence to the dietary regimen and achieving targeted blood glucose levels with successful improved diabetes control outcomes.

Dietitians who are credentialed as Certified Diabetes Educators (CDE) also have expanded roles in diabetes care, education, and management. Others are certified in nutrition support, pediatric nutrition, metabolic nutrition, health/fitness, and the like.

The term "nutrition therapist" describes dietitians who practice personalized, long-term, client-centered nutrition counseling in which the dietitian and client work as partners in solving problems related to dietary and lifestyle changes (29). Often the dietitian is part of a multidisciplinary team. Reiff and Reiff are "nutrition therapists" specializing in behavioral change in clients with eating disorders. The psychotherapy model is used, involving the following (30): (a) long-term care, (b) a relationship that is a key part of the therapeutic process, and (c) a highly individualized treatment plan evolving over time. Additional education and training in basic counseling skills through course work and supervision by a psychotherapist are needed for the role of nutrition therapist in eating disorders in order to have the qualifications to discuss the emotional issues related to weight, food, and body image (31). Nutrition therapists are a subunit of the Nutrition Entrepreneurs dietetic practice group.

All dietetics professionals need to be knowledgeable in the concepts, processes, and techniques of counseling, although they may apply them in different settings in professional practice. A comprehensive approach to counseling that considers lifestyle, environments, culture, and psychological and social factors is needed. Some clinical dietitians, with added training, are expanding their roles dealing with long-term health behavior problems in addition to diet, and they are counseling to achieve patient adherence. Other chapters discuss the behavior modification approach to counseling and the importance of cognitions to change.

REVIEW AND DISCUSSION QUESTIONS

1. Explain the steps in the nutrition counseling process.
2. Explain the steps in the process of goal setting.
3. What should be included in documentation of nutrition counseling?
4. What are some of the newer roles that dietitians are assuming?
5. What is included in medical nutrition therapy?
6. What is the relationship between nutrition counseling and health promotion?

SUGGESTED ACTIVITIES

1. During the next week, make arrangements to observe a dietitian's counseling session. Afterwards, discuss her philosophy of nutrition counseling.
2. Write both a paraphrase and empathic comment to the following comments made by a counselee:
   A. I feel awkward discussing my obesity. I feel I must be disgusting to you.
   B. People tend to think I'm fat, and I don't believe they take me seriously.
   C. I am at a point now where I don't believe I will ever control my blood sugar.
3. Form triads consisting of a counselor, counselee, and observer. Each individual should take a turn in each of the roles for 7 minutes. The counselee should play the role of a diabetic client, and the counselor should use paraphrasing and empathizing, along with open and closed questions, to facilitate disclosure and problem solving. After each round, the observer

CASE STUDY

Len Howard is a 48-year-old male executive in a Fortune 500 company. In a recent physical exam, he was 5'11" tall and 175 pounds. His serum cholesterol was 290 (desirable 200 mg/dl) with HDL of 50 (desirable 35–70 mg/dl) and LDL 220 (desirable <139 mg/dl). On the recommendation of his physician, he made an appointment with the dietitian in the corporate wellness program.

His family history revealed that his father and older brother both died of heart disease. His wife is employed as an attorney and they have a 15-year-old son.

Dietitian: You mentioned that the doctor wants you to try modifying your diet before considering medication for your cholesterol level?

Len: He said to reduce the fat and cholesterol in my diet.

Dietitian: Did you know that the saturated fat in your diet is especially bad in raising your blood cholesterol?

Len: I've heard of it, but don't know much about it.

Dietitian: Then let's talk about what you are eating now. Then we can identify what you are eating that is OK, and what, if any, changes that you need to consider making.

His nutrition history revealed the following information:

Breakfast: Orange juice, 2 slices of toast with peanut butter, and black coffee.

Mid-AM Snack: Coffee and doughnut.

Lunch: Beef sandwich or bacon cheeseburger, French fries, and Coke.

Mid-PM Snack: Coffee.

Dinner: 6–8-oz. Steak, baked potato with butter and sour cream, green vegetable, salad with blue cheese dressing, cookies, and wine.

Evening snack: Beer and pretzels.

1. What is he doing that is OK and that he can continue to do (foods low in cholesterol and saturated fatty acids)?
2. What are possible short-term goals for change for him to consider with you?
3. How would you assess the importance of the choice of goals with him?
4. After he selects two goals, how would you discuss any obstacles he sees to reaching the goals?
5. How would you discuss the steps he needs to take to reach the goals, such as discussions with his wife, shopping at the grocery store, or selecting restaurant meals at lunch?
6. What type of follow-up would you like to have with him?

should share his reactions to the counselor's approach and encourage feedback from the counselee to the counselor. From the counselee's perspective, what did the counselor do that helped their interaction; what did he do that hindered it?

4. Write an open-ended question for each of the statements below:
   A. I never enjoy eating at restaurants anymore. Being on this diet has taken the fun out of my life.
   B. Since I developed high blood pressure, it seems that all I do is think about my diet.
   C. It seems easy every morning to promise myself that today I will eat low fat foods and exercise. By noon, however, I begin thinking that I'll never be able to comply with the diet for the rest of my life, so why bother?

5. In groups of two, take turns discussing a lifestyle problem and restating it as a goal for change.
   A. Think of a lifestyle problem the counselee would like to change, such as eats too much, eats the wrong foods, exercises too little, doesn't study enough, needs to budget better, drinks too much, smokes too much, and the like.
   B. Help the person discuss the problem and the conditions and circumstances surrounding it. Then have the counselee restate the problem as a positive goal for change, i.e., "I will . . . ."
   C. Assess the importance of the goal on a scale of 1 to 10, with 10 being the highest importance. Revise the goal if necessary.
   D. Ask about and discuss the obstacles and barriers to accomplishing the goal and try to have the person resolve these.
   E. Have the person list the steps to achieving the goal. What will the person do, and when will it be done?

REFERENCES

1. Identifying patients at risk: ADA's definitions for nutrition screening and nutrition assessment. J Am Diet Assoc 1994;94:838.
2. Olendski MC, Tolpin HG, Buckley EL. Evaluating nutrition intervention in atherosclerosis. J Am Diet Assoc 1981;79:9.
3. Seidel MC. The consulting nutritionist in an employee health office. J Am Diet Assoc 1983;82:405.
4. Hyman DJ, Clark M, Houston-Miller N, et al. Cholesterol-related counseling by registered dietitians in Northern California. Prev Med 1992;21:746.
5. Dolecek TA, Olson MB, Caggiula AW, et al. Registered dietitian time requirements in the Modification of Diet in Renal Disease Study. J Am Diet Assoc 1995;95:1307.
6. Franz MJ. Practice guidelines for nutrition care by dietetics practitioners for outpatients with non–insulin-dependent diabetes mellitus: consensus statement. J Am Diet Assoc 1992;92:1136.
7. Pastors JG, Barrier P, Rich M, et al. Facilitating lifestyle change: a resource manual. Alexandria, VA: American Diabetes Assoc, and Chicago: American Dietetic Assoc, 1996.
8. Snetselaar LG. Nutrition counseling skills: assessment, treatment, and evaluation. 2nd ed. Rockville, MD: Aspen Publications, 1989.
9. Tinker LF, Heins JM, Holler HJ. Commentary and translation: 1994 nutrition recommendations for diabetes. J Am Diet Assoc 1994;94;507.
10. Curry KR, Himburg SP. Establishing an effective nutrition education/counseling program: skills for the RD. Study Kit 11. Chicago: The American Dietetic Assoc, 1988.
11. Position of The American Dietetic Association and The Canadian Dietetic Association: Nutrition intervention in the care of persons with human immunodeficiency virus infection. J Am Diet Assoc 1994;94:1042.
12. National standards for diabetes self-management education programs. Diabetes Educ 1995;21:189.
13. Gillis BP, Caggiula AW, Chiavacci AT, et al. Nutrition intervention program of the Modification of Diet in Renal Disease Study: a self-management approach. J Am Diet Assoc 1995;95:1288.
14. Laquatra I, Danish SJ. A primer for nutritional counseling. In: Frankle RT, Yang MU, eds. Obesity and weight control: the health professional's guide to understanding and treatment. Rockville, MD: Aspen Publications, 1988.
15. D'Augelli AR, D'Augelli JF, Danish SJ. Helping others. Monterey, CA: Brooks/Cole Publishing, 1981.
16. Laquatra I, D'Augelli AR, Danish SJ. Helping skills II: life development intervention leader's manual. New York: Human Sciences Press, 1983.
17. Bandura A. Social foundations of thought and action: a social cognitive theory. Englewood Cliffs, NJ: Prentice Hall, 1986.
18. Shenberger DM, Helgren RJ, Peters JR, et al. Intense dietary counseling lowers LDL cholesterol in the recruitment phase of a clinical trial of men who had coronary artery bypass grafts. J Am Diet Assoc 1992;92:441.
19. Burrows ER, Henry HJ, Bowen DJ, et al. Nutritional applications of a clinical low fat dietary intervention to public health change. J Nutr Educ 1993;25:167.
20. Bandura A, Cervone D. Self-evaluative and self-efficacy mechanisms governing the motivational effects of goal systems. J Personality Soc Psychol 1983;45:1017.
21. Gorbach SL, Morrill-LaBrode A, Woods MN, et al. Changes in food patterns during a low-fat dietary intervention in women. J Am Diet Assoc 1990;90:802.
22. Dolecek TA, Olson MB, Caggiula AW, et al. Registered dietitian time requirements in the Modification of Diet in Renal Disease Study. J Am Diet Assoc 1995;95:1307.
23. Franz MJ, Horton ES, Bantle JP, et al. Nutrition principles for the management of diabetes and related complications. Diabetes Care 1994;17:490.
24. Krasker GD, Balogun LB. 1995 JCAHO standards: development and relevance to dietetics practice. J Am Diet Assoc 1995;95:240.
25. Insull W. Dietitians as interventions specialists: A continuing challenge for the 1990s. J Am Diet Assoc 1992;92:551.

26. Schmidt L. A new career path for dietitians: study coordinators. J Am Diet Assoc 1993;93:749.

27. Mackey CS. New roles for RDs: diabetes case manager. J Am Diet Assoc 1993;93:401.

28. Powers MA, Wheeler ML. Model for dietetics practice and research: the challenge is here, but the journey was not easy. J Am Diet Assoc 1993;93:755.

29. Licavoli L. Dietetics goes into therapy. J Am Diet Assoc 1995;95:751.

30. Reiff DW, Reiff KKL. Eating disorders: nutrition therapy in the recovery process. Gaithersburg, MD: Aspen Publishers, 1992.

31. Position of The American Dietetic Association: nutrition intervention in the treatment of anorexia nervosa, bulimia nervosa, and binge eating. J Am Diet Assoc 1994; 94:902.

six

BEHAVIOR MODIFICATION

ANN B. WILLIAMS

There is one trait that is common to all living organisms, that is, engaging in behavior. The behavior of some organisms is simple, limited, and to many of us, quite unexciting. The behavior of other organisms, such as human beings, is complex, sophisticated, extensive, and to most people, quite exciting and interesting, however difficult it may be to understand. One of the first questions that a scientist asks in order to understand an organism is, "What does it do?"

Interesting and complex behaviors usually are based on a combination of inherited and acquired characteristics. The inherited characteristics cannot be changed—one does not have the option of choosing one's biological parents and thus, one's genetic inheritance. The acquired characteristics, those shaped by one's environment and experience, however, are amenable to change.

According to Stunkard and Berthold, "People are best described by their behavior—what they think, feel, and do in specific situations" (1). Since some behaviors are learned or acquired, these behaviors can be changed or modified. One of the challenges of the discipline of psychology is to establish the principles that underlie the process of behavior change or modification.

The approach of psychologists to this task has been primarily based on environmental analysis. Certain behaviors are thought to be acquired or learned through interaction with the environment. Because of this strong environmental emphasis, much attention has been devoted to the study of basic principles of learning. The position taken is that if many behaviors can be, and indeed, are learned, then these same behaviors also can be unlearned. There is tremendous potential for behavior change.

It has become recognized that major health problems are caused, precipitated, exacerbated, or maintained by lifestyle factors such as diet, exercise, and consumption of psychoactive substances. Alleviation of these health problems involve major lifestyle/behavior changes.

This chapter reviews the principles of learning and behavior modification, which are based on substantial research. Included are classical conditioning, operant or instrumental conditioning based on positive reinforcement or rewards, and observational learning or modeling after others. The role of cognitions, the individual's mental perceptions of events, and their effects on behavior, is considered and covered in more detail in the next chapter.

In behavior modification the therapist attempts to alter previously learned behavior or to encourage the development of new behavior. Food preferences and eating behaviors are deeply rooted within the individual and may be highly resistant to change (2). Furnishing information concerning *what* to eat often is insufficient in promoting alterations in eating behaviors or adherence to modified diets. In addition to information on nutrition, behavior modification principles may be used since they offer the dietetics professional another approach to counseling. Brownell and Cohen (3) report that "programs that integrate behavioral procedures such as self-monitoring, stimulus control, coping skills and relapse prevention appear to hold the most promise."

Applications of behavior modification principles as part of the treatment of various nutritional problems are examined in this chapter. One of the earliest and most frequently used applications was in the treatment of obesity. Therapy for eating disorders, such as anorexia nervosa and bulimia, and inappropriate eating behaviors related to diabetes mellitus and cardiovascular diseases are other potential uses of behavior modification.

In human resource management, supervisors may be interested in altering the behavior of subordinates and encouraging the development of new behaviors. More effective interaction between peers and superiors may also be a goal. Although the term behavior modification in the context of human resource management may sound manipulative, the principles may be used by an honest and understanding supervisor who has shared with employees the goals of the process. These learning principles are the basis for the advice in the book, *The One Minute Manager* (4). Modeling is a technique that frequently is used in employee training programs.

CLASSICAL CONDITIONING

The methods of behavior modification are based on principles of learning that, for the most part, have been discovered in the experimental laboratory. According to Hill, the best known animals in the history of psychology were the dogs housed in the laboratory of Ivan Pavlov, the Russian physiologist, who was conducting research on digestive processes (5). Serendipitously, Pavlov noted that his laboratory animals salivated not only when food was presented, but also when the laboratory assistant who regularly fed them came into the room; at times they even salivated at the sound of the laboratory door opening. Pavlov spent the rest of his life investigating a type of learning based on association, now known as classical conditioning.

Pavlov realized immediately that the response of salivation to laboratory assistants and noisy doors was not a part of the physiological makeup of the dog. The dogs were salivating when events occurred that had regularly and repeatedly come before the presentation of their food. An association was apparently being formed between some event and the future appearance of food.

Pavlov noted that certain environmental events or stimuli would reliably trigger or elicit a particular behavioral response. For example, food in a dog's mouth would reliably produce saliva. The triggering event (food in the mouth) became known as the unconditioned stimulus (US), while the response triggered (salivation) was called the unconditioned response (UR). This relationship was built into the organism, and hence, unconditioned. Conditioning occurs, then, when some other stimulus (a neutral stimulus) that originally does not trigger the particular response (salivation), eventually comes to produce that response. This occurs by pairing the originally neutral stimulus with the unconditioned stimulus. When conditioning has occurred, the conditioned stimulus (CS), which was originally neutral, produces the same, or a very similar, response as does the US. In the example, the CS was the presence of the laboratory assistant. Pavlov showed that bells, tones, lights, and many other stimuli could serve as the CS and could come to elicit the response of salivation, which is labeled a conditioned response (CR) once it is triggered by or produced by a CS.

Many different types of responses have been found to be subject to classical conditioning principles. Not only reflexive responses, such as salivation and eye blink, but complex emotional responses can be classically conditioned, as illustrated by the following example. The heart pounds and beads of perspiration appear on the forehead as one hears the siren of an ambulance approaching a neighbor's home. The same phenomenon may occur when the teacher passes out examination questions. Try to construct a scenario to account for this response in terms of classical conditioning principles, or think of other situations in which classical conditioning might play a part in human behavior or emotional responses.

OPERANT CONDITIONING

At about the same time that Pavlov was delineating the principles of classical conditioning, a young American scientist, psychologist Edward Thorndike, was pursuing the investigation of learning principles from another perspective. Thorndike used many types of animals in his research and designed and constructed "puzzle boxes" for cats. A hungry cat was placed inside the box with food located outside. To have access to the food, the cat had to solve the puzzle of how to escape from the box. Thorndike observed that the cats made trial-and-error responses until escape was achieved and the food consumed. Gradually, the time required to solve the puzzle decreased, and the behavior that achieved success in solving the puzzle became dominant, while nonsuccessful behaviors were eliminated.

Thorndike proposed an explanation for this phenomenon based on a principle he called the Law of Effect. The Law of Effect stated that behaviors could be changed by their consequences. Responses that were followed by satisfying consequences would be stamped in or strengthened. Behaviors not followed by satisfying consequences, or behaviors followed by annoying consequences, would be weakened and less likely to occur in the future. Thorndike's Law of Effect led to much research on principles of learning and formed the foundation for the study of operant or instrumental conditioning, which is learning or conditioning based on reinforcement or reward.

The focal point of research on the Law of Effect is the relationship between responses, or behaviors, and the consequences of those behaviors. Schwartz described four types of response-consequence outcomes (6). First, responses or behaviors may produce positive outcomes, a consequence known as positive reinforcement. An example would be the lavish praise and attention one might receive after achieving a svelte new figure. Second, responses may produce negative outcomes; this consequence is known as punishment. Punishment decreases the future likelihood of a response. Examples of punishment include the receipt of a traffic ticket for an improper left turn or the inability to fit into a favorite, expensive outfit after gaining weight. Third, responses may result in the elimination or removal of aversive stimuli that are already present. This consequence is known as negative reinforcement or escape, and it is similar to positive reinforcement in that it increases the future likelihood or probability of a response. Examples include escaping devastating cold by going into a heated building, escaping a poor television show by changing channels, and escaping unfavorable comparisons with others by shaping up and trimming down. Finally, responses may prevent an aversive event from occurring. Examples include avoiding the cold be staying indoors and avoiding unfavorable comparisons with others by maintaining body fitness. The avoidance of aversive events increases the future likelihood of the response, as does positive reinforcement. Behaviors that are not positively reinforced or negatively reinforced, and do not lead to escape or avoidance of aversive stimuli, should not increase in strength, and with continued nonreinforcement, should decrease in strength.

Later behavioral psychologists continued where Thorndike concluded. BF Skinner is best known for his championing of a set of methods and terms to explain behavior on the basis of the principles of operant conditioning. Skinner developed a situation in which behavior could be observed in discrete units and subsequently recorded. This situation was an operant chamber, which has been dubbed a "Skinner box." The lever presses of rats and key pecks of pigeons have been the most frequently studied responses. Skinner's enthusiasm for the behavioristic approach was not limited to lower animals, however, for he proposed wide application for the principles that were established. In recent years, the behavioristic approach has become an increasingly important practical technique in many settings, such as classrooms, mental hospitals, prisons, clinics, the work place, and self-management situations.

MODELING

In addition to classical and operant conditioning as means of behavior change, another form of learning is known as observational learning, or modeling. Learning by modeling involves the observation of some behavior or pattern of behaving, which is followed later by the performance of either the same or some similar behavior. Albert Bandura is associated with the study of learning by modeling (7).

The model being observed may be either another person or a representation of the pattern of behaving. The model, then, could be another human, an animal, or some symbolic representation that uses verbal or visual stimuli, such as films, television, or other media presentations.

The effectiveness of learning by modeling appears to be directly related to certain characteristics of the model. The two characteristics found to be most relevant are the observer's similarity to the model and the status of the model. The more similar the characteristics of the model are to those of the observer, the higher is the probability that learning by modeling will occur. Research has shown that models with greater status, prestige, or expertise are more likely to be imitated by the observer than models lacking these characteristics. Golfers, for example, are more likely to imitate the stance and swing of a player of the caliber of the young, hot new phenomenon on the professional tour, Tiger Woods, than the techniques of an unknown player. Certainly, this fact has been noted and capitalized on by movie and television stars and other well-known persons who have produced books and videotapes on their fitness/exercise/nutrition programs. Many people will model behavior after the person with "status" even though equally effective or superior programs could be developed by relatively unknown, but professionally trained, nutritionists and exercise physiologists.

To take advantage of modeling, dietetics professionals may try sharing success stories of people who have made permanent dietary modifications for the benefit of their health. In group therapy, clients who have followed their diets may serve as models for others. The counselor may be viewed as a model by the client. As a result, in counseling obese people, the counselor should be normal weight, and dietetics professionals should be following the normal nutrition recommendations that they give to others.

Behavior modeling is used in employee training programs to teach basic supervisory techniques, selling skills, and a variety of other skills through observation of films and videotapes. In assigning a new employee to work with a current employee, the latter serves as a model. Managers should make sure that their own behaviors are exemplary of what they expect of subordinates (8). If the supervisor adds an extra 10 minutes to the allowed time for a coffee break, for example, employees may model after the example set.

There is no doubt that a great deal of human learning or behavior change is due to modeling, even though traditionally, emphasis has been placed on the stimulus-response (or behavior-consequence) approach to explaining changes in behavior, or the acquisition and extinction of responses. These three approaches—learning through classical conditioning, operant conditioning, and modeling—form the basis for behavior modification. The behavioristic position is that many behaviors are learned or alterable through use of these three approaches to learning.

CHANGING EATING BEHAVIORS

As the principles that govern behavior and behavior change became more clearly defined, it was increasingly apparent that nutritionists and behavioral scientists should work together to provide methods of using these principles in applied settings in which changes in dietary habits are the primary goal. The most frequent application has been the behavioral management of obesity, but cooperative programs have led to application in such diverse area of concern as cardiovascular diseases, eating disorders, and diabetes mellitus.

As this collaborative approach became better established, comprehensive models for nutrition interventions were developed. One of these is the "Stages of Change" framework. This model is an approach to prepare the professional to develop realistic expectations of a prospective client's willingness and motivation to change behaviors. Once the person's stage is assessed the therapy can be more effectively matched to the person's situation, as noted in Chapter 1. According to this model, it is unrealistic to expect clients to move excitedly and effectively headlong into a program of action if they are not motivated nor willing to do so. Many of the behavior modification tactics can be used most effectively when the person is in the *Action* or *Maintenance* stage of this multistage model (9–11).

Dietary behaviors must be studied in terms of the client's total environment, which includes physical, social, psychological, physiological, and environmental factors, as well as all conditions and events which precede and follow eating. Several behavioral scientists have referred to this framework as the ABCs, derived from analysis of the **A**ntecedents (stimuli or cues), the **B**ehavior (response) itself (eating), and the **C**onsequences (reinforcement/reward or punishment) of the behavior (1).

$$A \rightarrow B \rightarrow C$$

For example, seeing a package of cookies left on the kitchen counter may be the antecedent or cue. The behavior could be eating half a package of cookies in the kitchen when one is home alone at 4:00 PM. The consequences may be pleasure from the taste of the cookies and reduced feelings of hunger or frustration, and increased feelings of happiness and satisfaction, which reinforce the behavior. The dietetics professional and the client must find ways to decrease undesirable eating behaviors and increase new, desirable ones.

Antecedents

Behavior modification techniques work by regulating the antecedents, the behavior of eating itself, and the consequences or rewards. Analysis of antecedents of behavior seeks to control or limit the stimuli or cues to eating. For example, a cue may be seeing or smelling food, watching television, arriving home from work or school, attending a social event, or noticing the presence of extra food on the table at mealtime. Behavior may be influenced by both internal and external factors. There may be internal cues, such as physiological feelings of hunger or psychological feelings of loneliness or boredom. A number of external variables may cue eating, such as noting the time of day or passing an ice cream shop in the street. Both internal and external factors may be mediated by cognitive factors, such as not caring about current weight levels or not wishing to dull one's appetite for the next meal (12).

The strategy involves decreasing the number of times the person is exposed to situations in which he consumes food. A list of suggestions for changing behavior that have been recommended by various authors for persons desiring to lose weight is found in Table 6.1 (1, 13, 14). To modify antecedents, the dietetics professional may suggest removing negative cues (not buying improper foods), introducing new, more positive cues (exercising instead of eating), restricting behavior to one set of cues (eating only at designated times), cognitive restructuring mentioned previously and in the next chapter, and role-playing new responses to old antecedents (telling a friend you would rather go to a movie than out to a restaurant for pizza). Breaking response chains and preplanning behavior are other strategies (15).

Some antecedents may be controlled by preplanning.

Preplanning meals and snacks and having only proper foods in the house is preferable to expecting one to maintain self-control when hungry. Preplanning social occasions and exercise is also helpful. Small portions of favorite foods may need to be included in the diet to avoid feelings of total deprivation leading to possible abandonment of dietary changes. Doing the right thing is enhanced by stimulus control. The goal is to decrease the number of times the person is exposed to tempting situations so that self-control is tested as rarely as possible.

In some instances responses occur in chains in which each response produces the stimulus for the next response. An example of a chain would be feeling tired, looking at the clock, realizing that it is bedtime, turning off the television, going to the kitchen, getting a snack, eating the snack, feeling satisfied (reinforcer), and going to bed. The components of the chain should be identified, and then a break in the chain should be planned, such as adding 5 minutes of stretching exercises after turning off the television.

Behavior

After identifying antecedents, one should explore the eating behavior itself, investigating the speed of eating, the presence of others, and activities carried on during meals or snacks, such as watching television. Breaking a chain of eating too rapidly, for example, is accomplished by introducing delays in eating. Members of the "clean plate club" need to leave some food on the plate. Concentrating on the act of eating and enjoying the flavors of the foods are recommended.

Consequences

Consequences of eating are described as reinforcements/rewards or punishments. According to Stunkard and Berthold, "Since behavior is believed to be maintained by its consequences, efforts are made to arrange consequences that will maintain desirable behaviors, such as adherence to the weight control program" (1). The consequences of eating may be positive, negative, or neutral. In general, positive consequences are more effective in promoting change than negative or punishing consequences. Alternatives to eating may be included, such as walking or exercising, writing a letter, cleaning a part of the house, partaking of a hobby, and so on. One recommendation related to sodium restriction was for the client to set aside a quarter (or dollar) as a reward for using a spice or flavoring in place of salt (13).

The client's current eating habits may be pleasurable, and if food is considered its own reward, then new and different rewards must be established. Eating is a powerfully motivated behavior, the occurrence of which is necessary to maintain the homeostasis of the organism. Without nutrient intake, the organism dies, so eating provides reinforcement of a powerful biological drive. The dietetics professional needs to identify new reinforcers with clients. Eating changes should be pleasurable to be self-

TABLE 6.1.

Techniques for Behavior Modification

I. Provide Incentives to Aid Patients in Maintaining Commitment
  A. Determine ways to focus attention on successful experiences. A positive comment by the counselor is helpful, and one can always find something positive to say.
  B. Encourage people to tell others about dietary goals. This public commitment often will aid in maintaining one's course of action.
  C. Have the person anticipate problems that might come up and consider possible solutions before a problem arises. Having a plan ready will make focusing on the goal easier.
  D. Concentrate on allowed foods and portions, rather than the disallowed. Be positive.
  E. Keep reminding the person that dietary change is a gradual process. Dietary habits were not developed in a brief period of time and probably will not be significantly changed in a short time. Set realistic goals for immediate and long-term change. Encourage successive approximations to the desired behavior.

II. Learn Eating Habits (and Exercise Habits) by Record Keeping
One cannot change a habit until one knows what it is. Self-monitoring with accurate records of the foods consumed is necessary for behavioral control of eating. Information to consider recording would be:
  A. What food was eaten.
  B. Quantity of each food.
  C. What the person was doing just prior to eating (to help identify cues).
  D. Place of eating (cue providing).
  E. With whom eating occurs, or alone (cue providing).
  F. How the person felt (cue providing).
  G. Time of eating (cue providing).
This record keeping exercise can identify the person's patterns of food intake and those cues that are associated with food consumption as well as the emotional outcome of eating. The person will become more aware of the environmental stimuli that are associated with eating behavior.

III. Control the Stimuli (Cues) and Restructure the Environment
  A. Physical environment
    1. Based on the records kept, have the person identify physical stimuli in the environment that are associated with, and therefore are cues to, inappropriate eating behaviors. Different stimuli become associated with the act of eating and can become signals for appropriate or inappropriate food consumption.
    2. Ask the person to identify physical stimuli that could remind him to eat properly. Examples of these would be charts or graphs, cartoons, signs, and the like. The presence of appropriate foods in the home will probably be the best cue to appropriate eating, supplemented by the elimination of inappropriate foods.
    3. Have the person specify a special place where food should be consumed, such as at the dining table, and not in front of the television set or kitchen sink.
    4. Make those foods that are acceptable in the nutrition plan as attractive as possible. Use good dishes, crystal, and so forth to make dining a pleasant event.
    5. Set up shopping trips based on the following suggestions:
      a. shop for food only after eating.
      b. use a shopping list.
      c. avoid ready-to-eat foods.
      d. do not carry more money than needed for shopping list.
    6. Set up specific plans and activities:
      a. substitute exercise for snacking.
      b. eat meals and snacks at scheduled times.
      c. do not accept food offered by others.
      d. store food out of sight.
      e. remove food from inappropriate storage areas in the house.
      f. use smaller dishes.
      g. avoid being the food server.
      h. leave the table immediately after eating.
      i. discard leftovers.

(continued)

TABLE 6.1. (continued)

    7. Regarding special events and holidays:
      a. drink fewer alcoholic beverages.
      b. plan eating before parties.
      c. eat a low-calorie snack before parties.
      d. practice polite ways to decline food.
      e. do not get discouraged by occasional setbacks.
  B. Social environment
    1. Have the person identify the types of social situations that contribute to poor eating habits. Examples of stimuli in the social environment that might contribute to difficulty for the person would be negative statements from family members or friends and social situations in which there are expectations for eating inappropriate or disallowed foods.
    2. Have the person identify the kind of social interactions that would be supportive of good eating habits and following the nutrition plan. Role-playing can be useful with the person practicing how he will ask others to help him change his eating habits.
  C. Cognitive or mental environment
    1. Have the person identify what thoughts and feelings are likely to make attempts to change eating habits unsuccessful.
    2. After the person has identified possible negative thoughts that could lead to discouragement, help him develop some positive thoughts that can be used to counteract the negative ones.
    3. Avoid setting unreasonable goals.
IV. Change Actual Eating Behavior
  A. Slow down.
    1. Take one small bite at a time.
    2. Put the fork down between mouthfuls.
    3. Chew thoroughly before swallowing.
    4. Take a break during the meal. Stop eating completely for a short period.
  B. Leave some food on the plate.
  C. Make eating of inappropriate foods as difficult as possible.
  D. Control snacks.
    1. Save allowable foods from meals for snacks.
    2. Establish behaviors incompatible with eating.
    3. Prepare snacks the way one prepares meals—on a plate.
    4. Keep a quantity of low-calorie foods, such as raw vegetables, on hand to use. Have them ready to eat and easy to get.
  E. Instruct the person that when he eats, he should not be performing any other act. The cues associated with eating should be restricted to that act, so one should not eat while reading, sewing, watching television, and so on.
  F. Have the person continue monitoring himself.
V. Change Exercise Behavior
  A. Routine activity
    1. Increase routine activity.
    2. Increase use of stairs.
    3. Keep records of distance walked daily.
  B. Exercise
    1. Begin supervised exercise program under specialist's direction.
    2. Keep records of daily exercise.
    3. Increase exercise gradually.
VI. Set up a Reward and Reinforcement System
  A. Have family and friends provide this help in the form of praise and material rewards.
  B. Clearly define behaviors to be reinforced.
  C. Use self-monitoring records as a basis for rewards.
  D. Plan specific rewards for specific behaviors. Use written contracts.
  E. Gradually make rewards more difficult to earn.
  F. Use creative reinforcers, such as dropping quarters in a bank, putting money away for each goal reached, and earmarked for something desirable. Take money back as a punishment if the goal is not reached.

Adapted from Stunkard A, Berthold, H. What is behavior therapy? Am J Clin Nutr 1985;41:821. Rabb C, Tillotson, JL, eds. Heart to heart. Washington, DC: US Dept of Health and Human Services, 1983; and Fensterheim H, Baer, J. Don't say yes when you want to say no. New York: Dell Pub Co, 1975.

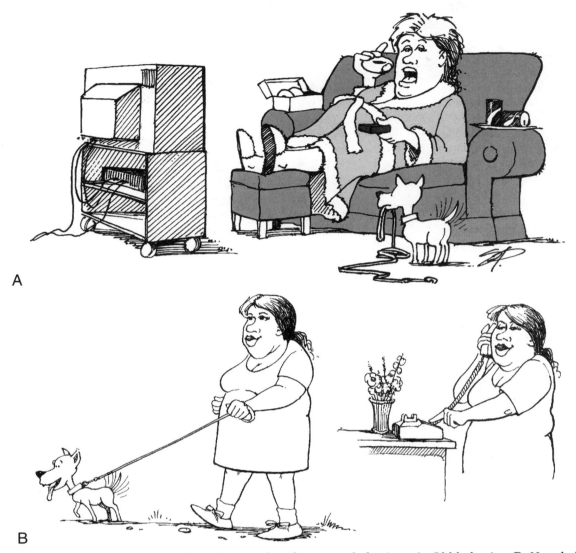

FIGURE 6.1. The counselor can assist the client in identifying new behaviors. **A.** Old behavior. **B.** New behaviors.

reinforcing. If new patterns are a chore and are disliked, they will fail to provide self-reinforcement.

The counselor can work with the client to establish reinforcers. The obvious approach is to ask people what they want as a reinforcer, but it is sometimes difficult for people to come up with concrete suggestions. This is an opportunity for the counselor to offer a list of suggested reinforcers for the client to select from. Another helpful approach is for the counselor to have ready a list of questions to ask the client. Activity reinforcers may be identified by asking, ''What do you like to do with your leisure time?'' Reinforcers may be walking, attending movies, plays, or sporting events, taking a bath, gardening, doing hobbies, playing cards, reading, or whatever the individual prefers. Social reinforcers may be found be asking, ''Who do you like to be with?'' Reinforcers may include visiting family or friends or phoning. Other questions are, ''What do you find enjoyable?'' ''What would you hate

to lose?'' ''What would be a nice present to receive?,'' and ''What do you like to buy when you have extra money?'' (other than inappropriate foods, of course) (16). Table 6.2 summarizes the identification of reinforcers.

The counselor is also part of the reinforcement and, rather than focusing on failures, should emphasize what the person has done right with verbal reward and praise. Remind clients to reward themselves cognitively by telling themselves they are making progress and have done something right. For the obese, the ability to fit into smaller-sized clothes hanging in the closet and the weight loss itself are reinforcing. New reinforcers, such as enjoyable activities, need to be established and introduced for weight maintenance, however. The reinforcement provided by significant others and self-monitoring are discussed later in the chapter.

After one or two eating changes or goals are identified, a schedule or reinforcement needs to be discussed and

---

TABLE 6.2.

Identifying Reinforcers

1. Make a list of leisure time activities and hobbies that you enjoy.
2. Make a list of people you like to be with.
3. Make a list of things you would like to purchase with small amounts of extra money.
4. What do you find relaxing?
5. What do you do for fun?
6. What are your favorite possessions?

---

established. The schedule specifies which behaviors, if any, will be reinforced and how frequently reinforcement will be provided. Continuous reinforcement is the simplest method, but this may lose its effectiveness if the reinforcer is used excessively. An alternative is intermittent reinforcement, such as reinforcement 3 times a day, or once a day. Eventually the time may be lengthened between reinforcements. The schedule should be appropriate to the behavior one is trying to strengthen, convenient for the person to apply, and applied immediately for the greatest effect. Never reinforcing a behavior should lead to its extinction.

In some cases, contracts may be desirable. Contracts are clear statements of target behaviors of the individual; they specify the type of reinforcers to be used, the person who will deliver the reinforcers, and the frequency of reinforcement. They may be signed and dated by the counselor and the client. Contracts ensure that all parties agree on the goals and procedures, and provide a measurement of how near the client is to reaching the goals. The signatures help to ensure that the contract will be followed, since signing is a commitment and may provide added motivation to change (13). Contracts may be very complex and elaborate or very simple and straightforward. A certain behavior may be followed by a certain reinforcer, for example, a certain amount of exercise will be followed by a shower before bed. No work, no shower. In other situations, a point system may be designed in which clients may earn many points per day and then use their points in exchange for a particular reinforcing item or activity (16). A sample behavioral contract is found in Figure 6.2.

Completion of behavioral assessment is needed prior to counseling. Examination of the ABCs by the dietetics professional and the client assists both parties in understanding current eating behaviors and allows discussion of what can be changed. The role of the counselor is to provide an integrated plan for the total nutrition program of each client. The therapist serves as a guide or facilitator of change rather than a director or controller of change, by suggesting behavioral techniques that are appropriate to the situation. The counselor should assist the client in learning to analyze the eating problems and should suggest possible goals, strategies, and techniques to deal with them (17).

Since clients are not in daily contact with the counselor (unless the telephone is used for follow-up), clients must be ready to assume personal responsibility for sound dietary changes, and must eventually become independent. They must learn to analyze and solve their own eating behavior problems. The therapist should have the client start with small, easy changes, which are most likely to be successful, and progress incrementally to more difficult ones in later sessions. To be self-reinforcing, the eating changes should be pleasurable ones. If clients enjoy potato chips, ice cream, pizza, and beer, they have to find substitutes they enjoy, such as crisp apples, fresh grapes, unbuttered popcorn, and dietetic beverages. It may be sufficient to start by reducing the quantity of favorite foods consumed. Needless to say, strategies must be highly individualized, and what is appropriate for one client may be inappropriate for another.

The client should be advised to expect difficult times and possibly some inappropriate eating binges, especially when under physical or emotional stress. Expecting total control over change is unrealistic and may lead to diminished self-esteem in clients who have problems following diets, with eventual abandonment of the dietary changes. Learning any new skill requires practice for a period of time. Analyzing high-risk situations and dealing with lapses is dealt with in Chapter 7, "Modifying Cognitions." Repetition of the same new behaviors gradually becomes reinforcing. Enthusiasm for change may drop rapidly after the initial period, especially if frustration and disappointments arise. The client must understand that as the behavior changes become consistent, satisfying emotions and thoughts will accompany the behavior. Weekly appointments with the counselor are probably needed at the outset of therapy.

SELF-MONITORING

Self-monitoring, or keeping records of eating behaviors to be controlled, was intended originally as a means of supplying the counselor and client with data for analysis. Clients record what, where, when, and how much they eat; the circumstances, e.g., watching television or feeling bored; and the persons present. Table 6.3 presents an example of a self-monitoring food record. The exercise of keeping records, however, was determined to have additional value of its own. It increased client awareness and understanding of current eating behaviors and the influences on them, and led to such realizations as "I'm eating too much during evening hours while I read." Data provided a basis for setting goals for change ("I'll eat a low-calorie snack instead") and finding ways to reinforce new behaviors ("I'll tell myself how well I'm doing"). Keeping records also served as a measure of commitment of the individual to change (1). Weight loss graphs for obese persons and records of physical exercise, blood

Behavioral Contract

Name _____   Date _____

During the next _____
                        (period of time, i.e., days, weeks)

I plan to do the following:

1. _____
        (specific behavioral goals, self-monitoring)

2. _____

3. _____

4. _____

If successful, I will reward myself _____
                                            (when—daily, weekly)

with the following: _____
                        (name of specific reward)

Signed: _____   Date: _____
            (client)

Signed: _____   Date: _____
            (counselor)

FIGURE 6.2.   Example of a behavioral contract.

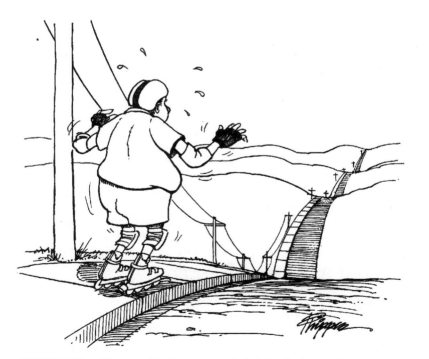

FIGURE 6.3.   The road to long-term behavioral change is not easy.

TABLE 6.3.						
Self-Monitoring Food Record						
TIME	FOOD/AMOUNT/METHOD PREP	ROOM PLACE	OTHERS PRESENT		HOW YOU FELT BEFORE EATING	ACTIVITIES SAME TIME
Example: 9:30 PM	8 cookies, 10-oz milk	family room	husband		bored, tired	watching TV

sugar, and blood pressure are other self-monitoring techniques.

SELF-MANAGEMENT

In most behavior modification programs for weight control, the client and counselor are together only for brief durations at specified intervals. Consequently it is not possible for the counselor to be continually in control of the dispensing of rewards and punishments, or withholding of rewards, for appropriate and inappropriate behavior, which is the basis of behavior modification. Therefore, self-regulation or self-management techniques are taught to clients so that they can regulate and control their own behavior. In this way progress may be achieved in the interval between meetings of the client and counselor.

Research has shown the importance of developing behavioral self-management techniques. Skinner explained that self-management or "self-control" occurs when the individual manipulates the variables on which the behavior depends (18). Self-management programs have been "designed to help persons become aware of and modify the social and physical antecedents of eating, to self-administer rewarding consequences for habit change" (or appropriate behavior), "or to self-administer aversive stimulation for inappropriate eating (behavior)" (12). As self-management programs have evolved, more emphasis has been placed on cognitive change. People have been helped to modify thoughts and beliefs that interfered with adherence to specific dietary regimens and to use self-reinforcing thoughts when appropriate behaviors occur.

For individuals in a weight reduction program, for example, it would be important for them to get in touch with their hunger. A simple exercise would be to rate hunger on a scale of 1 to 10, with 1 being ravenously hungry, 10 being filled to capacity verging on excess, and 5 being just comfortable. The individual should be encouraged to try not to eat unless hunger is at a 1, 2, or 3 level, and to try to stop eating when hunger is at a 4, 5, or 6 level. Becoming aware of one's inner state can be of assistance in achieving the desired self-management.

SOCIAL SUPPORT

The environment of clients often includes a number of people they contact daily. It is important to include the person's family and significant others when planning lifestyle and dietary changes. The dietetics professional should include family members in counseling for change whenever possible, since the changes in food plans at home may affect them as well. Social factors may be contributing factors to obesity. If the family system supports an obese lifestyle with high-calorie foods and little physical activity, change will be difficult for the client unless the whole family participates in the challenge (13). The involvement and support of spouse and family play an important role in weight loss (19).

Ideally, family and friends are supportive of the efforts of the client in changing eating behaviors. The counselor may need to discuss with clients the important role of support in achieving permanent change (20). In nonsupportive environments, the dietetics professional may suggest that clients request help from family or friends by seeking their agreements not to eat forbidden foods in front of them, or not to purchase or prepare the wrong foods. In addition, clients might ask their spouses, families, and friends to offer positive reinforcement for their efforts. Role-playing some of these situations with clients may be helpful.

When family members are present at the counseling session, they should be asked to discuss ways that they can contribute to the client's lifestyle change. Reinforcing proper behavior by the use of praise is an example. Controlling antecedents by having proper foods available is of great assistance. Family and friends should avoid acting the role of judge and jury. "You shouldn't eat that," "It's bad for you," and "I told you so," are not helpful remarks. Jealous and envious reactions may also appear. "You've lost enough weight," "Just this once won't hurt your diet," and "Your skin is getting to look awful" are remarks that the client may need to tolerate with humor or directly confront.

APPLICATIONS

Obesity

The most frequent application of behavioral principles and methods to the treatment of nutritional problems has

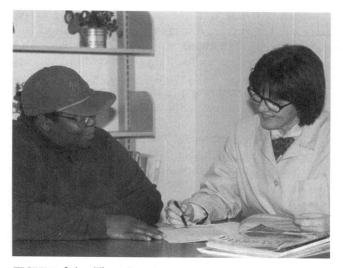

FIGURE 6.4. The client's current eating behaviors are the basis for developing changes.

been in the management of obesity. In 1959, Stunkard and McLaren-Hume noted that traditional psychotherapeutic approaches to obesity, as well as medical and dietary approaches, had not produced positive results. He reported that "most obese persons will not stay in treatment for obesity. Of those who stay in treatment most will not lose weight and of those who do lose weight, most will regain it" (21). Apparently, little has changed.

There is some difference of opinion regarding the efficacy of behavior modification techniques developed for use in treating overweight clients (22). Brownell has stated that behavior therapy is more effective than any other treatment with which it has been compared and is an essential part of any weight reduction program (23). Coates, in contrast, noted that "behavior modification has prospered under the protective shield of an especially good press" (12). These reports, while emphasizing differing evaluative statements regarding the outcomes of behavior modification, are not mutually exclusive and could indeed be accurate. Obesity is a complex state and is not treated easily. The obese person may be overweight for a variety of reasons, only one of which may be improper eating behaviors. The biology of weight control must be considered (2, 24). Stunkard, for example, recognizes that "there must be a very powerful biological pressure against losing weight" (25). This does not mean, however, that it is futile to attempt to control one's weight.

The American College of Sports Medicine, in a position statement, stressed that lifelong weight control requires commitment, an understanding of one's eating habits, and a willingness to change them (26). Realistic goal setting, combined with reduction of fat and caloric intake and a sound exercise program, is recommended. Behavioral methods have been used successfully in diet planning, nutrition education, and a strenuous physical edu-

cation program in a residential summer camp for obese boys. This combined approach resulted in significant improvement in body weight for the group (27).

In a study designed to include a 2-year follow-up to assess the effectiveness of a behavioral weight control program, the researchers found that after 2 years, 65.3% of the subjects were still below their baseline weights, 36.6% of the entire study group had maintained or enhanced the weight loss achieved during treatment, and 16.1% weighed at least 10% less than their baseline weight (28). These results, the authors felt, indicate that the behavior weight control program had an important and long-term impact on the weight status of a large sample of obese men and women. However, long-term weight loss remains a difficult task, and although weight loss may be achieved during the treatment period, many clients regain a portion of that weight during follow-up. Recent publications highlight an impressive long-term success story of behavior treatment of childhood obesity that stands in marked contrast to the sometimes disappointing long-term results obtained with obese adults. The author speculates that it may be easier to teach children healthy eating and activity habits or that strong parental involvement lessens the importance of self-control in weight reduction (29, 30). Clearly, improved methods to facilitate a higher level of success are needed. This search continues (31–34).

Motivation must be present for behavior change. This is particularly true for eating behaviors. There are several factors relevant to the prediction of success in weight control, one of which is motivation to reduce weight. Researchers have developed a cognitive inventory for use as a screening and counseling tool prior to entry into a behavioral weight reduction program (35). Brownell has also stressed the importance of screening patients adequately before the initiation of any weight control program. A behavioral test of motivation as a screening device has been suggested (23). Requiring a fee for treatment is one approach, but a deposit-refund system has been used also. In the latter system patients are asked to deposit money, which is later returned if the patient attends meetings faithfully and/or achieves a previously determined weight loss. This system appears to be effective in reducing the drop-out rate.

An added benefit of significant weight reduction based on cognitive-behavioral treatment in a long-term therapeutic setting has been the reduction in psychosomatic symptoms, anxiety, and depression in treated clients. More adaptive behavioral alternatives in longer goal-oriented programs seemed effective in promoting continued weight loss (36, 37). Research results, therefore, emphasize the fact that there is no "quick-fix" in weight reduction and the outlook must be long-term (38–43).

Eating Disorders

Anorexia and bulimia are disorders found most frequently among adolescent and young adult women, and are estimated to occur in up to 1 to 3% of these populations. Therapist errors in treating eating disorders have apparently contributed to patient resistance, treatment ineffectiveness, and premature treatment termination. A variety of medical and psychological approaches have been used in treatment. It is most important for the therapist to be aware of the alternatives for treatment. The behavior modification approach is one of these alternatives (44–46).

A now classic case study detailed the use of behavior modification techniques for the nutritional disorder, anorexia nervosa, a chronic failure to eat (47). A young woman who was 5'4" weighed only 47 pounds at the start of her behavior therapy. Before therapy commenced, the hospital environment provided many amenities and privileges. Because she appeared to enjoy them, these privileges and amenities were removed so that they could be used to reinforce appropriate behaviors, in this case, eating. All of the attention and sympathy that the hospital staff had used to coax the patient to eat were withdrawn. The therapist ate one meal a day with the patient, and the staff was allowed only to greet the patient on entering the room.

The social reinforcement that had helped to maintain noneating behavior was withheld so that it could be used later to strengthen eating behaviors. The therapist talked to the patient to reinforce her behavior when she picked up her fork, lifted food toward her mouth, chewed food, or performed any other eating behavior. She was then allowed the use of radio or television, but only after meals at which she increased her food intake over previous meals. As she gained strength and weight, other reinforcers were introduced, such as the privilege of choosing her own menu or inviting other patients to dine with her. Later reinforcers included walks, visitors, and mail.

The treatment was successful, and after 8 weeks of therapy, she was discharged to a program of outpatient follow-up weighing 64 pounds. Five years later, she had maintained her weight between 78 and 80 pounds and was successfully employed (16). Locating potential reinforcers or behavior strengtheners is an essential first step in any treatment program. What reinforces behavior for one person may not function as a reinforcer for another.

A later study reported the successful inpatient behavioral treatment of anorexia and bulimia (48). The treatment program was associated with increases in body weight and caloric consumption, which were generally maintained at 2-year follow-up. Self-monitoring of eating behavior, including caloric intake, emesis, and bulimia, proved to be a useful maintenance strategy. Other studies have noted the importance of self-monitoring and daily logging of intake, weight, and details of binge/purge episodes on progress and successful treatment of anorexia and bulimia (49–54). These reported successes of behavioral treatment of anorexia and bulimia have involved inpatient therapy and outpatient follow-up.

Another finding from the research on anorexia nervosa concerned the effect of size of food portions on eating behavior. The serving of larger portions was associated with increased food intake. Apparently the subjects had been eating a relatively fixed proportion of the amount of food presented, whether the portion was large or small. This pattern of eating has been noted in obese people as well, but not in normal adults or in young children (55).

Behavior modification has also been used successfully in the treatment of chronic food refusal in handicapped children. Records of conditions before treatment began indicated that all patients accepted little food, expelled food frequently, and engaged in disruptive behavior. Treatment methods used were social praise, access to preferred foods, brief periods of play with toys, and forced feeding. Marked behavioral improvement was noted for each patient as well as an increase in the amount of food consumed. Further improvements were noted at 7- to 30-month follow-up (56).

Participation in a behavioral treatment program proved useful when multiple problems were approached in the case of a 29-year-old married woman, hospitalized with anorexia following a diagnosis of multiple sclerosis at 21 years of age (57).

Many drug and hormonal therapies have been tried as treatments for this serious eating disorder. The most common treatment is behavior modification, combined with individual and family counseling (58). Under any treatment, however, a full return to normalcy in less than 4 to 5 years is rare (59, 60). The prognosis in anorexia is worse than that of bulimia and persons with anorexia appear more resistant than persons with bulimia to outpatient intervention (61).

In a comprehensive review of 30 studies on behavioral treatment of the eating disorder pica, results suggest that pica can be altered by manipulation of antecedent and consequent stimuli (62).

Diabetes Mellitus

Behavior modification methods have proven to be a useful component in the management of diabetes mellitus. Historically, poor patient adherence to dietary regimens has been a problem. Behavioral interventions such as cueing, self-monitoring, and reinforcement for appropriate behavior have been effective in promoting dietary adherence in patients with Type I diabetes. Success has not been as great, however, with behavioral techniques used in weight loss programs for obese patients with Type II diabetes (63, 64). A recent study showed that adolescents with insulin-dependent diabetes mellitus did not improve their weight loss percentages in a behavior-modification program when compared with the standard treatment in promoting long-term weight loss (65). As previously noted, however, the problem of control of obesity from the standpoint of any particular treatment is complex. An evaluation instrument (the Diabetes Self-Management Record) has been developed that provides a model for documenting behavior change associated with diabetes education programs. Research showed that the use of this self-monitoring instrument facilitated the persistence of positive behavior change associated with the education program (66).

Behavioral management techniques have also been used with young diabetic patients to improve adherence to prescribed medical regimens. Subjects were given training in behavioral self-management. In addition, they received training in negotiation and contracting, which allowed them to develop a contract to earn reinforcement from parents for using learned self-management skills. These behavioral procedures led to an increase in adherence to the prescribed medical regimen (67). Young adults with diabetes improved their ability to estimate their blood glucose levels after participating in a discrimination training program, in which they received feedback regarding the accuracy of their estimates. These resulting increases in accuracy of glucose level estimation have established the opportunity for better nutritional control of the disease (68).

A group intervention with elderly diabetic patients used behavior modification training as one component. These elderly individuals had experienced difficulty in managing their diabetic conditions because of poor compliance with diets. Participants in the intervention group had lower peak blood glucose levels and less frequent departure from their diets than the control group. Follow-ups at 12 and 24 weeks showed maintenance of lowered glucose levels; however, participants reported an increased number of diet deviations by 48 weeks (69).

Behavioral interventions, when used in the management of diabetes mellitus, should be geared to the developmental stage of the individual in treatment (70). An understanding of life span changes (i.e., preadolescence, adolescence, adulthood, and older adulthood) in relation to life role, peer conformity pressure, eating disorders, sexuality, pregnancy, and aging need to be taken into account. The strategy that is effective with a diabetic adolescent struggling with peer conformity pressures may well be markedly different from that which will be of assistance to a pregnant woman with diabetes, or an elderly person living alone. There is a definite need to individualize interventions directed toward behavior change (71-74).

Cardiovascular Diseases

In the Multiple Risk Factor Intervention Trial (MRFIT), behavioral scientists and nutritionists worked cooperatively with the aim of changing behaviors related to diet and smoking on a long-term basis to reduce the risk of cardiovascular disease. A self-evaluation system for monitoring food intake was developed so that the counselor could estimate the subject's progress in making appropriate dietary changes. A scoring system was used for classifying foods according to fat and cholesterol content as well as predicted effect on blood cholesterol. Subjects could use the system and select alternative food choices to meet appropriate eating goals. The self-monitoring records were employed as a method of measuring compliance, and also served to reinforce change and provide positive feedback for appropriate behavior (75). The behavioral contract was found to be a useful tool for changing eating behavior with the intent to reduce weight and blood pressure in families (76).

In a study concerning the dietary management of hypertension, Tillotson and coworkers identified steps in patients' behavior that were critical for the success of permanent dietary management (77). These steps are as follows:

1. The person acknowledges that he has high blood pressure.

2. The person considers diet as a sole or adjunctive method of helping to control high blood pressure.

3. The person participates in assessing his current dietary pattern, social environment, thoughts, beliefs, and feelings.

4. The person acknowledges that successful dietary change will require an extended period of time.

5. The person participates in developing an overall strategy and in setting long-term goals for blood pressure and diet.

6. The person participates in the planning of each step in dietary change.

7. The person makes each dietary change.

8. The person participates in assessing whether he has succeeded in making each change.

9. The person participates in assessing his attainment of blood pressure control.

10. The person participates in devising a plan for maintaining dietary changes as goals are approached.

In a review of the major behavioral interventions for hypertension, results suggested that behavior modification can prevent and reduce hypertension. Reducing weight, restricting sodium and alcohol use, and increasing physical activity showed the most promise (78).

Studies of healthy populations, of those at increased risk, and of patients with cardiovascular disease have shown that risk-related behavior can be altered and in some cases, the incidence of cardiovascular disease reduced (79-81). For example, a recent pilot study showed that university students profited from an intervention consisting of nutrition education and behavior modification techniques to reduce elevated low-density lipoprotein (LDL) cholesterol levels. The intervention group showed greater reduction in LDL cholesterol levels than the control group (82).

Since it is generally recognized that cardiovascular disease may result from voluntary behaviors such as smoking, inappropriate eating behaviors, and the pursuit of stress-prone lifestyles, it is most encouraging that we can emphasize the voluntary nature of the behaviors and hence the possibility of modifying these self-defeating behaviors. A recent study reports that dietetics professionals lag behind the ideal in the use of behavior modification compliance-enhancing techniques. Engaging social support was reported to be used more often than other behavioral strategies, such as goal setting, contingency contracting, reminder calls, follow-up visits, and self-monitoring techniques (83). Recent recommendations for promoting adherence to low-fat, low-cholesterol diets include providing patients with an adequate knowledge base to make dietary changes, using goal setting and self-monitoring techniques of behavioral self-management to assist patients to initiate needed dietary changes, enlisting the support of the patient's social group (family, friends, etc.) and encouraging in the patient a sense of confidence in his or her capability to succeed by mobilizing the motivation, cognitive resources, and courses of action necessary to succeed (self-efficacy) (84). Because certain risk factors are behavioral in nature, it is particularly appropriate to attempt to lower these risks using psychological methods based on behavior modification (85–89).

Human Resource Management

The behavior of employees is of major concern to supervisors interested in productivity and good human relations. Blanchard and Johnson's book, *The One Minute Manager,* provides examples of behavioral modification strategies (4). Goals begin new behaviors and in the "one minute goal," the manager uses observable, measurable behavioral terms to describe the discrepancy between the actual and desired performance. Supervisors need to convert ambiguous affective goal statements into a format that is useful for producing improved performance. For example, it is useless to encourage employees "to do better," if "better" is not defined and stated in behavioral terms (90). Because behaviors are maintained by their consequences, the "one minute praise" and the "one minute reprimand," examples of rewards and punishments, are recommended. Although most supervisors attempt to catch subordinates doing things wrong, Blanchard and Johnson suggest that they notice employees doing something right or approximately right and then gradually move them toward the desired behavior. The one-minute praise is used immediately to reinforce proper behavior. Eventually some employees begin to praise themselves for the proper behavior, which provides additional reinforcement. Table 6.4 lists positive reinforcers for employees. The one-minute reprimand is also used immediately and concentrates on the improper behavior, not on the person.

An important aspect of job satisfaction and performance is the employee's sense of personal control, so it is imperative that supervisors do not use behavior modification in ways that are seen as manipulative and degrad-

TABLE 6.4.
Positive Reinforcers
Praise
Positive feedback
Recognition (employee of the week, month)
Added responsibility
Compliments
Special assignments
Social events
Knowledge of results
Thank you letter
Salary increase
Bonus
Promotion

ing to employees (91, 92). Intrinsic motivation should be encouraged to emphasize the importance of a self-reinforcing loop.

IMPLICATIONS FOR THERAPY

Brownell has pointed out two major advantages of behavior therapy. Attrition from treatment programs is low, and patients in behavior therapy programs seem to show improved psychological functioning. Brownell and co-workers assert that such improvement has important implications for compliance and motivation, ingredients ultimately important for any type of treatment regimen (3, 23, 43).

Although eating behavior patterns are not altered easily, behavior modification therapy offers promising techniques that may be helpful to both the client and the counselor. Analysis of the ABCs—the **A**ntecedents of eating, the eating **B**ehavior itself, and the **C**onsequences of eating—by the counselor and client leads to understanding of the problems, the setting of goals, and the development of strategies for change. Efforts should be made to arrange consequences that reinforce and maintain desirable changes, with an ultimate goal being independent client self-management. Behavior modification may be used in conjunction with other counseling and education strategies.

REVIEW AND DISCUSSION QUESTIONS

1. Explain the Law of Effect.

2. Explain the 4 types of responses according to the Law of Effect.

3. What are some examples of the ways in which a dietetics professional may use modeling?

4. What are the ABCs? Give examples of how the dietetics professional may use them in counseling patients.

CASE STUDY

Ann Stevens, age 34, is an administrative assistant. She noticed that her clothes were feeling tighter. She stepped on the scale and found that she had gained weight, in fact she weighed 30 pounds more than she did when she finished school. She made an appointment with Joan Stivers, RD, who has a private practice.

On the day of the appointment, they discussed her current eating practices. Ann admitted that she had no time to cook breakfast, but stops at a fast food restaurant and eats in the car. She may send out for lunch and eat at her desk or go to a restaurant with coworkers. By the time she gets home, she is "starving" and heads for the kitchen for a snack. When her husband arrives, they frequently have a drink or glass of wine together and discuss their days activities while dinner is cooking. After dinner, she does housework or watches TV. They may have a snack during the evening or before bed.

1. What are Ann's cues to eating?
2. How can each be eliminated or changed to assist her in losing weight?
3. How can rewards (other than food) be planned for her?

5. How can self-monitoring assist a counselee?
6. What is the significance of social support?

SUGGESTED ACTIVITIES

1. Complete a food diary for 3 days following the format in Table 6.3. Identify your cues for eating. Identify your reinforcers. Set one goal for change with identified reinforcers.

2. Record and identify your own ABCs (antecedents, behaviors, and consequences) related to an activity other than eating, such as studying, exercising, smoking, and the like. How can these behaviors be made to occur more or less often by rearranging the antecedents and/or consequences?

3. Ask a friend or family member to keep a food record. Work with him or her to identify one goal for change and reinforcers. Follow up in 1 week.

4. Arrange to watch an adult interact with a child or children for half an hour. Tally the number of times the adult attends to desirable behaviors, which reinforces them, versus the number of times desirable behaviors are ignored, which may lead to their extinction. Note whether the adult responds to undesirable behaviors, which reinforces them.

5. Make a list of leisure time activities that you enjoy, people you like to be with, and things you would purchase with extra money, to identify your own reinforcers, following the format in Table 6.2.

6. You have been assigned two chapters to read (or a paper to write) during the next few days. Select an appropriate reinforcer for yourself, and identify a time schedule for dispensing the reinforcer.

7. Select an excessive behavior of your own that you would like to diminish. Record those situations in which it occurs for 3 days. Identify the controlling stimulus conditions just prior to the behavior and the reinforcement.

8. Identify situations in which modeling occurs.

9. In a social situation with friends, tally the number of times in one-half hour that you dispense social approval (smiles, nods, appreciative words) versus disapproval (frowns, disparaging words).

10. List 10 phrases of social approval or positive reinforcement that you are comfortable using with others.

11. Discuss your personal experiences at work and compare them with those of others. Does your supervisor praise or punish? What are the consequences of the supervisor's actions on your behavior and that of other employees?

REFERENCES

1. Stunkard A, Berthold H. What is behavior therapy? Am J Clin Nutr 1985;41:821.
2. Williams DF, Thompson JK. Biology and behavior: a set-point hypothesis of psychological functioning. Integrating personality assessment data and behavior therapy: toward a psychological behaviorism. Behav Modif 1993;17:43.
3. Brownell KD, Cohen LR. Adherence to dietary regimens 2: components of effective interventions. Behav Med 1995;20:155.
4. Blanchard K, Johnson S. The one minute manager. New York: Berkley Books, 1981.
5. Hill WF. Principles of learning. Palo Alto, CA: Mayfield Pub, 1981.
6. Schwartz B, Lacey H. Behaviorism, science and human nature. New York: WW Norton, 1982.
7. Bandura A. Social learning theory. Englewood Cliffs, NJ: Prentice Hall, 1977.
8. Sims HP, Manz CC. Modeling influences on employee behavior. Personnel J 1982;61:58.
9. Sigman-Grant M. Stages of change: a framework for nutrition interventions. Nutr Today 1996;31:162.
10. Prochaska JO. Why do we behave the way we do? Can J Cardiol 1995;11(Suppl A):20A.
11. Prochaska JO, Norcross JC, Fowler JL, et al. Attendance

and outcome in a work site weight control program: processes and stages of change as process and predictor variables. Addict Behav 1992;17:35.

12. Coates TJ. Eating—a psychological dilemma. J Nutr Educ 1981;13:S34.

13. Rabb C, Tillotson, JL, eds. Heart to heart. Washington, DC: US Dept of Health and Human Services, 1983.

14. Fensterheim H, Baer J. Don't say yes when you want to say no. New York: Dell, 1975.

15. Building Nutrition Counseling Skills. Vol. 2. Washington, DC: US Dept of Health and Human Services, 1984.

16. Reese EP, Howard J, Reese TW. Human behavior: analysis and application. Dubuque, IA: William C Brown, 1978.

17. Holli BB. Using behavior modification in nutrition counseling. J Am Diet Assoc 1988;88:1530.

18. Skinner BF. Science and human behavior. New York: Macmillan, 1953.

19. Abrahamson E. Behavioral treatment of obesity. Behav Therapist 1983;6:103.

20. Marcoux BC, Trenkner LL, Rosenstock IM. Social networks and social support in weight loss. Pat Educ Counsel 1990;15:229.

21. Stunkard A, McLaren-Hume M. The results of treatment for obesity. Arch Intern Med 1959;103:79.

22. Garner DM Wooley SC. Confronting the failure of behavioral and dietary treatments for obesity. Clin Psychol Rev 1991;11:729.

23. Brownell K. The psychology and physiology of obesity. J Am Diet Assoc 1984;84:406.

24. Westover SA, Lanyon R. The maintenance of weight loss after behavioral treatment: a review. Behav Modif 1990; 14:123.

25. Gurin J. Leaner, not lighter. Psychol Today 1989;23:32.

26. American College of Sports Medicine: Position statement on proper and improper weight loss programs. Med Sci Sports Exer 1983;15:9.

27. McKenzie TL. A behaviorally oriented residential camping program for obese children and adolescents. Educ Treatment Child 1986;9:67.

28. Lavery MA, Loewy JW, Kapadia AS, et al. Long-term follow-up of weight status of subjects in a behavioral weight control program. J Am Diet Assoc 1989;89:1259.

29. Duffy G, Spence SH. The effectiveness of cognitive self-management as an adjunct to a behavioural intervention for childhood obesity: a research note. J Child Psychol Psychiatry 1993;34:1043.

30. Wilson GT. Behavioral treatment of childhood obesity: theoretical and practical implications. Health Psychol 1994;13:371.

31. Wadden TA, Foster GD, Letizia KA. One year behavioral treatment of obesity: comparison of moderate and severe caloric restriction and the effects of weight maintenance therapy. J Consult Clin Psychol 1994;62:165.

32. Wadden TA, Foster GD, Letizia KA. Response of obese binge eaters to treatment by behavior therapy combined with very low caloric diet. J Consult Clin Psychol 1992; 60:808.

33. Forest JP, Goodrick GK, Reeves RS, et al. Response of free-living adults to behavioral treatment of obesity: attrition and compliance to exercise. Behav Ther 1993; 24:659.

34. Wing RR. Obesity and related eating and exercise behaviors in women. Ann Behav Med 1993;15:124.

35. Granlund B, Johansson H, Sojka P. Problematic obesity thoughts: an attempt to identify unsuccessful dieters prior to treatment. Scand J Behav Ther 1991;20:75.

36. Goldwurm GF, Jerich D, Colombo F, et al. Cognitive behavioral treatment for obesity: methods, results and consideration after one year's work. Act Nerv Super 1988;30:114.

37. Wade JB, Hart RP, Kirby DF, et al. An evaluation of the Garren-Edwards diet and behavior modification program. Group 1988;12:172.

38. Bennett GA. Cognitive behavioral treatments for obesity. J Psychosom Res 1988;32:661.

39. Perri MG, Nezu AM, Patti ET, et al. Effect of length of treatment on weight loss. J Consult Clin Psychol 1989; 57:450.

40. Hjordis B, Gunnar E. Characteristics of drop-outs from a long-term behavioral treatment program for obesity. Int J Eat Disord 1989;8:363.

41. Kalodner CR, DeLucia JL. The individual and combined effects of cognitive therapy and nutrition education as additions to a behavior modification program for weight loss. Addict Behav 1991;16:255.

42. Spiegel TA, Wadden TA, Foster GD. Objective measurement of eating rate during behavioral treatment of obesity. Behav Ther 1991;22:61.

43. Lissner L, Steen SN, Brownell KD. Weight reduction diets and health promotion. Am J Prev Med 1992;8:154.

44. Yager J. The treatment of eating disorders. J Clin Psychiatry 1988;49:18.

45. Thompson RA, Sherman RT. Therapist errors in treating eating disorders: relationship and process. Psychotherapy 1989;26:62.

46. Cox GL, Merkel WT. A qualitative review of psychosocial treatments for bulimia. J Nerv Ment Dis 1989;177:77.

47. Bachrach A, Erwin W, Mohr J. The control of eating behavior in an anorexic by operant conditioning techniques. In: Ullman L, Krasner LP, eds. Case studies in behavior modification. New York: Holt, Rinehart, and Winston, 1965.

48. Cinciripini P, Kornblith S, Turner S, et al. A behavioral program for the management of anorexia and bulimia. J Nerv Ment Dis 1983;171:186.

49. Leitenberg H, Gross J, Peterson J, et al. Analysis of an anxiety model and the process of change during exposure plus response prevention treatment of bulimia nervosa. Behav Ther 1984;15:3.

50. Cullari S, Redmon W. Treatment of bulimorexia through behavior therapy and diet modification. Behav Therapist 1983;6:165.

51. Smith G, Medlik L. Modification of binge eating in anorexia nervosa. Behav Psychotherapy 1983;11:249.

52. Fairburn CG, Hay PJ. The treatment of bulimia nervosa. Special section: eating disorders. Ann Med 1992;24:297.

53. Steel ZP, Farag PA, Blaszczynski AP. Interrupting the binge-purge cycle in bulimia. The use of planned binges. Int J Eat Disord 1985;18:199.

54. Treasure J, Todd G, Brolly M, et al. A pilot study of randomized trial of cognitive analytical therapy vs. educational behavioral therapy for adult anorexia nervosa. Behav Res Ther 1995;33:363.

55. Barlow DH, Tillotson JL. Behavioral science and nutrition: a new perspective. J Am Diet Assoc 1978;72: 368.

56. Riordan MM, Iwata BA, Finney JW, et al. Behavioral assessment and treatment of chronic food refusal in handicapped children. J Appl Behav Anal 1984;17:327.

57. Touyz SW, Gertler R, Brigham S, et al. Anorexia nervosa in a patient with multiple sclerosis: a case report. Int J Eat Disord 1989;8:231.

58. Hsu LKG. The treatment of anorexia nervosa. Am J Psychiatry 1986;143:573.

59. Crisp AH, Hsu LKG, Harding B, et al. Clinical features of anorexia nervosa. J Psychosom Res 1980;24:179.

60. Schwartz DM, Thompson MG. Do anorectics get well? Current research and future needs. Am J Psychiatry 1981;138:319.

61. Yates A. Current perspectives on eating disorders. Treatment, outcome and research directions. J Am Acad Child Adolesc Psychiatry 1990;29:1.

62. Bell KE, Stein DM. Behavioral treatment for pica. A review of empirical studies. Int J Eat Disord 1992;11:377.

63. Wing R, Epstein L, Norwalk M. Dietary adherence in patients with diabetes. Behav Med Update 1984;6:17.

64. Smith DE, Wing RR. Diminished weight loss and behavioral compliance during repeated diets in obese patients with Type II diabetes. Health Psychol 1991;10: 378.

65. Thomas-Dobersen DA, Butler-Simon N, Fleshner M. Evaluation of a weight management intervention program in adolescents with insulin-dependent diabetes mellitus. J Am Diet Assoc 1993;93:535.

66. Bielamowicz MK, Miller WC, Elkins E, et al. Monitoring behavioral changes in diabetes care with the diabetes self-management record. Diabetes Educ 1995;21:426.

67. Gross A. Self-management training and medication compliance in children with diabetes. Child Fam Ther 1982;4:47.

68. Gross A. Discrimination of blood glucose levels in insulin-dependent diabetics. Behav Modif 1983;7:369.

69. Robinson FF. A training and support group for elderly diabetics: description and evaluation. J Specialists Group Work 1993;18:127.

70. Hartman-Stein P, Reuter JM. Developmental issues in the treatment of diabetic women. Psychol Women Q 1988; 12:417.

71. Morgan BS, Littell DH. A closer look at teaching and contingency contracting with type II diabetes. Pat Educ Counsel 1988;12:145.

72. Peveler RB, Fairburn CG. Anorexia nervosa in association with diabetes mellitus: a cognitive-behavioral approach to treatment. Behav Res Ther 1989;7:95.

73. Cox DJ, Gander-Frederick L. Major developments in behavioral diabetes research. Special issue: behavioral medicine: an update for the 1990s. J Consult Clin Psychol 1992;60:628.

74. Perri MG, Sears SF, Clark JE. Strategies for improving maintenance of weight loss. Diabetes Care 1993;16:200.

75. Remmell PS, Gorder DD, Hall Y, et al. Assessing dietary adherence in the Multiple Risk Factor Intervention Trial (MRFIT). J Am Diet Assoc 1980;76:351.

76. Johnson CC, Nicklas TA, Arbeit ML, et al. Behavioral counseling and contracting as methods for promoting cardiovascular health in families. J Am Diet Assoc 1992; 2:479.

77. Tillotson JL, Winston MC, Hall Y. Critical behaviors in the dietary management of hypertension. J Am Diet Assoc 1984;84:290.

78. Dubbert PM. Behavioral (life-style) modification in the prevention and treatment of hypertension. Clin Psychol Rev 1995;15:187.

79. Patterson TL, Sallis JF, Nader PR, et al. Direct observation of physical activity and dietary behaviors in a structured environment: effects of family-based health promotion program. J Behav Med 1988;1:447.

80. Dressler WW. Type A behavior and the social production of cardiovascular disease. J Nerv Ment Dis 1989;177:181.

81. Johnston DW. Prevention of cardiovascular disease by psychological methods. Br J Psychiatry 1989;154:183.

82. McGowan MP, Joffe A, Duggan AK, et al. Intervention in hypercholesterolemic college students: a pilot study. J Adolesc Health 1994;15:155.

83. Gilboy MB. Compliance-enhancing counseling strategies for cholesterol management. J Nutr Educ 1994;26:228.

84. McCann BS, Retzlaff BM, Dowdy AA, et al. Promoting adherence to low-fat, low-cholesterol diets: review and recommendations. J Am Diet Assoc 1990;90:1408.

85. Oldenburg B, Owen N, Parle M, et al. An economic evaluation of four work site based cardiovascular risk factor interventions. Health Educ Q 1995;22:9.

86. Gomel M, Oldenburg B, Simpson JM, et al. Work site–cardiovascular risk reduction: a randomized trial of health risk assessment, education, counseling, and incentives. Am J Public Health 1993;83:1231.

87. Hamm VP, Bazargan M, Barbre AR. Life-style and cardiovascular health among urban Black elderly. J Appl Geront 1993;12:155.

88. Carleton RA, Sennett L, Gans KM, et al. The Pawtucket hearth health program: influencing adolescent eating patterns. Ann NY Acad Sci 1991;623:322.

89. Kashani IA, Langer RD, Criqui MH, et al. Effects of parental behavior modification on children's cardiovascular risks. Ann NY Acad Sci 1991;623:447.

90. Stuart JA, Wallace SG. Analyzing "affective" goal statements. Performance and Instruction 1988;27:10.

91. Greenberger DB, Strasser S, Cummings LL, et al. The impact of personal control on performance and satisfaction. Organ Behav Human Decision Processes 1989;43:29.

92. Klein HJ. Control theory and understanding motivated behavior: a different conclusion. Motivation Emotion 1991;15:29.

seven

MODIFYING COGNITIONS

Based on learning principles, behavior modification examines the influence of external environmental factors on an individual's behaviors as discussed in the previous chapter. A person's eating responses are linked to stimuli or cues in the environment, and behaviors are shaped by their immediate consequences or reinforcement without requiring conscious thought. A second approach by psychologists, which can be classified as internal, is exploring the relationship between cognitive processes and eating behaviors. Cognitions may be defined as thoughts or perceptions at a particular moment in time. Thinking patterns can profoundly influence how people behave and the way they feel (1). Strategies for dealing with cognitions are frequently incorporated into behavioral programs.

Since behavior is molded and changed through the interaction of both a person's environmental influences and cognitive processes, there is a role that cognitions can and do play in explaining people's behaviors. In addition to examining external environmental cues and reinforcement, the dietetics professional needs to assess the client's internal cognitions when teaching clients to implement coping strategies for promoting better dietary adherence. Combining several approaches to treatment holds the promise of better results. Weight control programs, for example, may include treatment components of behavior modification, cognitive change, exercise, social support, and nutrition (2, 3).

This chapter explores three interrelated areas—cognitions and cognitive restructuring, self-efficacy, and relapse prevention. Assessing a client's cognitions can provide valuable information about the maintenance of adaptive and maladaptive behaviors, since negative thoughts inhibit behavioral change. The dietary counselor and client need to identify distorted thoughts, to discover their effect on behavior, and to modify them into more positive, coping cognitions.

Self-efficacy, another cognitive process, deals with people's judgments about their competence to perform specific behaviors. These perceptions, not necessarily

one's true capabilities, influence the initiation and maintenance of health and other behavior changes.

Relapse prevention is a self-management program with both cognitive and behavioral components. To prevent relapse from a dietary regimen, the counselor works with the client to anticipate and prevent dietary lapses that may occur during high-risk situations and to help the individual recover from minor slips before they become a full relapse or total breakdown in self-control.

Negative cognitions and low self-efficacy ratings are predictive of relapse. Individuals with positive cognitions and perceived self-efficacy tend to call upon their coping skills and regulate their behavior better. Albert Bandura does not believe that appropriate behavior, such as eating what one should, is achieved by a feat of willpower. When people do not behave optimally even though they know what they should do, thoughts or cognitions may be mediating the relationship between what one knows and what one does (4, 5).

COGNITIONS

Cognitive events are conscious thoughts that occur in one's stream of consciousness. Beck refers to them as "automatic thoughts," since they run through the mind automatically, and Meichenbaum calls them "internal dialogue" (6). An individual's thoughts, also referred to as "self-talk," can influence how one behaves, feels, and appraises the outcomes of a behavior. Although one's actions are not governed solely by thought, thought does enter into the determination of many actions.

While people do not engage in self-talk all of the time, on some occasions they do. Times at which individuals are more likely to engage in self-talk include when they are integrating new thoughts and actions, such as making lifestyle and dietary changes or performing a new job; exercising choices and judgments as in novel situations; and anticipating and/or experiencing intense emotional experiences (6). According to Bandura, cognitive processes play a major role in the acquisition and retention of new behavior patterns (5).

The client's internal dialogue is viewed as a learned response that, in turn, may be a cue for succeeding responses (8). This self-talk may be positive, negative, or

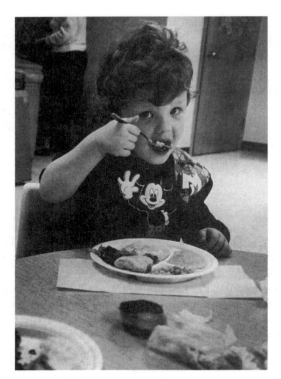

FIGURE 7.1. "This tastes good" is a positive cognition.

neutral. Positive cognitions support behaviors, as for example, "This diet isn't so bad." Negative cognitions, such as, "This diet looks difficult" inhibit behaviors. Cognitive variables are important in modifying dietary habits and in maintaining eating disorders, such as anorexia nervosa and bulimia (7). Dysfunctional thoughts and beliefs about "fattening" foods, fear of weight gain, and body image require examination and restructuring (8). In managing subordinates, an employee may be thinking: "I like my job," or "This job is boring".

Since cognitions are learned responses, the counselor may view the client's cognitions as behaviors to be modified or restructured. Counselors want to achieve desired changes in the client's behavior by altering thought patterns, beliefs, attitudes, and opinions. Many people cannot change their eating habits until they change their thoughts about food, eating, and drinking. Overeating and drinking can be an individual's way of coping with stress. The approach is to help the client by getting rid of unproductive, debilitating thoughts or beliefs and adopting more constructive ones.

Cognitive Distortions

Since negative thoughts inhibit behavioral change, it is necessary for individuals to first become aware of distortions in their thought patterns. Faulty thinking almost always contains gross distortions, often has little to do with actual reality, and may be self-defeating and destructive. Burns identified 10 common cognitive distortions (1).

1. **All-or-Nothing Thinking.** This refers to the tendency to evaluate personal qualities in black and white and is the basis of perfectionism. Performance is either perfect, or one is a failure. For example: "I ate this piece of pie, and I shouldn't have. I'm a failure."

2. **Overgeneralization.** One concludes that if one negative event happens, it will happen over and over again. For example: "I shouldn't have eaten that. It's no use. I will never be able to follow the diet."

3. **Mental Filter.** A negative detail in a situation is dwelt upon, and the whole situation is perceived as negative. For example: "If I can't eat whatever I want at the party, the party won't be any fun."

4. **Disqualifying the Positive.** Some individuals transform neutral and even positive experiences into negative ones. For example: "I am following the diet now, but this is a fluke. I probably won't be able to do it later."

5. **Jumping to Conclusions.** A negative interpretation is made even though there are no facts to support it. *(a)* Mind Reading. People assume that other people are looking down upon them. For example: "People don't want to be my friend because I am so fat." *(b)* Fortune Teller Error. One predicts that things will turn out badly and assumes that this is a fact. For example: "I don't think I can follow the diet." A positive prediction is: "I'll feel less lonely if I eat this bag of cookies." This is not entirely true, and later the person may feel guilty and have less self-respect. These negative feelings may lead to more binge eating. "I'll only eat one chocolate candy" is another prediction.

6. **Magnification and Minimization.** One either blows things up out of proportion, called "catastrophizing," or shrinks them into the small and unimportant. For example: "I goofed up. Everyone will hear about it. I'm ruined." Or, "I did it this time, but that is such a small gain that it doesn't amount to anything." The anorexic client, for example, overinterprets small increases in weight (9).

7. **Emotional Reasoning.** Negative emotions are taken as evidence of the truth. For example: "I feel inadequate. Therefore, I must be inadequate." Or "I'm so bored that I deserve a hot fudge sundae."

8. **Should Statements.** Individuals try to motivate themselves with "should," "must," and "shouldn't" statements. For example: "I should eat fruit," and "I shouldn't eat cake." When behavior falls short of one's personal standards, guilt results. To assert their independence when others tell people what they "should" or "shouldn't" do, some individuals feel rebellious and do just the opposite.

9. **Labeling and Mislabeling.** Instead of describing

TABLE 7.1.

Log of Cognitions

DATE	TIME	PLACE	FOOD EATEN	THOUGHTS ABOUT EATING BEFORE/DURING EATING	THOUGHTS ABOUT EATING AFTER EATING
1/10	2:15	Home	6 cookies, coke	"I feel hungry and tired. The cookies taste great."	"I'm not hungry any more. I feel better."

an error, individuals attach a label to themselves. Instead of thinking that a lapse occurred on the diet, for example, the person thinks, "I'm a pig."

10. **Personalization.** One sees oneself as the cause of some negative external event when one is not. For example: "What happened was my fault because I am inadequate."

Cognitive distortions are faulty thinking habits that have been learned. These negative thoughts create feelings that may lead to a negative self-image or sense of worthlessness. In addition, they can become a self-fulfilling prophecy. Because they have been learned, they can be changed or relearned with practice. However, since some people have had these thoughts for years, change may require extended effort and counseling.

To improve dietary adherence and outcomes, the dietetics practitioner should ask clients to keep records of their thoughts, should reinforce positive and coping thoughts, and should help clients recognize and restructure the negative ones. Cognitive assessment allows one to examine the role of thoughts and thinking processes in the development of adaptive and maladaptive behaviors. An example of a client log of cognitions is found in Table 7.1.

Cognitive Restructuring

Cognitive restructuring techniques refer to a variety of approaches involved with modifying the client's thinking and the assumptions and attitudes underlying their cognitions (6). The focus is on the false thoughts, inferences, and premises. Thus the counselor attempts to become familiar with the client's thought content, feelings, and behaviors and to understand their interrelationships. One needs to help the client identify specific misconceptions and distortions and to test their validity and reasonableness (6).

PHASES OF COGNITIVE BEHAVIOR MODIFICATION

Cognitive behavior modification consists of three phases, not necessarily in progression. The first step is concerned with helping the client understand the nature of the problem (6). A basic principle is that one cannot change a behavior without increasing one's awareness,

raising one's consciousness, or noticing a pattern in how one thinks, feels, behaves, and affects others by one's behavior. The client's recognition is a necessary first step, although not a sufficient condition to bring about change.

Rarely does the client recognize that thinking processes are a source of the dietary problems. The counselor should enlist clients in a collaborative, investigative effort to understand. The client needs to keep a written log of self-observations to heighten the awareness of the relationship between dysfunctional thoughts, feelings, and maladaptive behaviors.

Burns suggests having the client keep written, self-monitoring records with three columns, including first the false thought or self-criticism, then the type of cognitive distortion or thinking error it represents, and finally a self-defense response or the substitution of a more objective, coping thought (1). (See Table 7.2 for an example.)

In addition to written records, the counselor can discuss in an interview the range of eating situations, past and present, during which the client has false thoughts, such as thoughts about previous attempts to lose weight or follow a specific diet. The dietetics professional should ask clients to verbalize their thoughts and feelings concerning food, eating, and the dietary goal or change during the counseling session by asking: "How do you feel about . . .?" and "What do you think about . . .?" to determine what individuals are thinking to themselves, about the eating behavior to be changed, about their ability to change it, and at follow-up appointments, about their progress. In group counseling, cognitions can be discussed as, for example, the negative self-talk of the obese. Clients need to realize the false, self-defeating, and self-fulfilling aspects of their self-statements.

During the second phase, the counselor helps the client to explore and consolidate the conceptualization of the cognitive problem. As the client reports negative, self-defeating, and self-fulfilling prophecy aspects of thoughts, the counselor can ask how these affect overt behavior. The client needs to interrupt the automatic nature of negative self-talk and appraise the situation. The negative cognitions are viewed as hypotheses worthy of testing rather than as facts. The client should be encouraged to ask the following questions (1):

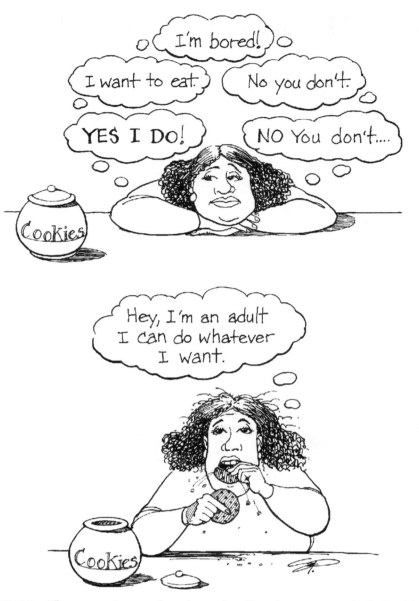

FIGURE 7.2. The counselor needs to have the client keep a record of cognitions.

What good does it do to focus on negative thoughts?

What is the worst that could happen versus the likeliest?

What is the factual evidence for thinking this thought?

What can I say about myself in self-defense?

Asking clients questions about their thoughts, rather than providing answers, promotes self-discovery (10).

In the third phase, actual change takes place. The counselor helps clients to modify their internal dialogue or self-statements and accompanying feelings and to produce new, more adaptive thoughts and behaviors. Clients are encouraged to control negative self-destructive statements, to offer positive self-statements as a coping strategy, and to reinforce themselves for having coped. An obese woman who is following a dietary change, for ex-

ample, can tell herself how well she is doing and to keep it up. The "power of positive thinking" enhances results greatly.

Besides these techniques, it may be necessary to teach the person other coping skills, such as problem-solving skills, mental rehearsal, and "thought stopping." Problem-solving approaches will help to teach a client to stand back and systematically analyze a problem situation. A problem-solving method called "STOP" requires the individual to: *(a) S*pecify the problem; *(b) T*hink of options; *(c) O*pt for the best solution; and *(d) P*ut the solution into practice (11). Cognitive rehearsal with visual imagery permits attention to the important details of a future, desired behavior. A client may rehearse, for example, his menu order at a restaurant or the amount of food

TABLE 7.2.

Assessing and Altering False Thoughts

DAILY RECORD OF		DATE:
FALSE THOUGHT OR BELIEF	TYPE OF DISTORTION	SELF-DEFENSE, COPING THOUGHT
"I shouldn't have eaten those cookies. I'm a failure."	All-or-none thinking	"Eating 3 cookies does not make me a failure. I can improve."
"I ate the pie. I'm a pig."	Mislabeling	"Pigs are animals and I am human. I don't have to be perfect."
"I don't have time to eat right."	Fortune teller error	"I have just as much time as anyone else."

and beverages to consume at a party. If individuals think about or imagine themselves overcoming barriers and performing adequately, actual performance is likely to improve.

Another behavior therapy procedure is "thought-stopping." Clients are trained to self-instruct themselves by saying "stop" whenever they are having false thoughts or negative self-talk. In addition, some of the same behavioral techniques used to modify overt behaviors discussed in the previous chapter, such as modeling and operant conditioning, can be used for covert thoughts. More suggestions are offered in a cognitive behavioral therapy package for obesity including six lesson plans (12).

Besides the role of cognitions in acquiring and regulating behaviors, motivation is partly rooted in cognition. The ability to represent future consequences or outcomes in positive thoughts provides a source of motivation (5). For example, positive thoughts that one will feel better, look better, or be in better health may contribute to motivation.

SELF-EFFICACY

In addition to correcting faulty ways of thinking, the actual mastery of new ways of behaving, including eating and exercise habits, may disconfirm faulty thought patterns and lead to heightened self-perceptions of efficacy. Bandura recognized that learning and behavior change are influenced not only by external environmental influences, including rewards and punishments, but also by

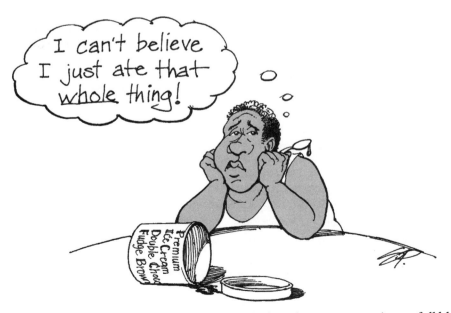

FIGURE 7.3.   Unless one's thoughts are redirected positively, a lapse can turn into a full-blown relapse.

the interaction of environmental demands and one's coping capabilities. In his view, successful therapies work by increasing an individual's confidence in his or her ability to engage in or practice a behavior, or self-efficacy (5). This, in turn, allows individuals to exercise greater control over their own behavior, motivation, and environment. Although it has received limited attention in the literature of health education research and practice, self-efficacy appears to play a critical role in the initiation and maintenance of health behavior change (13). There is overwhelming evidence that there is a close association between perceived self-efficacy and health behavior change and that self-efficacy is a powerful predictor of change (14).

Self-efficacy is a cognitive process dealing with people's judgments or beliefs about their capabilities to perform a behavior or set of behaviors adequately in specific situations and the influence of their self-percepts of efficacy on motivation and actual performance (5). An individual's competent functioning requires both a set of skills to organize and execute actions and self-beliefs of efficacy to use them effectively (5). Self-percepts of efficacy can affect people's choices of activities, how much effort they expend, and how long they will persist in the face of difficulties. The line, "I think I can" from the children's story *The Little Engine that Could,* for example, provides a vision of succeeding in performing a difficult task through sustained effort.

Bandura distinguishes between outcome expectancies and efficacy expectancies (4, 13). An outcome expectancy is a person's estimate or belief that a given behavior will or will not lead to a certain outcome. For example, reducing dietary sodium will lead to an outcome of lower blood pressure and better health; following a dietary regimen will lead to an outcome of weight loss; reducing dietary fat will lead to a lower cholesterol level in the blood; or successfully completing a project for one's superior will lead to a salary increase or promotion.

A self-efficacy expectation is the belief that one is or is not capable of performing the behavior required to lead to the desired outcome. A male client may or may not believe, for example, that he can reduce his dietary sodium intake sufficiently to attain the outcome. With staff, an employee may believe that performing work optimally will lead to the desired "outcome" of a promotion, but may or may not believe that he is capable ("self-efficacy") of optimum performance on a continuous basis. The two are differentiated because people may believe that certain actions can produce the outcomes, but they may have serious doubts about whether they can cope with the necessary changes to reach the outcome. One study defined self-efficacy toward nutrition behaviors as the ability to follow the dietary regimen, to follow general nutrition principles and practices, to select healthy foods, and to change food purchasing and preparation practices (15).

Choice Behaviors

Self-percepts of efficacy are generally good predictors of how people are likely to behave on specific tasks (5). Survey studies of self-efficacy by Strecher suggest a strong association between self-efficacy and progress in health behavior change and maintenance (13). Where the health practice is believed to lead to desired outcomes, but the change is difficult to make, self-efficacy considerations are probably paramount.

In addition, goal setting appears to enhance self-efficacy and satisfaction with one's performance. It can improve motivation to perform a task in part through cognitive self-evaluation of performance as compared with the adopted goal or standard. Enhanced self-efficacy increases effort and persistence in subgoals, which results in higher performance. Counselor feedback that a person is doing better compared with others enhances self-efficacy and actual performance (16).

People commonly have a higher sense of self-efficacy about one type of activity than another. For example, a woman may feel confident in performing in a theatrical production, but doubt that she can sustain the effort to maintain the dietary changes necessary to lose weight and/or increase exercise. A male employee may feel confident of his ability in one job, such as using a computer, but not another, such as giving a 30-minute oral presentation. People's judgments about their self-efficacy affect their behavior in a wide variety of situations, ranging from solving problems to making dietary and lifestyle changes.

Efficacy expectations are a major determinant of people's choice of activities (5). The client involved in a change of behavior, such as eating or exercise, must make decisions about whether or not to attempt a different dietary regimen, how long to continue, how much effort to make, and in the face of difficulties or aversive experiences, whether or not to persist. Bandura believes that these decisions are partly governed by judgments of self-efficacy. People tend to avoid situations that they believe exceed their coping capabilities, but are willing to undertake activities they judge themselves capable of executing (5). The stronger the perceived self-efficacy, or sense of personal mastery, the more persistent are the efforts, even in the presence of obstacles. When difficulties arise, those with lower perceptions of self-efficacy make less effort or may give up entirely.

Dimensions of Efficacy Expectations

The dietetics practitioner needs to assess the clients' thoughts about their abilities to make changes in eating and exercise behaviors or employees' thoughts about work behaviors. Different dimensions of thoughts may be examined, such as level and strength. When tasks have different levels of difficulty, efficacy expectations may limit some individuals to the simple tasks, while others may feel comfortable with the moderately difficult or difficult ones. Self-efficacy differs also in strength. Weak self-beliefs are easily extinguished by disconfirming experiences, whereas those with strong efficacy expectations will persevere in their coping efforts even through difficulties.

A two-step approach to measuring self-efficacy is suggested. First, given a group of tasks of varying levels of difficulty, ask clients which dietary goals or behaviors they can undertake. It is preferable to start off with the simpler ones in order to guarantee success. Then one can work up slowly to more difficult ones. Second, for each designated task in the behavior change, ask the individuals to rate the strength of their expectancy of success. Self-appraisals are reasonably accurate, and the individual's verbalized intentions provide a basis for predicting behavior. Using a four-point scale from 1, or very confident, to 4, or not at all confident, one study measured self-efficacy, or confidence in one's ability to change, regarding the ability to increase fruits and vegetables and to decrease dietary fat (17). People successfully execute tasks within their perceived capabilities, but shun those that exceed their perceived coping abilities. In relation to adherence to a diabetes self-care regimen by patients who did not view self-care as a high priority, self-efficacy appeared to be an important variable in relation to adherence, although it was unstable over different time frames (18).

According to Bandura: "Unless people believe they can master and adhere to health-promoting habits, they are unlikely to devote the effort necessary to succeed" (4). One study found that those with high initial self-efficacy had better outcomes in an intervention to lower serum cholesterol levels (19). Another reported that self-efficacy was a powerful correlate for vigorous activity in the overweight (20). Other studies have also found self-efficacy to be a key cognitive variable in behavior change (21, 22). Efficacy expectations and performance should be assessed periodically during the dietary change process, as the stronger the perceived efficacy, the more likely people are to persist in their efforts until they succeed.

Sources of Efficacy Information

One's expectations of personal efficacy are based on four major sources of information: (*a*) actual performance accomplishments, (*b*) vicarious experiences (modeling) by observing the performance of others, (*c*) verbal persuasion, and (*d*) physiological and emotional states (5). While verbal persuasion is used commonly be counselors, it is among the least effective approaches in influencing another's capability for coping with change.

ACTUAL PERFORMANCE

The most influential source of efficacy information is based on performance accomplishments or personal mastery experiences. "Nothing succeeds like success" reinforces this idea. Personal successes raise mastery expectations while failures lower them, especially early in the course of a change. Repeated successes in overcoming obstacles through perseverance strengthen expectations. People also perfect their coping skills and lessen their vulnerability to stress. Success begets success; failure begets failure.

VICARIOUS EXPERIENCES

A second source of efficacy information comes from modeling followed by guided performance. Clients can learn how to handle situations by observing a model demonstrating the appropriate behavior, such as ordering the proper food from a restaurant menu. The vicarious experience of seeing another perform, which relies on inferences from social comparison, can generate expectations that if another can do it, "so can I." To enhance self-efficacy, the model should be perceived as similar to oneself or possessing competencies to which one aspires. Clients should then be given an opportunity to perform the modeled behavior successfully. Employees also learn by observing and modeling after other employees. Stronger efficacy expectations, however, are produced by personal performance accomplishments than by only observing a model.

VERBAL PERSUASION

A third approach, verbal persuasion, is widely used by counselors in attempts to influence behavior. Telling people both what to do and that they possess the ability to do it, and informing them of the benefits is not as effective, however, especially if the individual has had a previous disconfirming experience, such as a failure to follow dietary changes or perform a task at work. The impact of verbal persuasion, or counselor "cheerleading," may vary greatly depending on the perceived credibility of the persuaders, their prestige, trustworthiness, and other factors. An added approach to verbal persuasion is to structure goals and situations in ways that will bring the person success.

PHYSIOLOGICAL AND EMOTIONAL STATES

Finally, people partly judge their capabilities from physiological states or emotional arousal. Situations in which the individual has to cope with changes may produce anxiety, stress, hunger, fatigue, and tension, which elicits emotional arousal. Whether or not one can perform in the face of negative signals provides personal information concerning one's competency. Individuals susceptible to anxiety may become preoccupied with their perceived inadequacies in the face of difficulties rather than with the task at hand. Stress-reducing exercises and discussion of correct interpretation of body signals may be of help when these problems arise.

The dietetics practitioner may use one or more of the four sources of efficacy information to raise or strengthen self-perceptions of clients and employees. Personal mastery of a dietary change or accomplishment of a goal is compelling. Small "wins" build confidence for additional changes (23). Models, such as former clients, may be enlisted to explain how they overcame difficulties by determined effort. Persuasive information is given by informing people that they are capable. The meaning of physiological information, such as anxiety, hunger, and stress, should be explained to make sure that the individual does not misread body signals and abandon efforts.

With employees, personal accomplishments give better efficacy information than telling people that they are capable of performing a job. Modeling after the performance of others, such as seeing that hard work leads to a promotion, is another source of efficacy information. Behaviors are adopted from seeing what others are doing.

Cognitive Appraisal of Efficacy Information

Many factors affect successful performance. The extent to which success raises self-efficacy depends in part on the amount of effort expended. Laborious effort connotes less self-efficacy than success achieved through minimal effort. A performance suggests higher self-efficacy if attained through continuous progress rather than through discouraging reversals and plateaus.

In addition, a number of factors enter into personal appraisals. Some individuals underestimate their self-efficacy. If people are not fully convinced of their personal efficacy, they abandon the skills they have been taught when they fail to get quick results or when they experience obstacles to success. People with high self-efficacy attribute failure to lack of effort while those with low self-efficacy may attribute it to low ability. Those with negative self-beliefs do not discard them readily. Even when actual performance attainments are beyond their previous expectations, they may discount their importance through faulty cognitive appraisal or credit their achievements to extreme factors rather than to their own capabilities.

The counselor may guide individuals to increased self-efficacy by guiding them through small, manageable steps or goals that gradually lead them to do more than they ever thought they could. Attainment of proximal subgoals indicates personal mastery, which can enhance self-efficacy and motivation, while distant future goals are not as good, as they are too far removed to have an effect (5). For example, attaining the subgoal of following the dietary regimen today is an immediate commitment rather than a future goal of never eating desserts again. With employees, a goal of improving performance today is better than a more distant goal of improving during the month.

In a study of dropouts from obesity treatment, it was found that self-efficacy at the beginning of treatment was an important predictor of the decision to drop out (24). Dropouts had lower expectations of success and were more likely to have doubts about whether they would ever reach their goal weights, while stayers felt confident that they would.

In the obesity study, perceptions of success proved more important than actual success in predicting who would drop out. Although it might seem that actual success in weight loss would have an important relationship to dropout, little relationship was found. Success results in greater increases in self-efficacy only when the subjects' successful experience is appropriately evaluated. People are influenced more by how they read their performance successes than by the successes per se, and this determines the course of cognitive and behavioral change. Thus efficacy expectations reflect a person's perceived rather than actual capabilities, and it is these perceptions and not one's true abilities that often influence behavior (13). Effective weight control as well as other regimens may need to include program elements aimed at higher participant perceptions of success.

If one ascribes success to one's ability or one's effort, self-efficacy is reinforced. Cognitive appraisal of the difficulty of the task accomplished further affects self-efficacy. Even in the face of a setback, if relative progress is perceived, efficacy may be raised.

Thus, in their daily lives, people will approach, explore, and try to deal with situations within their self-perceived capabilities, but will avoid situations they perceive as exceeding their ability. The theory posits a central processor of efficacy information. People weigh and integrate various sources of information about their capabilities. They regulate their choices of behaviors and the effort they put forth accordingly (5). Efficacy expectations are presumed to influence the level of performance by enhancing intensity and persistence of effort. Thus the dietetics professional needs to inquire of clients and employees regarding their judgment of their capabilities to perform a variety of tasks and the strength of the belief.

RELAPSE PREVENTION

The problem of relapse is a challenge for clients engaging in dietary changes and for the practitioners who counsel them. Relapse rates on dietary regimens are high, varying from 50 to 100%, and people cycle through various stages of change as noted in Chapter 1. The likelihood of relapse may be increased by social or psychological provocations, emotional reactions to initial slips, and problems in reestablishing control.

Marlatt and Gordon define relapse prevention as a self-management program designed to enhance the "habit-change process" (25). The change process is one in which old habits are unlearned and new adaptive behaviors are gradually learned and acquired to replace previous eating responses. Errors may occur, but each mistake is viewed as an opportunity for new learning, not a personal failure. The goal is to teach the individual involved in a behavior change program how to identify situations with a high risk for lapse and relapse, to use problem solving and coping strategies when confronted with these situations, and to deal with the negative thoughts that accompany a lapse.

Marlatt does not view relapse as an all-or-none phe-

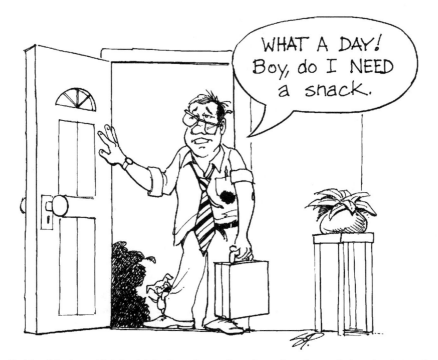

FIGURE 7.4. The individual is in a "high-risk" situation related to the time of day (arriving home from work) and the cognition.

nomenon in which there is either absolute control and total restraint or in the other extreme, loss of control and total indulgence. He makes a useful distinction between a "lapse" and a "relapse" (25). A "lapse," such as eating the wrong food or skipping exercise, is a single act, a slight error, a temporary fall, a reemergence of a previous habit or behavior, or a slip, not a total failure. Control is not lost and corrective action can be taken. A lapse may provide a learning experience if one examines the immediate precipitating circumstances and how to correct them in the future. After a lapse, one may continue with positive change or proceed to total relapse. A "relapse" may be defined as the individual's response to a series of lapses or a loss of control. A lapse does not necessarily become a relapse.

Relapse prevention is based on the principles of social learning theory and includes both behavioral and cognitive components (25). In the social learning view, behaviors may be viewed as overlearned, maladaptive habits that can be analyzed and modified. The eating behavior of individuals with anorexia nervosa, bulimia, and obesity, for example, may be viewed as overlearned, maladaptive habit patterns with maladaptive coping mechanisms (7). These maladaptive behaviors are generally followed by some sort of immediate gratification, such as feelings of pleasure or the reduction of anxiety, tension, boredom, or loneliness. When eating takes place before or during stressful or unpleasant situations, it represents a maladaptive coping mechanism.

Habits or behaviors are assumed to be shaped by prior

learning experiences. Changing these habits involves the active participation and responsibility of the client, who eventually becomes the agent of change. In a self-management program, the individual acquires new skills and cognitive strategies so that behaviors are under the regulation of higher mental processes and responsible decision making. As applied to a program to prevent relapse, the goals are *(a)* "to anticipate and prevent the occurrence of a relapse after the initiation of a habit change" and *(b)* "to help the individual recover from a 'slip' or lapse before it escalates into a full-blown relapse" (25).

Dietary counselors need to advise clients of the possibility of lapses and relapse and how to handle them. Failure to do so deprives the client of the opportunity for developing skills to cope with these situations and/or minimizing damage if one occurs. Using the term "lapse" avoids the value judgment associated with a term like "cheating" on the diet (26).

A Relapse Model
Marlatt and Gordon have defined a cognitive-behavioral model of relapse based on the coping response process in high-risk situations. They believe that an individual's control continues until the person encounters a high-risk situation, defined as "any situation that poses a threat to the individual's sense of control and increases the risk of potential relapse" (25). Examples of high-risk situations for a person on a dietary regimen are attendance at a social gathering, interpersonal conflicts, feelings of anxiety, boredom, fatigue, or hunger, and the like. When

high-risk situations, temptations, and urges occur, relapse prevention techniques are designed to enhance self-efficacy in coping (27).

There are two possibilities when a person is in a high-risk situation—a coping response or lack of a coping response (see Fig. 7.5). If the individual copes, self-efficacy is increased and there is less probability of a lapse or relapse. On the other hand, if there is no coping response and the person feels unable to exert control, the person experiences a decrease in self-efficacy, sometimes coupled with a sense of helplessness and passive giving in to the situation. ("It's no use. I can't stop myself.") If the person has positive outcome expectancies from eating ("It will taste delicious. I will feel better if I eat this.") and ignores the delayed negative health consequences, the probability of lapse or relapse is enhanced. The individual experiences a conflict of motives between a desire to maintain control and the temptation to give in (28, 29). The person consumes less desirable foods and a slip or lapse has occurred (Fig. 7.5).

Abstinence from less preferable foods is frequently viewed by individuals from an all-or-nothing perspective.

Marlatt postulates a cognitive "abstinence violation effect" when a person moves from control or restraint and consumes a food that he should not eat (25). This brings elements of guilt and of blaming oneself for the loss of control or indulgence. ("I shouldn't have, but I did. I'm guilty.") The obese individual may continue to eat to relieve the guilt ("I ate one cookie and I blew it. I might as well eat the whole bag") or alter his cognition from being a restrainer to an indulger. ("I never could follow the diet anyway.") The reward of instant gratification may far outweigh negative health effects in a distant future. People may even justify the action by rationalizing, "I deserve a break today. I owe myself this food," or change their commitment to save face, as "I changed my mind about following this dietary regimen and decided to eat whatever I want" (28). Thus, a single lapse, or series of lapses, may snowball into a full-blown relapse from which it is more difficult to recover. Figure 7.6 is an example of failing to cope at the grocery store and at home in the presence of the external cue of potato chips. The loss of control and dysfunctional self-talk result in binge eating and relapse.

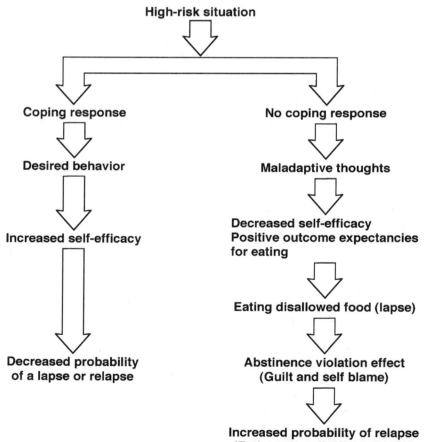

FIGURE 7.5. Cognitive-behavioral model of the relapse process. (Modified from Marlatt GA, Gordon JR, eds. Relapse prevention. New York: Guilford Press, 1985.)

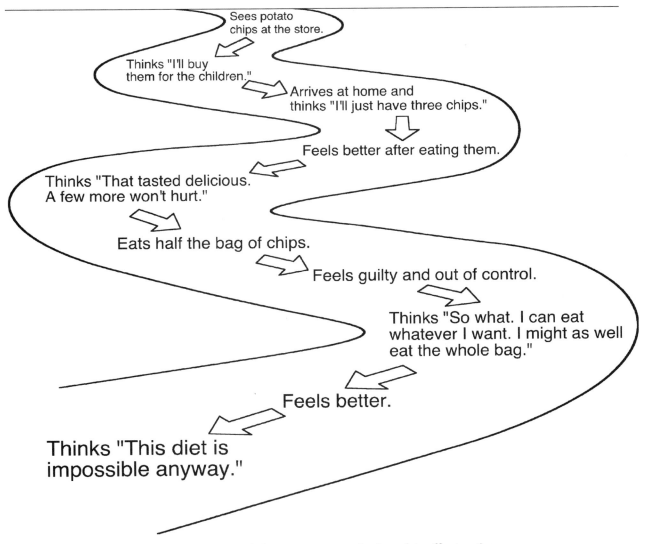

FIGURE 7.6.   In failing to cope, one's thoughts affect eating.

Determinants and Predictors of Lapse and Relapse
High-risk situations may be classified as individual, situational (environmental), and physiological (30, 31). Individual factors are within the individual or are reactions to environmental events. They include negative or unpleasant as well as positive emotional states, moods or feelings, inadequate motivation, responses to treatment, and coping skills. Table 7.3 summarizes examples.

Negative emotional states, such as depression, anxiety, stress, frustration, anger, boredom, feelings of deprivation, and the like, before or at the time of the lapse are related to relapse. Uncontrolled eating is a common response when a person is alone. The emotions increase the chance that a slip will occur and become a relapse. Positive emotional states in which one desires to increase pleasure and/or celebration are also a problem. A study of dieters found that negative emotional states occurring when the individual was alone and positive emotional states involving other people, such as social gatherings,

were both difficult high-risk situations to handle, suggesting that emphasis on managing these situations should be incorporated into counseling programs (31).

Clients initiate dietary changes with varying degrees of motivation. In addition, some who appear to be highly motivated initially may discover that long-term change is more difficult than first imagined. Initial response to treatment may predict later success. Patients on weight reduction diets who lose some weight, for example, and those who struggle but adhere to their dietary regimens, may be able to cope with temporary setbacks. Coping skills include cognitive responses, such as positive self-talk ("I can do it."), behavioral responses, such as calling a friend instead of eating less preferable foods, and beliefs about self-efficacy, or judgments concerning whether or not one can respond effectively in a situation.

Besides individual factors, situational or environmental factors also play a role in relapse. These include social support and environmental stimuli. The support of fam-

---

TABLE 7.3.

Examples of High-Risk Situations

Physiological feelings of hunger, fatigue, food cravings

Attending social affairs, parties

Holidays

Eating in restaurants

Inadequate motivation

Low self-efficacy

Stress

Negative self-talk

Lack of social support

Interpersonal conflicts

Positive emotional states, i.e., joy and celebration of an event

Negative emotional states, i.e., depression, anxiety, frustration, anger, boredom, loneliness, feeling deprived

---

ily, friends, or self-help groups is associated with better success in several studies, while the opposite situation, interpersonal conflicts with family, friends, or the employer are a sign for relapse (20, 21, 32). In addition, events in the environment may provoke a relapse. Eating cues in the environment, for example, may include holidays, restaurants, and parties where overeating is socially acceptable or where social pressure from others occurs. Social pressures from verbal interactions with others ("Eat it. Just this once won't hurt you.") and seeing others as role models when they are consuming foods not on the person's dietary regimen ("Everyone else is eating it. Why shouldn't I?") are problems.

Finally, negative physiological factors may contribute to relapse. Genetic factors, urges and cravings for foods, feelings of hunger, fatigue, or headache, changes in metabolic rate during weight loss, and metabolic tendencies toward weight regain when lapsing from a diet may increase the likelihood of relapse.

Identification and Assessment of High-Risk Situations

Assessment of high-risk situations may be viewed as a two-stage process (33). In the first stage an attempt is made to identify specific situations that may pose a problem for a client in terms of lapse or relapse. The use of self-monitoring records is helpful in identifying high-risk situations as well as in raising the individual's level of awareness of choice points. Eating may be an automatic response that cannot be dealt with until there is a conscious awareness that one is eating without any conscious decision to do so. Self-efficacy ratings in which the client is given a series of descriptions of specific situations and asked to rate how difficult it would be to cope, autobiographical statements about the history and development of the dietary problem, and descriptions of past relapses are other techniques that may be used (33).

Problem situations creating obstacles to dietary adherence in adults with diabetes were studied. Twelve types of situations were identified: negative emotions and stress, which tempted people to overeat; food, food cues, or cravings, which made it difficult to resist temptation; eating in restaurants; feeling deprived; time pressures; tempted to give up; lack of time for advance planning of what and when to eat; competing priorities; social events; lack of family support; inability to refuse inappropriate food offered; and lack of support of friends. An individual's ability to cope in these high-risk situations should be assessed so that problem-solving strategies can be a part of counseling (34).

In adolescents with diabetes mellitus, ten obstacles were found including being tempted to stop trying; negative emotional eating; facing forbidden foods; peer interpersonal conflict; competing priorities; eating at school; social events and holidays; food cravings; snacking when home alone or bored; and social pressures to eat. The counselor can assist clients in dealing with these situations (35).

The second stage is an assessment of the client's coping skills or capacity to respond in a high-risk situation. One can evaluate these in simulated situations with role playing or in written form. The individual can role play responses to high-risk situations with the counselor or fellow group members. Videotapes of these sessions may be helpful it they are available.

Treatment Strategies

The counselor needs to prepare the client for the possibility of a lapse and of relapse. Lapses are inevitable. Everyone will, on occasion, overeat or make less desirable food choices. Marlatt and Gordon use the metaphor of a fire drill. A person practices to escape a fire even though fires are rare (25). Brownell prefers the metaphor of a forest ranger whose responsibilities include not only preventing fires but also containing fires that start (30).

Relapse prevention strategies are important both in initial treatment or action phases and in maintenance phases of change. The cornerstone of the relapse prevention approach is to teach the client coping strategies with skill-training procedures (33). Skill training implies the actual acquisition of a new behavior through overt prac-

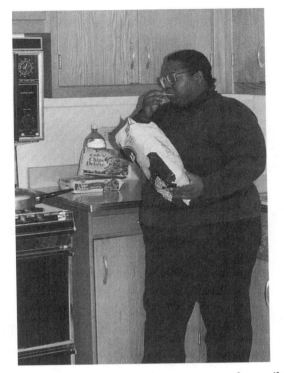

FIGURE 7.7. When one is hungry or upset, the availability of high-calorie foods presents a high-risk situation.

tice and rehearsal. One does not acquire a new skill, such as playing tennis, by verbal instruction alone. Actual practice of coping skills is essential (33). Both cognitive and behavioral coping strategies may be needed. "Practice makes perfect," as an old saying goes. Baseball players do not hit a home run every time they are at bat. In fact they may not even get a hit. If they strike out once, they just try again the next time.

Modeling, behavioral rehearsal, direct instruction, and coaching and feedback from the counselor are useful. Role reversal with the client teaching the dietary counselor how to cope with a high-risk situation and how to handle a lapse will give the client more convincing arguments than any counselor could provide. Increasing self-efficacy and modeling of positive self-statements are recommended, such as "I can do it" (33).

Relapse rehearsal through imagined scenarios in which the client engages in coping responses when temptations are present, which is called covert modeling, may be used to cope with reactions to a slip or lapse (33). Marlatt uses a strategy called "urge surfing." When confronted with an urge to binge, the clients are asked to imagine their urge is an ocean wave building to a crest. The challenge is to "surf" the wave and remain in balance without being "wiped out" (36). One continues until the urge has passed.

Relaxation training, meditation, exercise, visualization of relaxing, pleasant scenes and of carrying out coping behaviors when tempted, and stress management proce-

dures may be needed as an antidote to stress. In visualization, clients can be asked to think ahead of a situation in which they might at some point find themselves. With their eyes closed, the counselor can help them create a mental image of the situation by asking questions that create a visual picture of the situation and the accompanying emotions. If imagining a party, for example, the counselor may ask: "What do the surroundings look like?" "What are you doing?" "What are other people doing?" "Where are the foods and beverages?" "What will you choose?" "Who can you turn to for support?" "What will you say?" "How do you feel?"

Adopting a problem-solving orientation to stressful situations or modeling problem solving by thinking out loud with clients are helpful. When lapses are discussed, it is preferable to discuss how the individual might have succeeded in preference to focusing on the failures.

Cognitive restructuring teaches people to interpret events, attitudes, and feelings rationally, and to respond in high-risk situations. Cognitive restructuring may be used also to counter the cognitive and affective components of the "abstinence violation effect" (35). Instead of seeing the first lapse as a sign of failure characterized by conflict, guilt, and personal attribution, the client is taught to see it as a single event or small mistake rather than a total disaster, and that it is possible to resume the dietary regimen right away and learn from mistakes.

When the individual's high-risk situations are identified, one can teach the person to look for cues, such as an upcoming party, vacation, or stressful time at work. The client can take preventive action and make advance decisions about how to cope.

Chronic problems may require long-term treatment even in the maintenance stage of change (7, 30, 37). Just as Rome was not built in a day, neither is successful dietary change established in a short period of time. It may not be sufficient to teach new ways of eating and turn people loose and unaccountable on a maintenance program. They need to learn strategies to cope with the normal urge to lapse into old habits. They should be more successful when they keep in contact with a counselor, at least by phone, for a year or more. The model of lifelong treatment is used by several groups, such as Alcoholics Anonymous, Overeaters Anonymous, and the lifetime membership offered in Weight Watchers (30).

Counselors should give clients a summary or overview of the relapse prevention model. Together they should identify the individual's high-risk situations and coping skills. If clients have a level of awareness in high-risk situations, they are better prepared to use their coping skills and take remedial action. People need to see themselves as capable agents of control rather than as helpless victims in situations beyond their control.

REVIEW AND DISCUSSION QUESTIONS

1. What effect do negative cognitions have on behavioral change?

CASE STUDY

Carol Jones is a 50-year-old woman recently diagnosed with Type II diabetes mellitus. Her maternal grandmother had diabetes. Mrs. Jones was an overweight child and is an overweight adult at 5'4" and 180 pounds. She is married and works part-time at a retail clothing store.

Dr. Smith referred her for counseling to lose weight. The dietitian, Joan Stivers, notes in her conversation that Mrs. Jones seems to have a low self-image with negative cognitions. As a result, the counselor's current priority is cognitive restructuring.

Directions: Complete the dietetics professional's response to each of the client's statements.

Professional: "The doctor referred you because losing weight will help to improve your blood sugar levels."

1. Mrs. Jones: "I don't think I can lose weight."

    Professional:

2. Mrs. Jones: "My husband likes me the way I am. He does not think I am overweight."

    Professional:

3. Mrs. Jones: "I lost 10 pounds once before. But it was just a fluke. I couldn't do it again."

    Professional:

4. Mrs. Jones: "When I go out to eat at a restaurant, I won't get my money's worth if I don't eat the food they serve."

    Professional:

5. Mrs. Jones: "When the holidays come, my friends bring me candy and other goodies. So my husband and I eat them. We can't waste food."

    Professional:

2. What types of cognitive distortions do people have?
3. Explain the 3 phases of cognitive restructuring.
4. What are examples of coping skills the counselor may teach to the client?
5. What is the relationship between an outcome expectancy and an efficacy expectancy?
6. How do self-percepts of efficacy affect people's choice of activities?
7. Explain an individual's sources of efficacy information.
8. What is the difference between a lapse and a relapse?
9. Explain the relapse model.
10. What are examples of high-risk situations?
11. What strategies can help to prevent relapse?

SUGGESTED ACTIVITIES

1. Keep a log of what you eat during one day, noting your thoughts about food before eating, during eating, and after eating.
2. Identify your own high-risk situations for eating and how you respond.
3. For each of the following client cognitions, forecast how the client will behave. Then develop a more positive, coping thought.
    A. "I've never been able to stick to any low-calorie diet for more than a week."
    B. "The food doesn't taste any good without salt."
    C. "There are chocolate chip cookies in the cupboard, and I sure could use a few after the day I've had. I deserve a treat."
    D. "This television show is boring. Here is a commercial break—a good time to see what's interesting in the kitchen."
    E. "That leftover pie looks good, but I don't need it."
    F. "I've blown my whole diet eating that apple pie with ice cream. What's the use?"
    G. "I don't have time to prepare all of that special food today."
4. For 2 days, keep a tally of the number of times people use the terms "should," "shouldn't," "must," "have to," or "ought to" in statements about themselves. Or keep a tally of the number of times you use these terms.
5. For 2 or more days, consume a modified diet (low-fat, low-calorie, restricted sodium, high-fiber, etc.). Keep a log of your thoughts. Identify any high-risk situations.

REFERENCES

1. Burns DD. The feeling good handbook. New York: Wm. Morrow, 1989.
2. Brownell KD, Wadden TA. Behavior therapy for obesity: modern approaches and better results. In: Brownell KD, Foreyt JP, eds. Handbook of eating disorders. New York: Basic Books, 1986.

3. Foreyt JP, Goodrich GK. Evidence of success of behavior modification in weight loss and control. Ann Int Med 1993;119:698.

4. Bandura A. Social foundations of thought and action: a social cognitive theory. Englewood Cliffs, NJ: Prentice-Hall, 1986.

5. Bandura A. Exercise of personal and collective efficacy in changing societies. In: Bandura A, ed. Self-efficacy in changing societies. New York: Cambridge Univ. Press, 1995.

6. Meichenbaum D. Cognitive-behavior modification. In: Kanfer FH, Goldstein AP, eds. Helping people change, 3rd ed. New York: Pergamon, 1986.

7. Mines RA, Merrill CA. Bulimia: cognitive-behavioral treatment and relapse prevention. J Counsel Dev 1987;65:562.

8. Wilson GT. Cognitive-behavioral and pharmacological therapies for bulimia. In: Brownell KD, Foreyt JP, eds. Handbook of eating disorders. New York: Basic Books, 1986.

9. Garner DM. Cognitive therapy for anorexia nervosa. In: Brownell KD, Foreyt JP, eds. Handbook of eating disorders. New York: Basic Books, 1986.

10. Holli BB. Using behavior modification in nutrition counseling. J Am Diet Assoc 1988;88:1530.

11. Glasgow RE, Tooberi DJ, Mitchell DL, Donnelly JE, Calder D. Nutrition education and social learning interventions for type II diabetes. Diabetes Care 1989;12:150.

12. Fremouw WJ, Heyneman NE. Obesity. In: Hersen M, ed. Outpatient behavior therapy. New York: Grune & Stratton, 1983.

13. Strecher VJ, DeVellis BM, Becker MH, Rosenstock IM. The role of self-efficacy in achieving health behavior change. Health Educ Q 1986;13:73.

14. Schwarzer R, Fuchs R. Changing risk behaviors and adopting health behaviors: the role of self-efficacy beliefs. In: Bandura A, ed. Self-efficacy in changing societies. New York: Cambridge Univ. Press, 1995.

15. Matheson DM, Woolcott DM, Matthews AM, Roth V. Evaluation of a theoretical model predicting self-efficacy toward nutrition behaviors in the elderly. J Nutr Educ 1991;23:3.

16. Strecher VJ, Seijts GH, Kok GJ, Latham GP, Glasgow R, DeVellis B, Meertens RM, Bulger DW. Goal setting as a strategy for health behavior change. Health Educ Q 1995;22:190.

17. Campbell MK, DeVellis BM, Strecher VJ, Ammerman AS, DeVellis RF, Sandler RS. Improving dietary behavior: the effectiveness of tailored messages in primary care settings. Am J Public Health 1994;84:783.

18. Skelly AH, Marshall JR, Haughey BP, Davis PJ, Dunford RG. Self-efficacy and confidence in outcomes as determinants of self-care practices in inner-city, African-American women with non–insulin-dependent diabetes. Diabetes Educ 1995;21:38.

19. Van Beuren E, James R, Christian J, Church D. Dietary self-efficacy in a community-based intervention: implications for effective dietary counseling. Austral J Nutr Diet 1991;48:64.

20. Hovell MF, Barrington E, Hofstetter R, Sallis J, Rauh M. Correlates of physical activity in overweight and not overweight persons: an assessment. J Am Diet Assoc 1990;90:1260.

21. DeWolfe JA, Shannon BM. Factors affecting fat consumption of university students: testing a model to predict eating behaviour. J Canad Diet Assoc 1993;54:132.

22. Littlefield CH, Craven JL, Rodin GM, Daveman D, Murray MA, Rydall AC. Relationship of self-efficacy and bingeing to adherence to diabetes regimen among adolescents. Diabetes Care 1992;15:90.

23. Kayman S. Applying theory from social psychology and cognitive behavioral psychology to dietary behavior change and assessment. J Am Diet Assoc 1989;89:191.

24. Mitchell C, Stuart RB. Effect of self-efficacy on dropout from obesity treatment. J Consult Clin Psychol 1984;52:1100.

25. Marlatt GA. Relapse prevention: theoretical rationale and overview of the model. In: Marlatt GA, Gordon JR, eds. Relapse prevention. New York: Guilford Press, 1985.

26. Wylie-Rosett J, Swencionis C, Stern J. Nutritional and behavioral strategies for the obese individual with diabetes. Top Clin Nutr 1988;3:9.

27. Marlatt GA, Baer JS, Quigley LA. Self-efficacy and addictive behavior. In: Bandura A, ed. Self-efficacy in changing societies. New York: Cambridge Univ. Press, 1995.

28. Marlatt GA. Cognitive factors in the relapse process. In: Marlatt GA, Gordon JR, eds. Relapse prevention. New York: Guilford Press, 1985.

29. Marlatt GA. Cognitive assessment and intervention procedures in relapse prevention. In: Marlatt GA, Gordon JR, eds. Relapse prevention. New York: Guilford Press, 1985.

30. Brownell KD, Marlatt GA, Lichenstein E, Wilson GT. Understanding and preventing relapse. Am Psychol 1986;41:765.

31. Sternberg B. Relapse in weight control: definitions, processes, and prevention strategies. In: Marlatt GA, Gordon JR, eds. Relapse prevention. New York: Guilford Press, 1985.

32. McCann BS, Retzlaff BM, Dowdy AA, Walden CE, Knapp RH. Promoting adherence to low-fat, low-cholesterol diets: review and recommendations. J Am Diet Assoc 1990;90:408.

33. Marlatt GA. Situational determinants of relapse and skill-training interventions. In: Marlatt GA, Gordon JR, eds. Relapse prevention. New York: Guilford Press, 1985.

34. Schlundt DG, Rea MR, Kline SS, Pichert JW. Situational obstacles to dietary adherence for adults with diabetes. J Am Diet Assoc 1994;94:874.

35. Schlundt DG, Pichert JW, Rea MR, Puryear W, Penka MLI, Kline S. Situational obstacles to adherence for adolescents with diabetes. Diabetes Educ 1994;20:207.

36. Mindfulness and metaphor in relapse prevention: an interview with G. Alan Marlatt. J Am Diet Assoc 1994;94:846.

37. Marlatt GA. Lifestyle modification. In: Marlatt GA, Gordon JR, eds. Relapse prevention. New York: Guilford Press, 1985.

eight

COMMUNICATING AND THE NEW DIVERSITY

A changing cultural climate in the United States has created an increased awareness of the part cultural diversity plays in people's behaviors and attitudes (1). There is an undisputed need among health professionals for culturally sensitive information (2). Nutrition educators are faced with the challenge of providing nutrition education and assistance to people who come from a variety of cultures and are of diverse ages (3).

Ethnicity beyond the date of immigration and into second, third, and later generations is a matter of discussion, decision, and degree. No one can say for sure who consider themselves ethnics or where they live. Some people claim that existing counseling strategies are effective for all people and categorizing traits of different subcultural groups perpetrates stereotypes; others believe that existing models, based on a white dominant middle-class, are ineffective when used with people from other cultures (4).

The United States' population is heterogeneous, with each of the many groups represented in the country having its own traditional foods and food habits, and they often vary significantly from the so called "typical" American diet. Effective counseling and education require that these variations be acknowledged and understood within the context of culture. Cultural training for dietetics students typically consists of a background course in a related social or behavioral science, combined with dietetics education about food preferences and associated health problems of certain racial and ethnic groups. Although such instruction is valuable for introducing students to basic information, it does not adequately prepare them to incorporate cultural concepts into dietetics practice (5).

The term "culture" is often used to describe very large social groupings based on a shared national origin of people. It includes a set of beliefs, assumptions, and values widely shared by a group that structures behavior of group members from birth until death. Within cultural groups variations exist owing to differences in socioeconomic status, social class, religion, age, education, location, and length of time in the United States. People from a given culture, nevertheless, do tend to have experiences that are culturally patterned and similar in nature, although not identical (6).

Contemporary nutrition educators will need both to understand the meaning of "culture" and know how it affects their clients. Culture includes many aspects of peoples' lives—the language they speak, their values, the way they dress, the music they like, the way they interact, their health beliefs, and the food they eat. Although specific foods mean different things in different cultures, most cultural groups use food for similar purposes. People from virtually all cultures, for example, use food during celebrations, and many cultural groups use food as medicine or to promote health. Nutrition educators must recognize the strong preferences that people have for the food they eat and their special uses of food. There are numerous books written on the subject of food and culture (2, 4, 7–12).

It is the purpose of the opening section of the chapter to limit the discussion to the communication aspects of the phenomenon, providing dietetics professionals both with enough of a cultural overview so that they are able to avoid ethnocentric assumptions and to provide an awareness of the volume of data concerning the foods and food habits of various minority groups. The second section of the chapter discusses the implications of the diversity issues for dietetics professionals. The third section of the chapter examines the implications for dietetics practitioners of the changing American workforce. The chapter concludes with a discussion of counseling through the life span.

The foods and food habits of Americans are as diverse as its population. It was, in fact, never true that the typical American ate meat and potatoes. Recent census figures indicate that the majority of the population is rapidly being made up of minority groups, and each minority group has its own culturally based foods, food habits, and beliefs about health. The American diet, therefore, encompasses the numerous varied cuisines of the U.S. population (13). It has become necessary for those helping professionals who work with these minority populations to learn about their food habits.

What may appear illogical initially to a professional is,

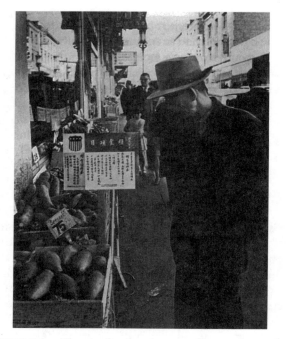

FIGURE 8.1. The professional counseling various ethnic groups needs a knowledge of their foods.

nevertheless, a valid reflection of the complex symbolic, economic, sociologic, ecologic, and physiologic realities of another culture. There already exists an extensive literature written for dietetics professionals to assist in working with people of different culture (13–22). It is not within the scope of this book, however, to discuss the dispositional and unique characteristics of the many varied cultures of individuals who are currently the clientele of dietetics professionals; rather, it is to discuss generally how the diversity itself should influence the way these individuals are counseled and taught.

Dietetics practitioners need today to expand beyond knowing their client's eating behaviors and lifestyle habits; they need to encourage their clients to come to new awareness about their food habits, particularly those culturally determined. In the management of patients with chronic diseases, such as diabetes, culture is important because of the lifelong course of the disease. Identifying cultural barriers to action is an important part of intervention planning (23). The professional, therefore, is expected to do more than design meticulously calculated diets. She is, in addition, expected to model a sensitivity to multicultural and other client-specific uniqueness.

The goal for health care providers is to accompany knowledge of the culture with awareness, respect, and acceptance of the client's cultural beliefs and practices. Monsen has pointed out that dietetics professionals are trained in the physiological effects of nutrients, but to translate their knowledge into recommendations useful to clients, these professionals need to be experts in the cultural and social roles of food as well (24).

The development of cultural competence in counsel-

ing has four stages, according to Campinha-Bacote (25). First, cultural awareness is the process that requires self-assessment. The dietetics practitioner needs to learn her own biases and prejudices toward other cultures, while making an effort to become sensitive to the views of clients. Second, cultural knowledge is the process of learning about the world views of other cultures. This can be done through books, workshops, self-study, audio-visual presentations, classes, etc. Third, cultural skill develops as providers learn to assess relevant factors related by the client that will affect nutrition education. Fourth, cultural encounters comprise the stage where providers are encouraged to get involved in culturally diverse interactions (16).

CONTEMPORARY CHALLENGES FOR DIETETICS PRACTITIONERS

Nutrition educators face major challenges in the 21st century as they attempt to communicate about food with their culturally diverse clientele. Practitioners are called upon to provide guidance to people who have recently joined the community, for whom everything—language, living accommodation, economic status—is new and different. According to the 1990 census, almost one in four Americans has African, Asian, Hispanic, or American Indian ancestry. That figure is projected to rise to almost one in three by the year 2020 and almost one in two by the year 2050 (12).

Additional time generally is needed to work effectively with culturally diverse clients, and this can present a challenge for both educator and client. When people are of different cultures, it takes time for trust to develop between them. The dietetics practitioner may need to spend extra time becoming familiar with the client's culture. A newly arrived immigrant family needs time to learn new ways. Language barriers slow communication, and different views of time occasionally cause misunderstandings between educator and client. The challenge for nutrition educators is to make the best and most effective use of time for all involved (12).

Besides providing quality time to clients, the dietetics practitioner needs exemplary communication skills as she attempts to focus on each family's background and present situation—without making assumptions. To do this, nutrition educators should learn about their client as an individual and about the client's family and culture as a whole, place the food habits of the individual or the family within a cultural context, and consider how the family's eating patterns are likely to change in a new environment.

Nutrition educators have suggested various techniques and ideas to create a common ground with clients, using food as the topic to open the dialogue (12). One way to get to know the client and her culture is to ask about food experiences. Everyone has memories related to food, and for many people, these memories are connected with family, celebration, and caring. Practitioners are encouraged to ask questions with an open mind, keeping a sense of humor; to tell their own food stories from their family history; to find out what foods are used as medicine or to promote health; and finally to ask about the client's favorite foods, meals, or recipes. Communication about food can be used to encourage involvement, active participation, and joint planning with the client.

Client Acculturation

"Acculturation" is the process of adopting the beliefs, values, attitudes, and behaviors of a dominant, or mainstream, culture, and it is a variable that must be considered during the assessment and treatment of the multicultural groups attended to by dietetics professionals (10). Part of this process includes changing some traditional dietary patterns to be more like those of the dominant culture. Practitioners must understand how acculturation affects the families with whom they communicate. There are many factors that influence acculturation, and they do not only involve immigrants. Acculturation is an ongoing process that affects anyone who moves from one community to another.

Acculturation occurs differently for everyone. People adjust at different rates, and the rate may vary among different families from the same cultural background. Acculturation may also occur at different times among members of the same family. It is affected by such things as education, exposure to the mainstream culture, length of time the individual or group has been in the community, involvement of the individual with his ethnic group in the community, ties with family, family structure, language, employment, age, and opportunities for exposure to new ideas. Acculturation ultimately affects dietary patterns because individuals tend to reevaluate the food in their diet and make changes by adding, substituting, or rejecting foods. These changes result in repatterning of the diet, sometimes causing major changes in nutrient intake.

Acculturation of groups into the larger society tends to be a two-way street. Whenever people from two or more cultures interact, they influence each other. When new members of the community adopt typical "American" food, generally they also contribute some of their favorites to the American diet. The variety of ethnic restaurants in all major cities and the growing ethnic sections of traditional American supermarkets affirm this contribution.

There are many factors that affect the food choices people make every day, and these factors apply no matter what one's cultural background. For new arrivals to a community, however, an even greater number of factors play a part in determining food choices. Factors that affect everyone's food choices include such things as availability, cultural eating patterns and family traditions, exposure to new foods and new methods of food preparation, economics, ability to get to the market, living arrangement (including the presence of specific food preparation equipment), convenience of preparing food,

and skill at preparation. For new arrivals to a community the additional factors include access to traditional and nontraditional foods and beverages, length of time in the community, time and skill required to prepare new dishes rather than traditional ones, availability of low-cost ethnic restaurants, level of comfort shopping (ability to ask for items, drive to stores, etc.), and ties with family or ethnic groups in the new community (12).

Communicating With Clients and Families

Communication provides an opportunity for persons of different cultures to learn from each other. It is the key to the dietetics practitioner's role as an educator. To keep the lines of communication open, the professional must build skills that enhance communication between cultures. These skills will help overcome any real or perceived differences with clients or their families.

Although this point has been made in other chapters, it bears repetition here: establishing rapport with clients is always the first priority. Only after rapport has been established is the client likely to lower barriers and engage in authentic interaction. In many cultures, moreover, until rapport is established, it is inappropriate to discuss business. The few extra minutes taken to do this may save many hours of work in the long run. Learning to communicate effectively with individuals and families is a very important part of nutrition education. Rapport is enhanced when clients sense the professional's interest in the community in which they live, the places where they buy their food, and their sources of information. This information, furthermore, will have an effect on the kind of approach the professional uses and on the way messages are received (12).

In addition to being open, honest, respectful, nonjudgmental, and willing to learn, dietetics practitioners need to develop listening and observation skills. Barriers can be broken down by listening to people and letting them know that the professional is interested in what they have to say. This is the single most important way to make people feel that their interactions with health professionals have been successful. When cultural experts are available, the practitioner should take advantage of those knowledgeable to help interpret people's actions. Relying on one's own point of view may lead to misinterpretation.

While in the process of learning about her clientele, the practitioner should be sensitive to feedback from them, looking for cues to determine if and when communication has shut down. Should this occur, the best strategy for getting back on track is to avoid overexplaining while encouraging a give-and-take discussion. There are cultural and language barriers to communication, and the rules of proper professional behavior vary dramatically the world over. Dietetics professionals must be cognizant of the client's expectations regarding professional treatment and attempt to meet the expectation (26).

Practitioners should both anticipate and be prepared

for identifying the "teachable moment." Allowing clients to tell the professional what she needs to know is a special skill in itself, the skill of nonjudgmentally listening and nonverbally encouraging clients to disclose their concerns. The professional who learns to start by accepting the clients' subjective reality and relates to them on their own level provides them with the opportunity to bring up related topics. This may mean that the professional will have to set aside her own agenda, being flexible, in order to take advantage of any opportunity to teach someone about nutrition. People tend to learn what and when they feel the need to know and to understand. Addressing their concerns or confusion first, increases considerably the likelihood of their learning. Furthermore, when communicating with clients for whom the American English lexicon is foreign, simple, directed, and repeated messages are preferred, teaching one idea at a time.

Another suggestion for practitioners to enhance their communication and teaching with clients is to create opportunities to combine nutrition with social events. Whenever possible the professional should plan social occasions that allow people from different cultures to interact and share food experiences. This "fun" activity provides an opportunity for nutrition education, not only with one another but with the professional as well. The professional might, for example, teach about nutritious snacks by hosting a tasting party at the WIC, Head Start, or some other appropriate facility. This not only gives people a chance to try new or unfamiliar foods but also allows participants to become receptive to new foods used as snacks.

Learning experiences in the area of nutrition tend to be enhanced when they occur in a social or "party-like" atmosphere. Wellness parties are effective teaching vehicles, allowing the professional to focus on healthful eating. Success of the project increases when community members are either paid or rewarded in some other way and when men in the community are included as well (12).

Practitioners encouraging situations where they have access to the entire family is an excellent teaching strategy, providing an opportunity to strengthen nutrition education. Each family member tends to influence the foods and dishes eaten by others in the family. In fact, clients often want to check with their family before making decisions or agreeing to try something new. When practitioners attempt to identify the decision-makers in the family and invite the client to discuss important decisions with these members, they enhance their long-term chances of being effective. Many cultures, including Asians and Hispanics, see the oldest male as the head of the family. In African American families and in American Indian families, an elderly male or female may be the most respected. Ideally, all interested family members should be invited to take part in counseling or nutrition education. Children too may be an avenue for getting nutrition information to parents. There are times when they are the only vehicle available for getting nutrition information into the home. Children can take home what they learn in school, Head Start, or some other nutrition program, often acting as translators for parents when educative materials are brought into the home.

The Multilingual Environment

The clients for whom health practitioners care are frequently people who are newcomers and who are neither acculturated nor assimilated into the cultural values of the dominant culture. Language becomes an issue because the probability is high that the new immigrants do not speak English, and the phonics of some languages do not easily convert into English (27).

Professionals who do not speak the same language as their clients face a big challenge. There are, however, many things that can be done to compensate. Practitioners enhance their credibility, for example, when they learn key phrases in the client's language, and this allows the client to infer both the practitioner's interest and caring. Because most people learn both by listening and watching, the professional can provide nutrition information without written words. Pictures, food models, videotapes, and print materials (especially those in the person's native language), hands-on food demonstrations, flip charts, and games can all be effective learning methodologies.

When working with people who speak another language, practitioners should remember to applaud them for making an effort to speak in English. In addition to learning greetings, titles of respect, and their attitudes toward touching, the sensitive practitioner will provide print materials in a variety of foreign languages. When asking questions, the practitioner should remember to phrase them in a variety of different ways. People often have a limited understanding of the meaning of certain words, and they may use only the words they do know in English to answer questions. In addition to learning the proper pronunciation of people's names and being friendly, accepting, and approachable, above all the practitioner needs to remember that EVERYONE relates to a smile—perhaps the most intense communication vehicle of all.

When serving a person or group whose language the practitioner is unable to speak, the question arises of whether or not an interpreter or translator is necessary. The skills needed to be a good interpreter are different from those of a good translator. When dealing with written information, a translator is more critical, but when dealing with the spoken word, an interpreter is preferred. Interpretation is the conversion of the spoken words into another language, and translation is the conversion of the written word into another language.

When dealing with interpreters, the practitioner needs to remember to speak clearly in short, simple sentences, avoiding technical terminology and professional jargon.

The professional should look at and speak to the client rather than to the interpreter. While listening carefully to the client and watching for nonverbal cues, the professional can often respond intuitively. Sessions with an interpreter take longer, so extra time needs to be allotted. Persons who are experienced speaking the language and who understand its subtle meanings can be enormously helpful to the professional dietetics practitioner. Generally it is not a good idea to ask clients' family members or friends to be interpreters. Using them may cause problems, such as breach of confidentiality. Practitioners should also be sensitive to the fact that by asking a child to interpret, difficulties may be triggered because of the reversal of authority in the household.

Although the practitioner most certainly will encourage positive cultural food habits, she should also be teaching clients about "American" foods. People want and need to learn about American foods. A need to find substitutes for traditional foods that are not available in the United States, a desire to know what their children are eating at school and with friends, and exposure to unfamiliar restaurant menus are a few situations where the newcomer wants knowledge about the foods of his new country. When people are motivated to learn about these "new" foods, the professional should be prepared to provide information about food selection, preparation, and storage (12).

MANAGING DIVERSE EMPLOYEES

In spite of the period of downsizing, merging, and outsourcing that the United States experienced in the 1980s and 1990s, with accompanying unemployment of large portions of the traditional corporate workforce, a labor shortage and a dramatic shift in the American labor market is anticipated by the early 21st century (8). The tiny baby-bust generation, born between 1964 and 1975, as well as the oldest of the baby boomers, may not be able to fill all the jobs vacated by the retiring pre-World War II employees and the millions of new jobs being created each year as a result of the new technologies.

The labor mix of the 21st century will continue to be ethnically diverse. In the year 2000, women will compose about 47% of the labor force, and minorities and immigrants will hold 26% of all jobs. As is certainly evident among dietetics professionals, it is no longer a white man's world, given that he accounts for only 32% of the entering workforce. In the health care environment, the ability to attract and retain good employees is the key to maintaining a competitive advantage. Jobs are being created without an adequate supply of trained people to fill them, and competition for qualified professionals is becoming increasingly intense. Ironically, of the three factors that lead to increased productivity, capital investment, new technology, and workforce performance, the latter has received the least attention and made the smallest contribution to improved productivity. Faced with a rapidly shrinking labor pool, American businesses, including health care, are realizing that their ability to meet corporate goals is going to depend on how well they can attract, develop, and retain today's workers for tomorrow's jobs.

The term "browning of America" has been used to describe the reality that the labor of the country is being provided primarily by people of color and the management ranks will eventually come from people who call themselves "African Americans," "Asian Americans," "Native Americans," "South and Central Americans," "Mexican," and "Latin Americans." As the levels of formal education rise among these groups, it goes without saying that the health professions generally and the area of dietetics practitioners specifically will eventually reflect this pattern.

The successful dietetics practitioners/managers of the 21st century need to develop the following skills: first of all, they need an understanding of how their own assumptions regarding their own cultural norms do, in fact, form the basis of their perceptions of what's "right." In other words, managers need to be taught about their own ethnocentricity and the harm it can do if left unchallenged. Second, they need to accept that their own biases do affect their decision making and judgments about others. They need to acknowledge any prejudices. Beyond that, contemporary health care professionals need training in the customs, work attitudes, and values of the various groups they work with or manage.

Most health care professional management texts have not yet begun to include extensive guidelines for managing diversity, perhaps because the "guidelines" are in process and still emerging. Listed below, however, are recommendations for those expecting to manage others different from themselves.

Orientation of minority employees should be tailored for specific groups, with the new hire being given clear explanations of the ways in which the business culture may vary from the employee's expectations, based on his or her past cultural experiences.

Management training programs typically deal with such issues as delegation, motivation, communication, and participatory management, and although training in these areas is critical, managers and supervisors for the 21st century need intensive education regarding the cultural differences related to attitudes toward authority, competition, women as supervisors, and openness.

The Chinese, for example, are very uncomfortable challenging authority, and Asians, as well as Native Americans, prefer rewards that are less public and more personal. In Eastern cultures, people are less expressive. They think a lot more before they say something. Americans are very direct and tend to be impatient.

Management at the World Trade Center has found that, in general, people from hotter climates tend to be more casual about punctuality. When training such employees, it becomes key that explicit guidelines regarding time be communicated. For individuals coming from cultures where long midday breaks are the norm, training programs need to explain that in America a brief period for lunch is the norm.

Although the process has begun, health care corporations and dietetics practitioners need to develop a means of assuring upward mobility for women and minorities through attention to their careers. Mentoring programs, for example, have been developed to raise the retention rate of new employees, especially for women and people of color. A bilingual individual, for example, from the same ethnic group may be asked to mentor an employee whose English is still weak. Mentoring goals might include an introduction to the department's culture, explaining norms of the work group, and communicating and providing basic support. The organization can foster support groups to provide opportunities for minorities to mentor one another as well as forums for discussing problems and developing solutions.

Organizations can act as a catalyst for cultural awareness by encouraging ethnic celebrations of food and dance. These alone, however, would not be nearly enough to promote cultural awareness. Real awareness and appreciation will come primarily with an appropriate number of qualified minorities in visible positions of leadership, authority, and power.

The suggestions above could easily be expanded; however, the point is that the 21st century managers need to become familiar with the cultures of their employees and either adjust their own behavior, where feasible, or explain why acceptable behavior in another culture may need to be modified in the new culture.

As the need for educated and competent labor increases, other "minorities" are actively sought as well. Organizations face the challenge of attracting untapped or underutilized sources of labor. This category includes older or retired workers, teenagers, people with disabilities, part-time workers, people who work at home, and job-sharing employees.

Every day, 5200 Americans celebrate their 65th birthday. They are healthier, better educated, and live longer than previous generations, yet they are leaving the workforce at younger ages. In 1950 almost 50% of the men 65 and older were working, while today less than 20% work. These retirees account for a vast pool of knowledge and skills that are being underutilized. Given a severe shortage of younger workers, it is predictable that older workers will continue to be sought after. In order for them to be mainstreamed into the workforce, however, attitudes currently prevalent about older workers need to be altered. Many supervisors feel uncomfortable supervising older workers and often do not recommend them for hiring or training. They perceive the older employee as incapable of learning new skills and mistakenly assume that older workers are frequently absent, are safety hazards, or are just putting in time. The truth, however, is that, in general, older workers are on time, on the job, and as productive as younger employees.

Another challenge for the management group of the 21st century is to bring younger employees, another distinct minority, into the workforce. Not only is this group of workers in short supply, but, for them, the rewards of work lie outside the job. They tend to be motivated by personal needs and material rewards. The fast-food industry, which traditionally employs the 18–24-year-old group, has discovered that linking work with educational goals has helped to reduce their turnover rate. Some firms offer a choice of a cash bonus or a scholarship upon completion of a set number of hours of work. Strategies for recruiting and retaining this minority group need to be developed now.

People with disabilities are America's largest minority group, cutting across racial, ethnic, religious, economic, and social lines. They comprise about 13% of the entire U.S. population. Unfortunately, they are often more seriously impeded by human barriers created out of ignorance, prejudices, stereotyping, or fear than by the effects of their own disability. The key word for people with disabilities is "accessibility." Inaccessibility is a form of discrimination, even when it is unintentional. The Americans With Disabilities Act is forcing business, as well as individuals, to examine the value system regarding persons with disabilities. Organizations need to promote accessibility to jobs as well as to services.

Americans have a tendency to be uncomfortable with difference. Those barriers can be eliminated through communication of facts, understanding, and common sense. Disability means that one or more things most people can do, a person with disabilities cannot do as easily, or cannot do at all. The persons affected, however, prefer to emphasize what they can do, not what they cannot do, just like a person without disabilities. The most significant difference for persons with physical disabilities is that they have to adapt to an environment designed for the nondisabled. When their environment is designed to accommodate their needs, their disabilities are relatively unimportant. Under the Americans With Disabilities Act, the number of these environmental barriers should decrease. Physical disabilities are almost never "total" and usually affect a surprisingly narrow range of activities.

Flextime can provide an alternative to having to choose between work and family. Flextime programs, which are widely used by men too, may vary in their specific construct, but they all generally share three common features: core hours, flexible hours, and a bandwidth. Core hours are the specific hours of a day that an employee must be at work. Flexible hours are ranges of hours at the beginning and end of the day during which the employee may or may not choose to work. The bandwidth is the total number of hours between the earliest permitted start time and the latest permitted stop time. The larger the bandwidth, the more flexible the program.

Changing a rigid schedule structure to a more flexible one is both useful to the employees and advantageous to employers. In addition to the decrease in absenteeism and increase in productivity, companies offering flextime can expand their labor pool while allowing employees to function more efficiently in their roles in and out of work.

In summary, nearly one-third of all new entrants into the labor force during the 1990s came from so-called minority groups. Immigrants, who present distinct training needs and multicultural issues, make up as much as 40% of the annual growth in the U.S. workforce. To compete, companies must learn to manage them successfully (28). Progressive companies are reshaping their own management style and culture to ensure that all employees are contributing to their full potential. Rather than play the equal opportunity numbers game, they are creating an atmosphere in which differences are nurtured and all employees' needs are considered. Developing supervisors who recognize these differences and can manage workers who not only look, but think differently than they do, is becoming a priority. Their first challenge is to make their company a place where people want to work, a place where minorities are comfortable.

Seeing diverse employees not as problems, but as assets can enhance an organization's effectiveness. Health care organizations are beginning to realize that the diversity of their workforce reflects the diversity of their suppliers, clients, and patients. Hiring a diverse staff, one that matches the demographics of one's patients, assures that one will have employees who understand how to respond to the market. Staffing one's office with English-speaking employees, for example, when most of the clients are Spanish-speaking is frustrating for both, and may well lead to a loss of business.

The competitive advantage of the 21st century will come from one source: people. Reaching these people will take ongoing commitment, resourcefulness, training, and sensitivity. Only by first meeting the needs of their employees can organizations assure themselves of an appropriate staff to meet the needs of their customers.

COUNSELING DIVERSITY THROUGH THE LIFE SPAN

Besides being diverse in their ethnic backgrounds, the clients of the contemporary dietetics professional will be diverse in their ages as well. Practitioners interact with people of all ages. While many of the communication and education principles and strategies in other chapters of this book are appropriate for anyone, this section focuses specifically on preschool-aged children, school-aged children, adolescents, older adults, and those with limited literacy skills. At all ages, the dietetics professional is concerned with promoting good nutritional practices for optimum health.

Preschool-Aged Children

Children's food habits are learned through family food experiences, through education, and through personal experiences. In the preschool years, family practices are a major influence on what children eat (29, 30). As children mature in language and social skills related to eating, meals become important social and family events (31). Another influence comes from watching television, and media pressures on food selection begin to develop early (30, 31). Professionals work with parents and other caregivers in influencing children's eating behaviors.

Some children may be in Head Start or other day care programs. Studies show that parents/families and teachers working together can mutually reinforce learning about nutrition and make more of an impact than either working alone (29). Recommended strategies for teaching nutrition include action stories, songs, tasting parties, food preparation, vegetable and fruit gardens, puzzles, and healthy snacks. Social modeling of healthful eating by adult role models and peers is helpful (30).

School-Aged Children

Childhood is the prime time of human development (32). It may be easier to establish healthful dietary and exercise habits during childhood than later in life. The American Dietetic Association takes the position that "all children and adolescents should have access to adequate food and nutrition programs," including "nutrition education, screening, assessment, and intervention" (33). In these years, nutrition education seeks to teach children the knowledge that they will need to select healthy foods and also the analytical and evaluative skills necessary to examine food and nutrition information (34). Since risk factors for some chronic diseases begin in youth, behaviorally focused nutrition education is appropriate. Studies show that interventions that focus on specific behavior changes result in more changes than a more general nutrition education approach (34).

The dietetics professional needs to spend time assessing the child's family, social, physical, and psychological environment when dietary changes need to be made. Since a 6-year-old is very different from a 9-year-old, an evaluation of the developmental stage of the child according to theories of child psychology and of the cognitive level will help in planning any intervention (34). The child's activity pattern, including number of hours spent watching television or playing video games daily, should be noted.

The professional should bear in mind that breakfast has to be planned around school bus schedules, and the noon meal may be at the school lunch program, requiring choices to be made by the child, such as selecting either whole or skim milk. After-school snacks are required to meet the child's energy needs. Children who become involved in competitive sports, such as Little League baseball, may be receiving nutrition advice from a coach (31). As the child gets older, peer influences on eating increase, yet the family is still a major influence on the child's early eating patterns.

Dietetics professionals commonly recognize the need to include the family in the counseling process. Family nutrition counseling involves people who live in the same household, not just relatives in traditional family structures (35). They may share common biological, social, psychological, and environmental spheres. The goal is to use the shared environment to influence nutrition and health for the better and to foster healthful food consumption practices. In some cases, the father, not the mother, is the person responsible for menu planning, purchasing, and preparation of food. Children may prepare some of their own snacks or foods in the microwave oven. With divorce, the children may live with each parent at different times. The professional must be sensitive to family relationships.

If the family cooperates, social, psychological, and environmental support will assist in fostering dietary changes in the child. In families dealing with obesity, diabetes mellitus, or atherosclerosis, for example, dietary changes often benefit everyone. Changes in food buying and preparation practices for all will influence the child's adherence to the regimen (30).

Children, and even adolescents, are obviously highly dependent on their parents who control, to a great extent, the food served in the home. They influence the child's eating patterns from day one. When only the correct food is in the home, environmental cues to eat are reduced, and following the dietary regimen is enhanced (35). Family members can serve as good role models for appropriate eating and can encourage and reward healthful habits in the child (30). Children frequently mimic their parents' food habits. If Dad refuses broccoli, for example, so will Johnny. Parents who want their children to drink milk instead of Coke need to set a good example. The counselor can negotiate changes in what is purchased and prepared by the family.

There are some barriers to family counseling. Some clients do not wish to involve certain family members; members may refuse to participate; spouses and parents may be overly controlling and negative in dealing with the child; and mutually acceptable times for appointments may be difficult to arrange for several people (35). Other sources of social support may have to be located if the family has problems.

Other problems may exist. Parents may not be good role models or supportive of their children. They may use sweets and desserts as a reward or bribe. Siblings may tempt and tease a brother or sister who is not supposed to eat certain foods. Parents who take a food plan too literally create a stressful environment in the family leading to food battles and conflicts. Nagging, criticism, and policing about food and weight should be replaced by positive reinforcement and praise when correct dietary behaviors are observed. One visit is insufficient for most family counseling (35).

For the nutrition education of children, national objectives have been identified by government agencies, including the Department of Health and Human Services, the Department of Education, and the Nutrition Education and Training (NET) program (36). Objectives, priorities, and strategies for promoting healthy eating in children are recommended by NET. All states mandate or have initiatives to promote nutrition education in schools as a component of the curriculum. Other agencies that commit resources to nutrition education of youth and adults include the National Cancer Institute (NCI) and National Heart, Lung, and Blood Institute (NHLBI).

In the earlier grades (K–3) family-based programs were found to be more effective, but not for middle or high school students (34). In one case, worksheets, games, and other activities were mailed to homes so that the child and family could work on them jointly; this has been found to be a successful method of intervention.

Another study reported a survey of students in grades

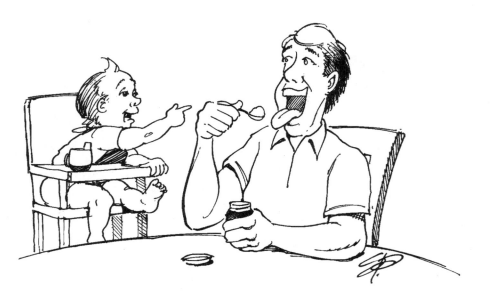

FIGURE 8.2. Parents should set a good example.

5, 8, and 11 (36). The three topics students were most interested in learning about were weight control, how to improve their diets, and nutrition and disease, but interest varied by grade level.

In selecting ways they would like to learn about nutrition, fifth graders preferred games and food experiments most and information presented by the teacher least. Eighth graders preferred food preparation, but interest in any method was low. Videotapes and information from teachers were least preferred. Students in eleventh grade expressed interest in videotapes, games, and food preparation. Least interest was expressed in individual projects. Interest in food preparation and guest speakers increased by grade level (36). The most popular methods and educational strategies actively involved students while passive techniques were undesirable.

Concerns about body image start early. About one-third of the students surveyed thought that their weight was too high. In the previous year, one-half had attempted weight loss (36). The number of students who skipped meals increased with grade level. The study concluded that children and adolescents wanted to learn about nutrition topics that were consistent with their developmental stage.

Children want learning to be fun (37, 38). What was fun for you during childhood? Was it riding a new bicycle, throwing stones into rain puddles, playing with a cat or dog, or spending time with Grandma? Childhood is a time for play exploration and opportunities for learning. The play approach to learning has been recommended as an alternative to the social learning theory and behavioral approach. The play approach, based on the theory of Jean Piaget, focuses on internal, rather than external, transaction, on intrinsic motivation, and on fun (37).

In the play approach, children actively explore and experiment with objects, materials, and knowledge. Active experimentation, hands-on experiences, and self-directed activities are recommended. Real-life situations, such as reading food labels, measuring quantities of food, recording and charting data, such as the amount of sugar in popular beverages or cereals, and communicating with others about food choices are examples. Experiments with new foods and methods of preparing them are appropriate (37). Partnerships of children, schools, and families can promote health and well-being and influence lifetime food habits.

Children who have medical problems present an educational challenge. In the management of children and adolescents with diabetes mellitus, involvement of families is essential. Parents can serve as resources and as support groups for other parents (39). Needs can be assessed through telephone contacts, formal questionnaires, or informal information supplied at clinic visits. Games for use with diabetes mellitus are found in the literature (40, 41).

When dietary modifications are needed, the dietetics professional should try to choose words that children use and understand. The word "diet," for example, turns off most children as well as adults (41). Food, food plan, meal plan, or menu are better choices. The office environment can be made attractive with colorful, plastic food models, magazine pictures, cardboard food models, posters, food packages of commonly eaten foods, and beverage glasses of various sizes and shapes. One group used food exchange playing cards, coloring placemats, and food models in teaching the diabetic exchange system (41).

Another study assessed the effects of a home-based, parent-child autotutorial (PCAT) program for 4–10-year-old children with elevated low-density lipoprotein cholesterol (LDL-C) (42). The PCAT program, based on social cognitive theory, included 10 talking-book lessons (audiotaped stories with accompanying picture books) and follow-up paper and pencil games for the children. A manual for parents was provided. The program was effective in helping children gain knowledge of "heart-healthy eating" and in reducing their dietary fat consumption and their plasma LDL-C levels.

A team approach using the classroom, school lunch program, athletic department, and activities in the home and in the community will help to teach children about nutrition. While school teachers spend about 10 to 15 hours per year on nutrition education, one study found that 15 hours could only bring about changes in knowledge and that 50 hours were required to change attitudes and behaviors (34). The school lunch menu, if available, may be used in teaching which foods to select.

Many successful programs include self-assessment of dietary intake to identify problem behaviors, setting personal goals for change, observing models (peers and adults) of desired behavior, enhancing self-efficacy through skill building, and providing incentives and reinforcement for change (34). All children enjoy incentives for reaching goals. Experiential, active, and hands-on educational methods are recommended.

Six elements of successful nutrition education programing have been identified. They include the following: (a) programs are behaviorally based and driven by theory; (b) for elementary school children, family members are involved in the program; (c) self-assessment of eating practices is included for middle school to senior high students; (d) behavior change programs intervene in the school classroom and lunchroom environments; (e) behavioral change programs also intervene in the larger community; and (f) intensive instruction time is included (43).

Adolescents

Increasing growth rates occur in girls between 10 and 12 years of age, and in boys, about 2 years later (31). Individuals vary in rates of physical growth and in the timing of the growth spurt. Physical activity patterns vary from little activity to active involvement in sports. The dietetics professional needs to assess each person individually as the first step before planning intervention, counseling, and education.

The teen years are a time for balancing freedom and responsibility, for experimentation, for questioning people in authority, and for independence (39). Food is often central to social life with peers. Adolescents have major problems with anything that makes them different from their peer group (41). This can affect foods eaten at parties, eating out, alcohol, after-school snacks, and sports events. Many teenagers have their own money to spend. Personal decisions related to self-care can be explored between the dietetics professional and the adolescent. In working with groups, one may ask them how they handle these situations.

The connections between dietary practices and health may be discussed. Intervention strategies should target the affective domain, or feelings and attitudes, not just knowledge (30). Adolescent attitudes and patterns related to diet and physical activity should be explored since they may persist into adulthood (32). The foundation for coronary heart disease prevention, for example, by the promotion and maintenance of healthy lifestyles is important in adolescence and young adulthood. Obesity is increasing in this age group.

A number of adolescent girls may become pregnant. If they have not completed the growth spurt, the nutritional needs of pregnancy are added to their normal needs (31). Nutrition is vital to the growth and development of the fetus and the outcome of pregnancy. Adolescents, however, are vulnerable to poor nutritional practices and pregnant teens are at particular risk of having low-birth-weight babies (34). Pregnancy may provide the counselor with an opportunity to encourage the vulnerable adolescent to improve her eating patterns (30).

Girls are susceptible to other health hazards. They diet frequently and as a result, may have marginal nutritional status (31). Dissatisfaction with one's body image and weight is more common in girls (30, 31). Idealized standards of attractiveness may make some refuse food, resulting in nutritionally inadequate intakes. In some, dieting may lead to anorexia nervosa and bulimia (30). Those who become vegetarians may be vulnerable to nutritional deficiencies if their diet is not balanced properly (29).

Many teens are involved in competitive sports activities. A coach may try to influence eating patterns as a way to improve athletic performance (31). The professional should look for nutrition misinformation and fads with this group. In some sports, such as wrestling, for example, males may be trying to lose weight by inappropriate means in order to wrestle at the top of a lower weight class. Adolescent boys may be highly motivated to learn about nutrition to improve their sports performance.

Promoting nutritional health over the life span can be a cooperative goal of many public and private agencies as it is in the earlier years (31). Many agencies have a nutrition education component. Examples are the Special Supplement Food Program for Women, Infants, and Children (WIC), the Food Stamp Program, the School Breakfast Program and National School Lunch Programs, the Nutrition Education and Training (NET) Program, and the Commodity Supplemental Food Program (CSFP) (44). Federal, state, and local public health agencies employ nutritionists. As members of a health care team, they assess the community nutrition needs as well as provide services, such as maternal and child health. Other agencies, such as the American Heart Association and the American Dietetic Association, also have educational materials.

Older Adults

The American population is growing older and the aging trend is expected to continue. In the future as many as one in four Americans will be age 65 or older (30, 45) (Table 8.1). The number of persons aged 85 years and older is also increasing. People are living longer. People who reach 65 can now expect to live into their 80s (32). Not all of these years may be active and independent ones. Adults aged 65 and over are a varied group.

Good nutrition is important in the promotion and maintenance of health in older adults. With existing health problems, good nutrition can improve the quality of life as age advances, and aid in the management of acute and chronic diseases (45). Eating nutritiously to maintain optimum health continues to be a goal as it is throughout the life span (46). As a result, nutrition interventions are important to consider.

The majority of individuals 65 years and older believe

TABLE 8.1.

Resident Population Projections by Age (in thousands)

AGE	1995	2010
Less than 5 years	20,181	20,017
5–13 years	34,262	36,213
14–17 years	14,591	17,388
18–24 years	25,465	30,220
65–74 years	18,963	20,978
75–84 years	11,087	13,157
85 years and older	3,598	5,969

Reprinted with permission from the American Almanac 1995–1996: Statistical Abstract of the United States. Austin, TX: Reference Press, 1995.

themselves to be in good to excellent health (45). A preponderance of these, however, have one or more nutrition-related medical problems, such as hypertension, cancer, cardiovascular disease, and arthritis. The nutritional problems affecting the elderly, as with other adults, include nutritional excesses, such as from overeating and obesity and from self-prescribed nutrition supplements. Others suffer underweight and malnutrition due to nutritional deficiencies of vitamins, minerals, protein, or calories (44). Yet many are not in poor health.

As with any client, individual assessment is the first step. A 65-year-old is different from a 75- or 85-year-old. Because they are such a diverse group, the dietetics professional has to individualize the dietary intervention based on the assessment (45, 46). Working with older people is no different than working with others. One must, however, recognize differences in sensory and physical abilities, the fear many older people have of losing their independence, and the increased role of storytelling.

Federal programs for older adults have a component of nutrition education. Examples are the Congregate and Home-Delivered Meals Program, the Child and Adult Day Care Program, the Food Stamp Program, and the Commodity Supplemental Food Program (CSFP) (44).

One needs to assess the various conditions that are negatively associated with food intake. Examples are low income, low educational level, living alone, bereavement, and ill-fitting dentures that make chewing difficult. The relationship between poor health and lower socioeconomic status has been well documented (32.) Physical inactivity may increase as one ages. What about the client's independence? Does the individual still drive a car, get to the grocery store, and prepare meals? These questions need exploration.

Needs assessment for older adults may be handled through personal interviews, self-administered questionnaires, or focus groups (47, 48). Assessment is important in ensuring that nutrition education is appropriate to the needs and characteristics of the individual or group, including educational level, socioeconomic status, physical ability or limitations, and cultural and ethnic background (45).

What changes should the dietetics professional look for during needs assessment? Physiological changes occur as age progresses. Sight and hearing may diminish. Print material and visuals should be large enough to be seen. At least 12 or 14 point type is needed. Greens, blues, violets, dark colors, and pastel colors may look alike to some older learners (48, 49). If one suspects that the client has his or her eyeglasses in a pocket or purse, the practitioner may wish to stop and ask the individual to read something in order to assess visual acuity. This may also give some indication of educational level. Short sentences are preferable. Slowing the pace of speech is helpful, so one should speak more slowly and clearly (48). Somewhat increased volume may be necessary and helpful, but not shouting. If one notices that the client

is watching the face intently, it may be an attempt to read lips to compensate for hearing loss. If so, the practitioner needs to face the client when talking. Reviewing frequently, repeating information, and allowing time for questions is recommended. Hurried instructions are likely to be ineffective and lead to client anxiety.

Older adults have their own food myths, as for example, that cheese is causing their constipation. As with others, many elderly are confused by the weekly, changing nutritional messages in the print and visual media (50). They may watch a lot of television and see exposés on "Prime Time Live," "20/20," and "60 Minutes." Every week the news carries the results of medical and nutritional research, often contradictory. They are then unsure of what to eat. A careful dietary history may identify categories of food that are avoided.

Educational programs for older adults should be planned with consideration of the characteristics of older learners. Studies have shown that older adults are able to change their behaviors and continue to learn in their 60s, 70s, and 80s (47). The old adage "You can't teach an old dog new tricks" is not true. The desire to learn is not extinguished in older learners. They may, however, require different learning conditions than younger adults, more modeling by peers, and reinforcement. Active practice is recommended. Making the most of the food dollars, shopping for one, and cooking easy-to-prepare, nutritious food for one are problems they need to solve (44, 48).

The framework for planning, implementing, and evaluating learning discussed elsewhere in the book is the same at all ages. Knowles' principles of "andragogy" also apply (see Chapter 10). Readiness to learn is based on the need to know something, such as the relationship of nutrition to health. Learning should be oriented to the present and to problems, such as menu planning or shopping, that the individual needs to solve, not to facts. One may ask "What would you do if you went on vacation? Ate in a restaurant? Had to read labels in the store? Wanted a snack?" Counseling should recognize the individual's vast prior experience. Many have had experience with dietary regimens already and a lifetime of pleasurable eating.

Since older learners suffer from physiologic, psychological, and social changes, the dietetics professional needs to adapt teaching and learning strategies to enhance learning and memory (47). As people age, memory may decline. The dietetics professional can assist learning by carefully organizing new material to be learned, using more visuals, and helping people to fit new material into their current knowledge networks, as mentioned in another chapter.

The physiological changes associated with long-term illness should also be assessed. Clients with arthritis, cancer, diabetes mellitus, renal disease, and osteoporosis, for example, may have changed their food habits. Lack of appetite may be a problem and the senses of taste and smell may be diminished. Fatigue may come on easily

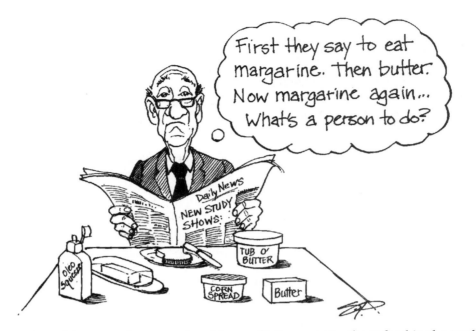

FIGURE 8.3.   Many people are confused by conflicting reports about food in the media.

with little activity. There may be loss of lean body mass as the weight distribution changes to fat (51). The individual may become chronically tired and increasingly immobile. Others, of course, walk every day, run, golf, and are physically active.

Socioeconomic status is likely to change after retirement. People live on fixed incomes and financial problems may occur (48). As time progresses, loss of spouse and/or long-term friends may lead to loneliness and depression. Feelings of lack of control and dependency are possible. Some venture out only during the day and will not attend evening sessions.

Some retirees eat lunch or the "early bird" dinner in restaurants every few days (49). It is a pleasant social event they look forward to. In counseling individuals with diabetes mellitus or hypercholesterolemia, for example, the dietetics practitioner needs to explore where meals are eaten.

Older adults are a heterogeneous group. The challenge is to fight the tendency to stereotype. The dietetics practitioner should not overestimate or underestimate the ability of older learners. When assessment is adequately performed, good teaching and learning can occur (45). Ample time should be allowed with active learner involvement. The result of better functioning and better health status can result.

Examples of nutritional issues facing older adults are the following (44, 48, 50):

Limiting fat, saturated fats, and cholesterol

Increasing fiber intake

Controlling sodium intake

Consuming adequate calcium

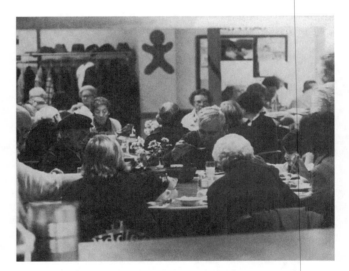

FIGURE 8.4.   Older adults enjoy eating together.

Maintaining energy balance and normal weight

Continuing fluid intake

Avoiding nutrient-drug interactions

Maintaining physical activity

One may recognize that some clients lived through the depression of the 1930s and rationing of food during World War II in the early 1940s. In those less affluent times, they may have learned a great deal about nutrition. They grew up eating a cooked cereal for breakfast instead of a doughnut or sugary cereal.

The risk of drug-nutrient interactions is greater in older adults. Many take self-prescribed over-the-counter medi-

CASE STUDY

Mrs. Hernandez, a 45-year-old Mexican woman, has hypertension. The doctor referred her to Joan Stivers, RD, for counseling about the sodium content of her diet. She cooks a great many ethnic dishes, including tortillas, refried beans, salsa, and the like. But she also eats at fast-food restaurants. Joan is unsure of the ingredients in some of the ethnic dishes mentioned. She wonders about the sodium content.

Question: What should Joan say to find out about Mrs. Hernandez's ethnic cooking practices?

cines, such as aspirin and laxatives, as well as multiple prescription drugs. Many are consumers of vitamin-mineral supplements and may shop at health food stores. There are times when a supplement is appropriate, but not megadosing (51).

Limited Literacy

The mean literacy level in the United Sates is at or below the eighth grade level. As a result, half of the adult population needs easy-to-read print materials (52). People under a great deal of stress also have limited ability to understand and prefer materials that are easy to read.

The poorly educated suffer the highest rates of morbidity and mortality from chronic diseases. As a result, improved communication is necessary. A gap exists between readers and available printed educational materials as well as in information given orally (52). The mismatch between the level of information delivered and the level of client understanding must be eliminated. Many clients with low literacy are also low income. When preparing written materials, one needs to consider segmenting the audience and targeting materials to defined populations. The use of two readability formulas, mentioned in another chapter, to check the level of written information is recommended (52). Resources are available for writing for audiences with limited literacy (53, 54).

Although various needs assessment methods may be used with clients who have limited literacy, focus groups have the advantage over quantitative surveys and questionnaires because of the nondirective process used. Focus groups allow members to offer opinions, insights, comments, and explanations (55).

Twelve focus groups of Expanded Food and Nutrition Education Program (EFNEP) participants, for example, were conducted, with different groups including participants with low literacy skills, teenaged mothers, and Hmong and Cambodian women who did not speak English (55). They thought lectures were an ineffective way to learn nutrition information. Their preference was for hands-on activities that allowed participants to share experiences and ideas. Four barriers mentioned to making changes in eating behaviors were the extra time and money to prepare healthful foods, the possible objection of family members to different recipes and cooking practices, the lack of interest and skill in cooking, and the lack of knowledge of what foods are healthful. Most were interested in recipes and in how fast foods and conve-

nience foods could fit into a healthful diet. They expressed preference for simple, convenient, and affordable ideas.

In all jobs, the dietetics professional may expect to work with a diverse group of clients, patients, employees, other professionals, and audiences. Many nutrition problems exist. The practitioner who has performed a careful assessment of needs is prepared to provide an appropriate nutrition intervention that can improve the quality of life.

REVIEW AND DISCUSSION QUESTIONS

1. Why do dietetics practitioners need to expand beyond knowing their client's eating behaviors and lifestyle habits?
2. What are Campinha-Bacotes' four stages of cultural competence in counseling?
3. How can a dietetics practitioner focus on each family's background and present situation without making assumptions?
4. What is acculturation?
5. How can practitioners anticipate and prepare for identifying the "teachable moment"?
6. What can professionals do to compensate for not speaking the same language as their clients?
7. What does family nutrition counseling involve?
8. What skills does the successful dietetics practitioner/manager need to develop?
9. What will the source of competitive advantage of the 21st century come from?
10. In dealing with children, what factors should be assessed?
11. What educational strategies are recommended for children?
12. In dealing with boys and girls in the adolescent years, what factors should be assessed?
13. What factors may impact on the diet of older adults?
14. What strategies are helpful in educating older adults?

SUGGESTED ACTIVITIES

1. Discuss the stereotypes of older adults as seen in the media, including both advertising and programs.

2. Watch children's programs on television and note what advertising is directed to them.

3. Plan a 15–30-minute presentation on nutritious snacks for fifth graders.

4. Interview a dietetics professional who works with children or adolescents.

5. Interview a dietetics professional who works in a public health nutrition education program.

6. Interview the mother of a child to discuss eating problems and practices.

7. Interview a teenager about eating practices.

8. Interview an older adult (aged 65 or older) about his food intake and nutrition problems. Decide what nutrition intervention you would recommend.

9. This activity is intended to help the participants understand experiences that may have made others feel "included" or "excluded" from a group.

   A. Write the word "Exclude" on a flip-chart. Have the group brainstorm and list on the flip-chart examples of when they or others may have been excluded from a group (i.e., being a minority or in some way being perceived as different from others).

   B. Now write "Include" on the flip-chart. Have the group brainstorm and list on the flip-chart examples of when they or others may have been included in a group (i.e., common interests, shared experiences, etc.).

   C. Using these two lists, discuss how easy or difficult it is to be included in a group or excluded from a group.

   D. After the discussion, ask each person to write a suggestion on actions he, she, or the organization might take to include employees, patients, or clients who may feel excluded from groups in which they must interact.

   E. Volunteers present their suggestions to the group. NOTE: Participants should not use actual names when presenting their suggestions.

REFERENCES

1. Peterson R, Smith J. A patient care team approach to multi cultural patient issues. J Nurs Care Qual 1996;10: 75.

2. Kittler PG, Sucher K. Food and culture in America. Minneapolis: West Publishing, 1995.

3. Bronner Y. Cultural sensitivity and nutrition counseling. Top Clin Nutr 1994;9:13.

4. Newman JM. Melting pot, 2nd ed. New York: Garland Publishing, 1993.

5. Terry RD. Needed: a new appreciation of culture and food behavior. J Am Diet Assoc 1994;94:501.

6. Cross-cultural counseling. Washington, DC: 1986; US Dept of Agriculture, FNS-250.

7. Kreps GL, Kunimoto EN. Effective communication in multicultural health care settings. London: Sage Publications, 1994.

8. Svehla T, Crosier G. Managing the mosaic. New York: American Hospital Publishing, 1994.

9. Geissler EM. Pocket guide: cultural assessment. St Louis: Mosby, 1994.

10. Paniagua FA. Assessing and treating culturally diverse clients. London: Sage Publications, 1994.

11. Sanjur D. Hispanic foodways. Boston: Allyn and Bacon, 1995.

12. Elides DC, Suitor CW. Celebrating diversity. Arlington, VA: National Center for Education in Maternal and Child Health, 1994.

13. Sucher K, Kittler P. Nutrition isn't color blind. J Am Diet Assoc 1991;91:297.

14. Olmstead-Schafer M, Story M, Haughton B. Future training needs in public health nutrition. J Am Diet Assoc 1996;96:282.

15. Keenan DP. In the face of diversity. J Nutr Educ 1996; 28:86.

16. Kittler P, Sucher K. Diet counseling in a multicultural society. Diabetes Educ 1995;16:127.

17. Natow S. Cross-cultural counseling. J Nutr Elderly 1994; 14:23.

18. Hays PA. Addressing the complexities of culture and gender in counseling. J Couns Dev 1996;74:332.

19. Sridaran G, Kolhatkar I. Ethnic food practices of Asia India. Top Clin Nutr 1994;2:45.

20. Wu-Jung, C. Understanding food habit of Chinese Americans. Top Clin Nutr 1994;2:40.

21. Bronner Y, Burke C, Joubert B. African-American/soul foodways and nutrition counseling. Top Clin Nutr 1994; 2:20.

22. Rodriquez J. Diet, nutrition, and the Hispanic client. Top Clin Nutr 1994;2:28.

23. Murphy B, Satterfield D. Diabetes educators as cultural translators. Diabetes Educ 1993;19:113.

24. Monsen R. Editor's outlook. J Am Diet Assoc 1991;91:90.

25. Campinha-Bacote J. The process of cultural competence. Wyoming, OH: Transcultural CARE Associates, 1991.

26. Thiederman S. Overcoming cultural and language barriers. Personnel J 1988;67:34.

27. Storti C. Cross-cultural dialogues. Yarmouth, ME: Smithborne, 1994.

28. Solomon CM. Managing today's immigrants. Personnel J 1993;72:57.

29. Contento I, Balch GI, Bronner YL, et al. Nutrition education for preschool children. J Nutr Educ 1995;27: 291.

30. Worthington-Roberts BS, Williams SR. Nutrition throughout the life cycle, 3rd ed. St Louis: Mosby, 1996.

31. Committee on Nutrition. Pediatric nutrition handbook. Elk Grove Village, IL: American Academy of Pediatrics, 1993.

32. Healthy People 2000: National health promotion and disease prevention objectives. Washington, DC: Superintendent of Documents, 1990; US Dept of Health and Human Services Pub. No (PHS) 91-50213.

33. Position of the American Dietetic Association. Child and adolescent food and nutrition programs. J Am Diet Assoc 1996;96:913.

34. Contento I, Balch GI, Bronner YL, et al. Nutrition education for school-aged children. J Nutr Educ 1995;27: 298.

35. Dwyer J. Focus on family nutrition counseling: new ways to reinforce and extend eating behavior changes. Nutr Update 1991;1:1.

36. Murphy AS, Youatt JP, Hoerr SL, et al. Nutrition education needs and learning preferences of Michigan students in grades 5, 8, and 11. J School Health 1994;64:273.

37. Rickard KA, Gallahue DL, Gruen GE, et al. The play approach to learning in the context of families and schools: an alternative paradigm for nutrition and fitness education in the 21st century. J Am Diet Assoc 1995;95:1121.

38. Evers CL. How to teach nutrition to kids. Tigard, OR: 24 Carrot Press, 1995.

39. McKelvey J, Borgeren M. Family development and the use of diabetes groups: experience with a model approach. Pat Educ Counsel 1990;16:61.

40. Barry B. Games and activities to teach children and diabetes and nutrition. Diabetes Educ 1995;21:27.

41. Connell JE. Pizazz in the pediatric population. Diabetes Educ 1991;17:251.

42. Shannon BM, Tershakovec AM, Martel JK, et al. Reduction of elevated LDL cholesterol levels of 4- to 10-year-old children through home-based dietary education. Pediatrics 1994;94:923.

43. Little L, Achterberg C. Changing the diet of America's children: what works and why? J Nutr Educ 1995;27:250.

44. Boyle MA, Morris DH. Community nutrition in action: an entrepreneurial approach. Minneapolis: West Publishing, 1994.

45. Position of the American Dietetic Association. Nutrition, aging, and the continuum of health care. J Am Diet Assoc 1996;96:1048.

46. Contento L, Balch GI, Bronner YL, et al. Nutrition education for older adults. J Nutr Educ 1995;27:339.

47. Kicklighter JR. Characteristics of older adult learners: a guide for dietetics practitioners. J Am Diet Assoc 1991;91:1418.

48. Magnus MH. What's your IQ on nutrition education for older adults? J Nutr Elderly 1993;12:59.

49. Templeton CL. Nutrition education: the older adult with diabetes. Diabetes Educ 1991;17:355.

50. Lach HW, Dwyer JT, Mann M. P.E.P.: a partnership to assess and modify nutrition behavior in older adults. J Nutr Elderly 1994;13:57.

51. Practical nutritional advice for the elderly, part I: Evaluation, supplements, RDAs. Geriatrics 1990;45:26.

52. Plimpton S, Root J. Materials and strategies that work in low literacy health communication. Public Health Rep 1994;109:86.

53. Shield JE, Mullen MC. Developing health education materials for special audiences: low-literate adults. Chicago: The American Dietetic Association, 1992.

54. Making health communication programs work. Bethesda, MD: National Cancer Institute; 1989. NIH Pub. No 89-1493.

55. Hartman TJ, McCarthy PR, Park RJ, et al. Focus group responses of potential participants in a nutrition education program for individuals with limited literacy skills. J Am Diet Assoc 1994;94:744.

nine

MOTIVATION

A major theme of this book has been the need for dietetics professionals to motivate clients and staff. It is important to acknowledge, however, that motivation is a hypothetical construct, an invented definition that provides a possible concrete causal explanation of behavior (1). Although it is an idea that helps to make sense of human behavior and performance, it cannot be directly measured or validated through the physical or natural sciences. The concept is powerful, the idea of determining the ingredients of influencing the behavior of others. Because the exact nature of motivation cannot be scientifically validated, however, there currently exists a myriad of differing opinions and definitions of motivation in the literature (1).

Applying what is currently known regarding human motivation is, nevertheless, vitally important in setting goals, planning behavior modification strategies, designing and executing educational curriculum and training seminars, counseling others individually or in groups, and defusing hostility or working through conflict situations. Professionals who understand motivational concepts and have the skills to adapt them to particular situations significantly increase their chances for being instrumental and influential in helping others.

Motivation can be defined as something that causes a person to act or the process of stimulating a person to action. It is concerned with the question of why human behavior occurs. The word itself is frequently used to describe those processes that *(a)* arouse and instigate behavior; *(b)* give direction and purpose to behavior; *(c)* continue to allow behavior to persist; and *(d)* lead to choosing or preferring a particular behavior (2). It is concerned not only with what people can do, but also with what they will do. Recent studies appearing among the medical literature indicate continuous and ongoing study into the applications of motivation theory to health care (3–9).

Individuals can be motivated in many ways. Some can motivate themselves, while others must be goaded, threatened, or challenged to act. Those in the first category are referred to as "motivation seekers" and are motivated primarily by the nature of the task or job they perform. Most people, however, need to be stimulated to act, particularly when a change in life-style, diet, or health practices is necessary (10, 11).

Motivation is complex, and there are a number of factors or variables, both intrinsic and extrinsic, that influence the process at any one moment in time. Today's motivational influences may differ from tomorrow's, and short-term goals may take precedence over the long-term ones. Having knowledge of how one should work to get the most accomplished, of what one should eat to become or remain healthy, or of what one should do to cope with a current physiological condition, such as diabetes, may easily be overpowered by other motivational factors. The problem is that being motivated to work, to become or remain healthy, or to learn what one needs for appropriate cardiovascular or diabetes care involves long-term goals, and eating something such as chocolate cake, or coming in late for work "just this once," meets a short-term goal of pleasure. Some people may delay the long-term for the immediate pleasure. Although there is a great deal of knowledge concerning motivation that is helpful, there are no miracle methods or universal answers to difficult motivational problems (2, 12).

Motivation can arise from factors that are either intrinsic or extrinsic, and these factors can affect the individual either positively or negatively. Intrinsic motivation arises from within individuals, owing to their needs, desires, drives, or goals. Individuals who desire to be promoted, for example, have internal goals that motivate their performance. A man who has recently suffered a heart attack may be intrinsically motivated to change his dietary practices. External or extrinsic factors may supplement intrinsic motivation positively, or they may serve as barriers having a negative impact on motivation. Examples of positive external factors enhancing motivation include support from others, praise, or material rewards. An individual's motivation toward achieving dietary goals, however, may be hampered by social occasions or by family or friends who are not supportive and offer improper foods (Fig. 9.1).

Dietetics professionals are involved daily in motivating

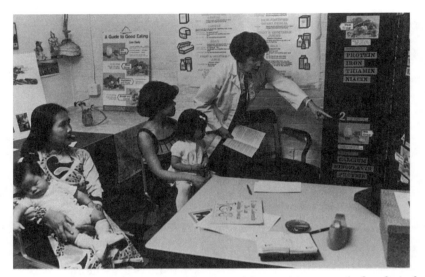

FIGURE 9.1.   Parents may be motivated to provide nutritious meals for their families.

employees and clients, and they need to understand this complicated concept and its multiple processes (13). The dietetics manager influences the motivation of employees, who must learn the procedures necessary to work effectively, do their jobs conscientiously without close supervision, and grow to improve in the work environment. The clinical dietitian must motivate not only staff, but also clients, who may need to learn about such things as the effects of diet on prenatal care, or the problems of sodium, cholesterol, or sugar in the diet. After they have been motivated to learn and to appreciate their problem or situation cognitively, motivation becomes a factor in obtaining their participation in dietary counseling and compliance with a dietary regimen.

This chapter discusses motivation in the three contexts

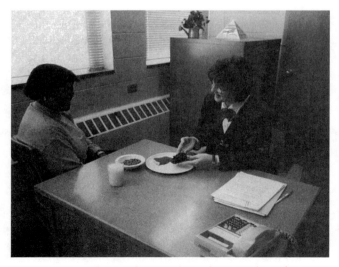

FIGURE 9.2.   The professional needs to explore the motivation of the client.

previously mentioned: as an aid to client compliance, as an aid to teaching, and as an aid to managing staff. Although these three areas are treated separately in the chapter, the same motivational principles and theories apply to all of them.

MOTIVATION OF CLIENTS AND PATIENTS

The goal of nutrition counseling and education is to change food and eating behaviors so that the individuals select healthier diets. Food selection is a part of a complex behavioral system, which is shaped by a vast array of variables. The food selection of children is determined primarily by parents and by the cultural and ethnic practices of their group. Early experiences and continuing interactions with food determine the food preferences, habits, and attitudes exhibited by adults. In addition to the profound role of family and culture in making dietary choices, influences include price of food, prestige value of food, religion, geography, peer and social influences, advertising, facilities, food preparation and storage, skills of the consumer in food preparation, time factors and convenience, and personal preferences and tolerances. All of these factors make food consumption a highly individual matter and resistant to change (14, 15).

In spite of problems associated with changing food behaviors, some people do change. People today are consuming less red meat and eggs than previously, for example. A summary of some of the motivational forces that influence the eating practices of clients is presented in Fig. 9.3. Practitioners and other health educators should consider these factors with their clients and possibly add others from their own experience. More detailed discussion of some of the variables are found in previous chapters (Fig. 9.3).

Knowledge of which foods to consume is a first step in influencing healthful food behaviors, but it is probably

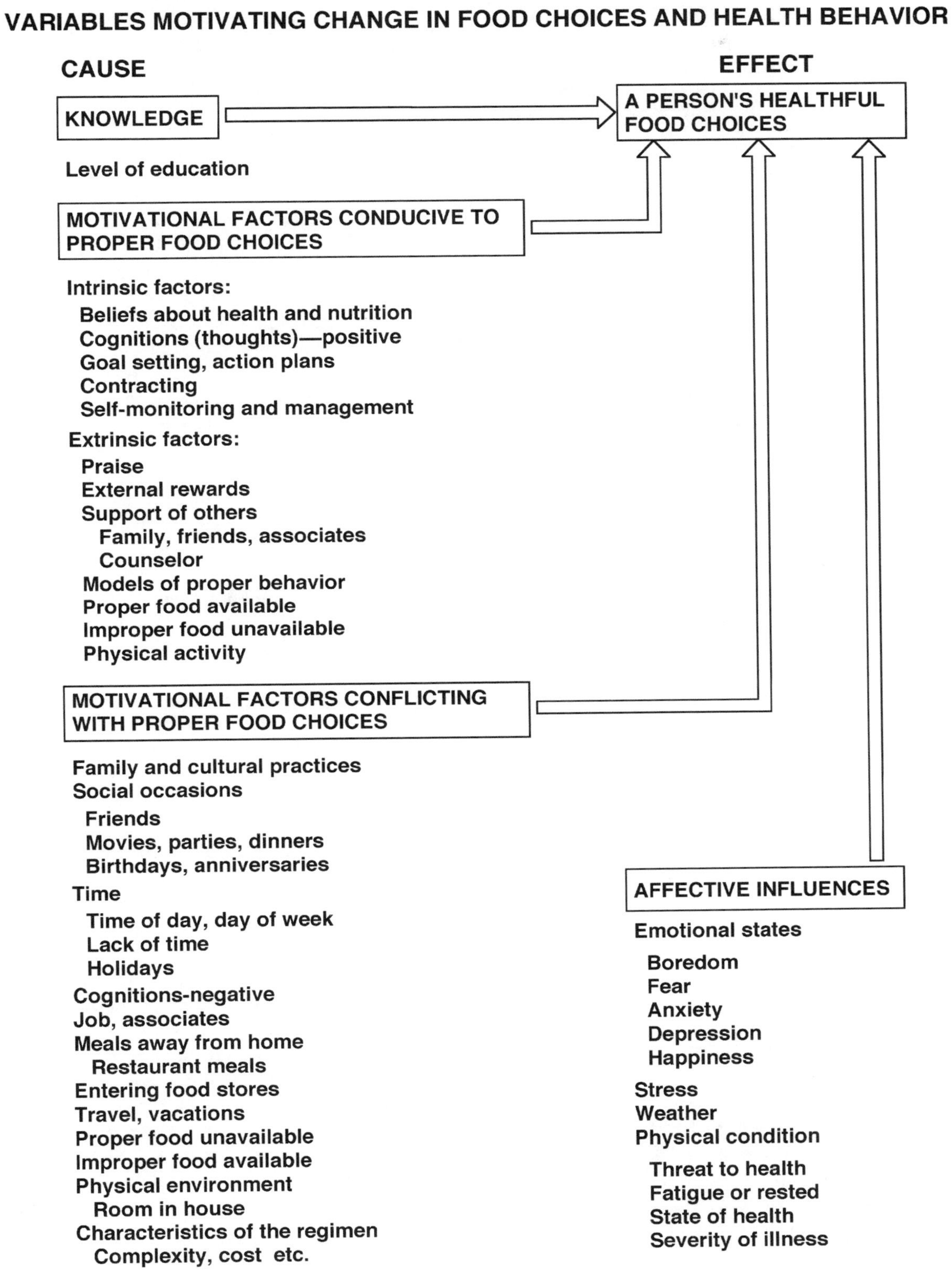

VARIABLES MOTIVATING CHANGE IN FOOD CHOICES AND HEALTH BEHAVIOR

CAUSE

EFFECT

| KNOWLEDGE |

Level of education

| MOTIVATIONAL FACTORS CONDUCIVE TO PROPER FOOD CHOICES |

| A PERSON'S HEALTHFUL FOOD CHOICES |

Intrinsic factors:
  Beliefs about health and nutrition
  Cognitions (thoughts)—positive
  Goal setting, action plans
  Contracting
  Self-monitoring and management

Extrinsic factors:
  Praise
  External rewards
  Support of others
    Family, friends, associates
    Counselor
  Models of proper behavior
  Proper food available
  Improper food unavailable
  Physical activity

| MOTIVATIONAL FACTORS CONFLICTING WITH PROPER FOOD CHOICES |

Family and cultural practices
Social occasions
  Friends
  Movies, parties, dinners
  Birthdays, anniversaries
Time
  Time of day, day of week
  Lack of time
  Holidays
Cognitions-negative
Job, associates
Meals away from home
  Restaurant meals
Entering food stores
Travel, vacations
Proper food unavailable
Improper food available
Physical environment
  Room in house
Characteristics of the regimen
  Complexity, cost etc.

| AFFECTIVE INFLUENCES |

Emotional states
  Boredom
  Fear
  Anxiety
  Depression
  Happiness
Stress
Weather
Physical condition
  Threat to health
  Fatigue or rested
  State of health
  Severity of illness

FIGURE 9.3. Variables motivating change in food choices and health behavior. A given behavior, such as healthful food choices, is affected by more factors than an individual's knowledge of what to do. Level of motivation is influenced by a number of interacting variables, which may differ on a daily basis.

overrated. When people do not follow their diets, some health educators tend to devote more and more time to teaching, redoubling their efforts and assuming that the problem is a deficit in knowledge, rather than exploring other motivational factors that may be more important. The relationship between what people know and what people do or how they behave has been described as a "highly tenuous one," with only a weak relationship, if any, between nutrition knowledge and dietary practices (16). Knowledge does not instigate change, but functions as an instrument if and when people want to make changes (17). Better educated people may rely more on facts and knowledge as motivators for changing behavior than those who are less educated (16).

Other motivational factors, both intrinsic and extrinsic, may encourage changes in food behaviors. People's interest in health, and their beliefs regarding nutrition as a factor in health promotion and disease prevention, may affect food choices. For example, a health belief that food was "good for them" correlated strongly with dietary practices among older women, but less so for those among younger women (14). Positive cognitions such as "Nutrition is important" and "This dietary change is worth the effort" are helpful. Since food's flavor, convenience, and cost are prime motivators of food choices, Hochbaum has suggested that a nutritious diet should offer these advantages, and that these aspects should be stressed more than potential health benefits (17). Dietetics practitioners, therefore, need to overcome the public's perception that nutritious diets are costly, insipid, and inconvenient to purchase and prepare. They must promote the perception that dietary changes are pleasurable and possible. Previous chapters have emphasized the importance of matching the intervention to the client's stage of change and of having clients set one or two short-term goals for change, and have suggested the use of self-monitoring of food intake and written contracts.

Motivation provided by intrinsic factors may be supplemented by extrinsic factors. Praise and material rewards are positive consequences for proper food behaviors, and they may serve to enhance motivation. The support of significant others—family, friends, and the health counselor—is helpful. People who model proper skills can influence others to follow. Needless to say, healthful foods should be made readily available while improper foods should not. Alternative activities, such as physical activity, may also serve to promote change.

In spite of positive motivational and life-style factors, barriers to motivation may arise. Clients should be told to expect problems. The health educator should examine these problems with clients and attempt to reduce or eliminate them. Social occasions, holidays, eating in restaurants, weekend activities, food shopping, and travel require preplanning. A particular time of day, a particular day of the week, or just a lack of time may be barriers to healthful food choices. Problems may also arise from a person's workplace and job associates, and from not having the right foods available. Negative cognitions such as "It's not worth it" and "I'd rather die young and happy than follow this diet" interfere with motivation. Some people discover cues to improper eating in their physical environment, such as in certain rooms of the house. The characteristics of the regimen, such as complexity and cost, are other factors.

Food choices are also influenced by several affective factors involving attitudes, beliefs, and values. Attitudes are thought to be predispositions to action (18). Such emotional states as boredom, anxiety, and depression may lead to eating the wrong food, but so may happiness and elation. Fear of illness or death can be a motivating factor, as can stress and the individual's physical condition. Whether people are tired or rested, whether their medical problem is new or not, the severity of their illness and its perceived threat to health may each influence motivation.

Motivation to make and maintain dietary changes is complex, for behavior is influenced by many motivational factors operating simultaneously. The interrelationships among knowledge, attitudes, and behavior are described as "more intricate than many of the studies of nutrition education acknowledge" (14). While knowledge of proper food choices is an essential first step in changing food behavior, knowledge may be easily overpowered by something that seems more important at the moment. Following a proper diet to promote health and prevent disease is a long-term goal with rewards situated in the future, which may do little to enhance motivation. More immediate rewards may take precedence, such as eating a luscious piece of chocolate cake right now for the pleasure of it.

Nothing is known about the relative importance of each of the variables involved in motivation, the possible interaction of the factors, or the strength of their effect on food selection. Motivational variables directing today's food choices probably differ from tomorrow's and next week's choices, owing to the changes in environmental dynamics. Behavioral change requires a major personal commitment, the setting of goals for change, support from others in one's efforts to modify long-standing practices, and reduction or elimination of barriers in the social, cultural, physical, and psychological environments of the individual. Although studies have focused on knowledge and attitude changes affecting eating practices, few studies have dealt with the complexity of all of the behaviors involved in food selection (17).

MOTIVATION IN TEACHING

Teaching is a job responsibility of most dietetics practitioners, and nutrition education of the public is viewed as an obligation of all practitioners. The clinical practitioner may teach an individual or a group such subjects as proper nutrition practices for senior citizens, recommended prenatal nutrition, preparing nutritious meals on a limited budget, losing weight, and so forth. The administrative dietitian's teaching responsibilities include providing orientation for new employees, training staff in new practices and procedures, and coaching subordinates on a one-on-one basis. One of the keys to successful teaching is learner motivation.

Motivation is complicated and multifaceted. There is no single element that controls success. The best lesson plans, optimal materials, a well-informed and highly motivated dietitian–teacher, and an interesting and current curriculum cannot continuously guarantee that individuals will want to learn (2).

Teachers do not motivate learners directly. They can, however, make learning attractive and stimulating, providing opportunities and incentives, encouraging the development of competence, and matching the learner's interest with learning activities. Because there is no direct line of control between teacher behavior and students' motivation, the intervening variables, including the learners' perceptions, values, personalities, and judgments, ultimately account for their degree of motivation (19).

This section is intended to enhance the professional's teaching and to facilitate learning by focusing on the practical use of knowledge about motivation. Though it is incomplete, the extant knowledge on motivation is considerable and can be applied logically and effectively through careful planning.

Time-Continuum Model of Motivation. Learning situations can be divided according to a three-period time continuum, consisting of a beginning, middle, and end, with motivation being facilitated during each of the stages through a motivational method (2). Wlodkowski discusses the critical periods and the factors that can be applied to motivational strategies within each period (2).

The first critical period (''beginning'') occurs when the learner enters the learning process. Two general motivational factors during this stage are (a) the learner's attitude toward the learning environment, teacher, subject matter, and self, and (b) the learner's needs at the time of learning. Needs are experienced by individuals as forces moving them in the direction of a goal. The second period (''during'') occurs when the person is involved in the body or main content of the learning process. The general motivational factors during this stage are (a) the stimulation process, which affects individuals as they become involved in the learning experience, and (b) the simultaneous affective or emotional experience of the learner. The third period (''ending'') occurs when the person finishes or completes the learning process. The motivational factors during this stage are (a) the sense of competence developed from the person's learning experience, and (b) the quality of the reinforcement that results from the learning experience.

To facilitate motivation, to prevent problems with motivation, and to diagnose potential for motivation in learning situations, the dietetics practitioner needs to understand and evaluate the six factors described in the preceding paragraph as they occur during the critical time periods of a learning event. The following example is intended to illustrate how the multiple motivational factors interact on a dynamic basis to help or hinder motivation along a time continuum (Fig. 9.4).

A woman receiving public assistance may have had little success in working with health professionals and as a result may feel defensive and have a poor ''attitude'' toward the subject matter. This same individual, however, may ''need'' the information the practitioner has to share to feed and properly nourish her family on a limited budget; thus, she may feel some sense of determination to complete the program. At this beginning stage, the practitioner has a client who is not enthusiastic but is willing to ''give it a try.'' If the professional provides material and experiences that are interesting and appropriate, the client may find the class ''stimulating'' and sincerely try to do well. If she enjoys the other participants in the program, and if they work well together in solving mutual problems, she may become even more motivated by the ''affective'' climate. At the end of the program, if the client feels that she has mastered the content and has a sense of confidence and ''competence,'' she will feel encouraged or ''reinforced,'' and will probably continue with this new interest in the future.

One might infer from Fig. 9.4 that the three phases of motivational impact are independent of one another. Wlodkowski points out, however, that the motivational influence constantly interacts with the learner. At the end stage, for example, the competence and reinforcement value interact with the previous factors to affect the learner's motivation at the moment. This interaction results in new attitudes and needs.

Any single motivational factor can have an overwhelming influence on a particular learning situation. The negative influence of one factor may be so powerful that it prevents involvement in learning. Alternatively, the positive influence of a factor may be so strong that it produces a desire to learn that supersedes the possible negative influence of the other factors. For example, a storeroom employee with a negative attitude may refuse to try to learn even though he needs the skills presented in the training for future advancement. The negative attitude may prevail even though he has peers in the course whom he enjoys, has the ability to master the material that is presented in a stimulating way, and knows that he will receive a wage increase upon successful completion. Another employee, whose desire for future advancement is strong, may learn in spite of course material that he believes is useless, instructors whom he experiences as boring, and a sense of isolation between himself and his peers. In most instances, however, influences of the motivational factors are more equally distributed.

Because dietetics professionals generally do not know which of the six factors is going to be the most critical for individuals, they should plan strategies for each factor,

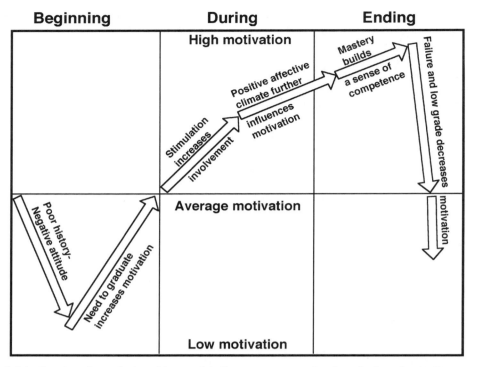

FIGURE 9.4. Model indicating the relationships and influences on motivation during three time periods (Reprinted with permission from Wlodkowski RJ. Motivation and teaching. Washington, DC: Nat Educ Assoc, 1984).

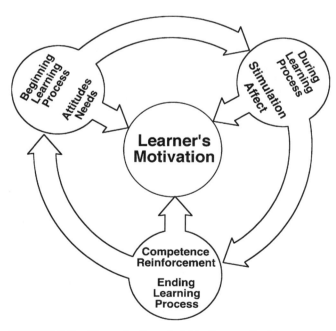

FIGURE 9.5. Organizational aid to be applied to groups of individuals. When the practitioner attends to the six factors, he can, in any learning situation, design motivation strategies for his clients and staff throughout the learning process (Reprinted with permission from Wlodkowski RJ. Motivation and teaching. Washington, DC: Nat Educ Assoc, 1984).

providing continuous and interactive motivational dynamics (Fig. 9.5).

Six basic questions useful in planning a learning experiences are listed below:

1. What can the instructor do to encourage a positive attitude toward the learning situation?
2. What can be done to satisfy an individual's needs through the learning activities?
3. Are there ways to stimulate the individuals continuously while they are learning?
4. What might increase the positive affective or emotional climate for this particular learning activity?
5. How can this learning activity be structured to increase the person's feelings of competence?
6. What reinforcement will this activity provide?

MOTIVATION OF EMPLOYEES

This section explores the concept of motivation as it relates to employees and examines theories of motivation and their behavioral implications for dietetics professionals. Although the concept of motivational forces was defined earlier in this chapter, the reader should keep in mind that the forces instrumental in motivation are usually multiple rather than singular, that they differ in strength, and that more than one may be present at a given time (20).

Maslow and Herzberg

Two theorists who have made major contributions to the study of motivation are Abraham Maslow and Frederick

Herzberg. Maslow correlated human motivation with individual desires. In his "hierarchy of needs" theory and "need-priority" model, he lists five universal needs to explain human motivation: physiological needs; the need for safety and security; social needs; the need for esteem; and the need for self-realization (Fig. 9.4). For each need to become active as a motivating factor, the desire immediately preceding the need must be fulfilled. In simplified terms, Maslow would say that the way to stimulate motivation in individuals is to determine which of their wants is most unsatisfied and then to structure their work so that in the accomplishment of the work goal, they satisfy their personal goals as well (21). Wlodkowski has described Maslow's theory as being the most holistic and dynamic approach offering an interrelated set of guidelines to enhance learner motivation (2) (Fig. 9.6).

The most basic human requirements are physiological. Sickness and hunger tend to take precedence over all other human needs. Only after they are satisfied does one experience the desire to satisfy the other needs. Indigent persons who are able to take care of only their physiological necessities may work regardless of the working conditions for their own and their families' sustenance and shelter. Once they have enough money to satisfy these basic essentials, however, working merely for nourishment and shelter is no longer adequate. At that point, the motivation to work arises from a drive to maintain safety and security. In most organizations today, these needs are satisfied through work contracts, unions, governmental regulations, and various insurance plans. With the fulfillment of biological and security needs, the individual's urge for social affiliation and activity becomes the dominant unsatisfied needs, and they should, therefore, be considered in designing work goals to motivate the employee. Social needs can be experienced as a desire to become a member of, and participate in, a recognized group: family, church, community, work, neighborhood business, union, and so forth. Should this need become satiated, the employees' motivation is stimulated by their desire for esteem and status, which is commonly experienced as the need to attain recognition for accomplishments.

Although each of the five areas of needs becomes dominant at some time, the strongest motivator at a given moment is the one immediately above the last need satisfied. Once the requirement for esteem is no longer lacking, for example, the desire for self-realization will become dominant. Self-realization is the highest human urge and most self-centered. This drive for self-realization and the opportunity to grow as a person can be fulfilled only when most other needs are met. This need is commonly experienced as an urge for personal and professional growth through the work experience.

It is difficult for dietetics practitioners to apply Maslow's theory with any degree of certainty, although social scientists still recognize his hierarchy of needs as fundamental to designing an effective structure to facilitate motivation (22). Unless, however, one has few others reporting to her, the task of getting to know subordinates well enough to infer their current need level accurately is not likely to be accomplished; furthermore, need intensity at each level can vary from day to day, and sometimes from

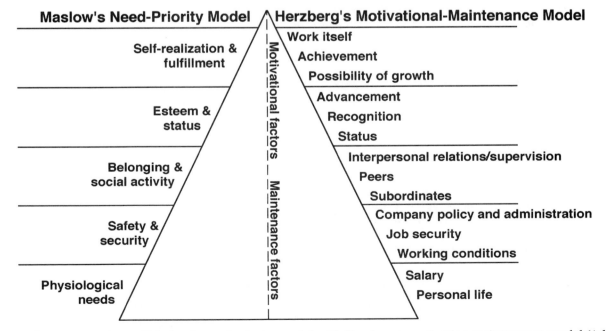

FIGURE 9.6. A comparison of Maslow's need-priority model with Herzberg's motivation-maintenance model (Adapted from Herzberg F. Work and the nature of man. Cleveland, OH: World Publishing Co, 1966; and from Maslow AH. Motivation and personality. New York: Harper and Bros, 1954).

hour to hour. One may be operating at the need level for increased esteem, suddenly have an accident, and become overwhelmingly concerned with the physiological needs of being able to feed the family if one is incapacitated and unable to work. In spite of the limited applications of Maslow's theory, however, it does provide insight into the process of motivation and can often be useful in designing jobs, selecting staff, and developing strategies to maintain enthusiasm and interest among employees.

Frederick Herzberg, a contemporary of Maslow's, is credited with the "two-factor theory of motivation" or the "motivation-maintenance model," which complements Maslow's theory and provides additional perspectives (23). Herzberg reviewed previous theories and studies and attempted to ascertain the essence of motivation by asking employees what they liked about their jobs and what they disliked about their jobs. After examining the data, he determined that the answers to the first question ("What do you like about your job?") were "motivation factors," while the answers to the second question ("What do you dislike about your job?") were what he termed "maintenance factors" (see Fig. 9.6). The five motivators he compiled in response to the first question were *(a)* the work itself, being personally involved in the work, with a sense of responsibility and control; *(b)* achievement, feeling personal accomplishment for having done a job well; *(c)* growth, experiencing the opportunity for challenge in the job and the chance to learn skills and knowledge; *(d)* advancement, knowing that the experience and growth will lead to increased responsibility and control; and *(e)* recognition, being recognized for doing a job well, resulting in increased self-esteem (24).

Herzberg called the answers to the second question maintenance factors because he found that they maintained but did not improve current levels of production. Maintenance factors were physical conditions, e.g., lighting in the office and food in the cafeteria; security, a feeling of certainty about the future and of contentment; economic factors, salary and fringe benefits; and social factors, relationships with fellow workers and the boss.

Herzberg found that when the maintenance factors were poor, productivity decreased. Inadequate maintenance factors, then, hindered production while adequate maintenance factors only maintained the current level. Thus, maintenance factors merely "satisfy" workers; they do not motivate them. Although Herzberg's theory first gained prominence in the 1960s, it remains the basis for current research in the area of motivation (25). As indicated in Fig. 9.6, Herzberg's motivational factors are similar to those at the top of Maslow's "need priority" model, and his maintenance factors are toward the bottom of Maslow's model.

CONTEMPORARY THEORIES OF MOTIVATION

The theories of Maslow and Herzberg are well known but have not consistently been validated empirically. Several contemporary theories, however, do have a reasonable degree of valid supporting documentation. They are called "contemporary theories" not because they are only recently developed but because they represent the current state of the art in explaining employee motivation.

David McClelland's Theory of Needs

David McClelland's theory of needs focuses on three needs: achievement, power, and affiliation. Some people are driven by the need to excel, to achieve in relation to a set of standards, to strive to succeed; others are driven by a need for power, the desire to make others behave in a way that they would not otherwise have behaved in; still others are driven by a need for affiliation, the desire for friendly and close interpersonal relationships. McClelland suggests that determining an employee's major need structure is key in fitting that person into the right position. Although this is somewhat oversimplified, the theory posits that persons with high achievement needs might do particularly well managing themselves in sales for example, but would not necessarily do well in management positions. Persons with high needs for power and recognition, however, would more likely be suited for management. Persons whose primary needs are in the affiliation area are the best suited for helping professions.

Although McClelland has conducted studies in the three need areas, most of the studies have concentrated in the area of achievement. McClelland has determined that high achievers prefer job situations with personal responsibility, feedback, and an intermediate degree of risk. When these characteristics are prevalent, high achievers will be strongly motivated. A high need to achieve does not necessarily lead to being a good manager, especially in large organizations. People with high achievement needs are interested in how well they do personally and not in influencing others to do well (26–29).

One promising phenomenon of McClelland's achievement theory is that employees have been successfully trained to stimulate their achievement need. Motivation specialists have been successful in teaching individuals to think in terms of accomplishments, winning, and success, as well as helping them to alter behavior so as to act in a high achievement way by preferring situations where they have personal responsibility, feedback, and moderate risks. Human resource professionals are optimistically hoping to learn that management can select a person with a high achievement need or develop its own candidate through achievement training (30).

Equity Theory

Equity theory is based on the belief that individuals compare their inputs and outcomes with those of others and then respond so as to eliminate any inequities. Employees might compare themselves to friends, neighbors, co-workers, colleagues in other organizations, or past jobs they themselves have had. Which referent an employee chooses will be influenced by the information the employee holds about referents as well as by the attractiveness of the referent. If a dietetics practitioner, for example, were hired right out of college with a fair salary, challenging work, and an excellent opportunity to gain important experience, she would most likely be motivated to excel in her position until and unless someone she viewed as less competent was also hired to do the same work but for more money.

Based on equity theory, when employees perceive an inequity they can be predicted to make one of six choices (30, 31):

1. Change their inputs (i.e., stop exerting as much effort).

2. Change their outcomes (i.e., individuals paid on a piece-rate basis can increase their pay by producing a higher quantity of units of lower quality).

3. Distort perceptions of self (for example, "I used to think I worked at a moderate pace but now I realize that I work a lot harder than everyone else").

4. Distort perceptions of others (for example, "Mary's job isn't as desirable as I previously thought it was").

5. Choose a different referent (for example, "I may not make as much as my brother-in-law, but I'm doing a lot better than my dad did when he was my age").

6. Leave the field (for example, quit the job) (30).

The primary distinction of equity theory is its contention that individuals are concerned not only with the absolute amount of rewards they receive for their efforts, but also with the relationship of this amount to what others receive. They make judgments as to the relationship between their inputs and outcomes and the inputs and outcomes of others. When individuals infer an imbalance in their outcome-input ratio relative to others, tension is created. It is this tension that provides the basis for motivation, as people strive for what they perceive as equity and fairness.

Expectancy Theory

The expectancy theory, formulated by Victor Vroom, is based on the belief that the strength of a tendency to act in a certain way depends on the strength of an expectation that the act will be followed by a given outcome and on the attractiveness of that outcome to the individual. Currently expectancy theory is one of the most widely accepted explanations of motivation. Although it has its critics, most of the research evidence is supportive of the theory (32, 33).

Expectancy theory would suggest that an employee is motivated to exert a high level of effort when he or she believes effort will lead to a good performance appraisal; a good appraisal will lead to organization rewards like a bonus, a salary increase, or a promotion; and the rewards will satisfy the employee's personal goals.

Three relationships are focused on in this theory.

1. Effort-performance relationship: The probability perceived by the individual that exerting a given amount of effort will lead to performance.

2. Performance-reward relationship: The degree to which the individual believes that performing at a particular level will lead to the attainment of a desired outcome.

3. Rewards-personal goals relationship: The degree to which organizational rewards satisfy an individual's personal goals or needs and the attractiveness of those potential rewards for the individual (30).

Expectancy theory can be a useful tool in understanding why some dietetics employees are not motivated on their jobs and merely do the minimum necessary to get by. If, for example, an employee's motivation is to be maximized, an affirmative answer would be required for the three questions below:

1. If I give a maximum effort, will it be recognized in my performance appraisal?

2. If I get a good performance appraisal, will it lead to organization rewards?

3. If I'm rewarded, are the rewards personally attractive to me?

If the answer to any question is negative, less than maximum effort could be predicted according to the theory.

This chapter has attempted to provide a brief background on numerous theories of motivation. Attempts to validate most theories, however, have been complicated by methodological, criterion, and measurement problems. As a result, many published studies that purport to support or negate a theory must be viewed with caution.

Motivation Through Enhancement of Self-Esteem

Key issues of the early 21st century are the attraction and retention of skilled workers. Shortages of human talent, rather than surpluses, will characterize United States business during the early part of the new century. As a result of the baby boom, those born between 1945 and 1964, and the following baby bust, there may be fewer entrants to the job market in the early 21st century. There may not be enough workers in the small cohort of people born in the 1964–1975 period to fill the bottom level of the typical corporate pyramid. The majority of the work force today is composed of baby boomers and their children or younger brothers and sisters. Both groups tend to define success in terms of power, prestige, and money, and this definition is generally supported by senior management as well. Managers face a challenge in responding creatively to these new demographics, and a major concern of the contemporary manager is to understand the new workforce and how to adapt its needs to those of the organization (34, 35).

Another employment issue results from the fact that the number of highly qualified people in the workforce is growing at a much faster rate than is the number of senior-level jobs. Consequently, supervisors must understand how to spot the plateau problem and deal with it effectively before the employees have no alternative but to quit the organization. The worker who has hit a career plateau suffers from losses in productivity and/or self-esteem. When employees' careers have reached a plateau and the company does not want to lose them, the company can redefine success so that the sense of having hit a plateau does not arise (36–38). Success can be redefined, for example, through various forms of public recognition, such as company awards, plaques, and so forth.

A third reality of the early 21st century, particularly in the health professions, is that organizations will have to continue to maintain as lean and as motivated a staff as possible to compete and to comply with governmental regulations. In the process of becoming "lean" by eliminating, "downsizing," "right-sizing," and combining as many positions as possible, those staff members who have survived may feel insecure, defensive, hostile, and fearful of losing their jobs, and may object to having had their former positions changed or enlarged without any monetary compensation. They may be unwilling to extend themselves because of the inference that the organization does not care about them. The manager or supervisor who is attempting to "motivate" staff under these conditions has a considerable challenge. While monetary increases are being kept to a minimum, the manager is expected to obtain more work from fewer people, who are already feeling unappreciated and overworked. Given this depressing but not unrealistic scenario, the manager needs to know and to exercise every motivational option available.

Many members of the current workforce differ from their predecessors. Recent surveys indicate that baby boomers' values are distinctly different from those of their parents (39–41). These younger employees generally are more affluent and educated, and are less willing to rely on authority figures. They have different perceptions of themselves and are generally unwilling to tolerate a disrespectful supervisory style. What today's workers indicate they want most are a heightened sense of self-esteem, realization, recognition, autonomy, responsibility, and managers who recognize their capacity for these achievements (42–45). Although some employees can always be motivated by the hope of merit salary increases, contemporary managers will benefit most from enhancing their staff's self-esteem and confidence as the prime method of increasing motivation to perform competently (46–48).

A great deal is known about the relationship between motivation and increased self-esteem or recognition. For more than half a century, social scientists have been aware of the phenomenon of the "self-fulfilling prophecy," which suggests that people perform and develop according to others' expectations of them. In one study, students and instructors were selected randomly, and some instructors were told that they had been selected to have all the brighter students in their classes. These instructors had students who performed statistically and significantly better than those in classes where instructors had no previous expectations (49). Individuals who are told that they are incompetent and will be unable to achieve a specific goal or task perform poorly as compared with those who are told that they are competent and will be able to achieve the task, even though neither group has had previous experience with the task. An individual's self-perceived ability, based on previous performance, is positively related to later performance. Success begets success, and failure begets failure (42).

Unfortunately, an appreciation of the implications of this phenomenon for business and industry has only recently become apparent. Whenever supervisors acknowledge success in subordinates, they add to the likelihood that subsequent tasks will be performed successfully. For this reason, supervisors need to select carefully the right worker for the task, to provide adequate training to ensure employee success, and to assign work tasks that are manageable and accomplishable.

Managers can enhance the self-esteem of employees by providing opportunities for their achievement, growth, recognition, responsibility, and control, which increase their motivation to improve or to continue to do well. Several specific suggestions are described in the following paragraphs. They include involving employees in decision making, showing them respect, building their confidence, providing them with achievement experiences, increasing their personal and professional growth, and sharing time with them.

Dietetics managers must seek opportunities to observe and acknowledge their staff performing tasks properly. Employees are motivated when their esteem is enhanced through recognition of their work. Once employees know what is expected of them, positive strokes for good performance yield more positive performance (50). The manner in which the work is recognized is a major factor in motivating employees. Simply saying "good job," for example, may be better than no comment at all, but it is not nearly as effective as a specific comment, such as, "the kitchen has never looked so organized. You did a splendid job of rearranging the storage cabinets." Needless to say, frequent reinforcement must be honest and must not sound patronizing.

Staff members can be motivated when they sense personal growth through their work. Learning new skills and exercising judgments can be motivating. When practitioners believe staff members are competent enough to succeed at special assignments—those that are perceived as "job enrichment" and that offer opportunities to develop skills—and they allow the employees adequate time to perform the new task successfully, they are, in fact, motivating them. Notice the qualifying comments in the preceding statement. A staff member should be selected only when the chances of success are high. Asking employees to perform tasks for which they are not prepared may decrease motivation. Adequate resources and time are critical to success.

Somewhat similar to the motivational effect of assigning special projects to staff is delegating responsibilities that had formerly been the supervisor's. When such assignments are made, it is important that they be given to employees who will not resent the added responsibility, but will see it as it is intended—a form of recognition.

Taking the time to interact with employees on a person-to-person basis and listening to their comments about their work can be motivating when the employee perceives such interaction as a sign of respect and caring. The professional may be busy and prefer to go on working without acknowledging the employee; however, just as being listened to is motivating, being ignored is nonmotivating and demoralizing.

When employees make suggestions that the manager intends to consider, writing them down in the presence of the employee acknowledges that intention and decreases the possibility of the comments being forgotten. As with the other motivational strategies, however, the motivational potential of this technique will be short-lived if the employee interprets it as manipulation. When dietetics managers write down a suggestion, the expectation is that within a reasonable time, they will act on it. Accumulating and ignoring a drawer full of such suggestions will eventually discourage motivation in employees.

Acknowledging the feelings of employees who are obviously unhappy or excited is a way of showing caring respect, as is recognizing important events in employee's lives. Attending funerals or sending flowers and greeting cards for specific occasions can be motivating if the employee perceives such acts as genuine signs of respect and recognition. Engaging in small talk with subordinates, visiting with them for a few minutes, and asking about their families or commenting on new clothes all tend to go beyond the content of the message and express caring and acceptance of the employee.

Documenting some exceptional success provides the employee with a sense of recognition among the entire staff. For example, sending copies to the organization's director of a letter sent from a grateful client who comments on the work of an employee, and pinning a copy on the bulletin board, can provide recognition and build esteem.

If there is occasion to support the actions of subordinates and defend them to others in the organization, the dietetics manager should do so. All organizations have informal communication grapevines, and employees will eventually hear that their supervisor extended herself on their behalf. Such actions have the potential to motivate many others as well, who, seeing themselves as members of the department's team, may vicariously feel defended as well.

The rationale for involving staff in decision making is discussed in detail in another chapter. When staff are consulted by their supervisor and involved in a decision, they not only tend to gain confidence from the experience, but also are motivated through the supervisor's appreciation of their worth.

Maintaining a motivated staff must be viewed as an ongoing process, and one that can be reinforced frequently through the quality of the professionals' and employees' interaction. The dietetics managers' admitting when they are wrong, for example, and saying to subordinates, "You are right," are actions that acknowledge respect for the subordinate. When problems arise in an employee's performance, the manner in which the assistance is offered or the employee is questioned is significant. Showing constructive concern in explaining the error adds to the employee's self-esteem; belittling, humiliating, or embarrassing an employee, especially in front of peers, diminishes it. Physical contact with subordinates can indicate caring and enhance self-esteem. Shaking hands with employees or patting them on the back for a job well done are examples of human respect, caring, and affection, not sexual harassment. Many of the foregoing suggestions may seem obvious and simple, but it is their frequent absence that erodes the self-esteem of employees and inhibits their motivation to improve.

High turnover rates, mediocre performance, and chronic absenteeism are symptoms of the erosion of self-esteem and the inability of supervisors to develop it in staff. Several supervisors, with whom one of the authors was working as a managerial consultant, were asked whether they would be willing to make a special effort to give recognition, or a word of praise, to one of their workers for something he did well. Although they all claimed to be willing to do this, a subsequent meeting of the group found that none carried out the assignment. The reasons given included, "You just don't praise men," "Workers will think you are setting them up for something," and "It's a sign of weakness to praise people for what they do." One group member acknowledged that he simply did not know how to give praise.

Smiling and looking pleasant can also be a factor in maintaining a supportive relationship with staff. Employees cannot read the dietetics manager's mind, so if she looks angry and upset, the natural tendency is for employees to infer that they, the employees, have somehow caused the unpleasant expression. Supervisors need to monitor their nonverbal behavior so that it does not suggest negative messages unintentionally. When the supervisor is genuinely upset and subordinates are not at fault, they should be reassured that they are not the reason for her negative demeanor.

Providing employees with new equipment or other resource materials is another way to show confidence in their abilities, and it reinforces the impression that the practitioner wants them to succeed. Dietetics managers should try to learn from the employees themselves what they believe they need to work more efficiently. Whenever possible, employees should be provided with the resources requested.

A way to acknowledge excellence in subordinates is to ask them to share their knowledge by teaching others. Giving the employee an assignment to train a new staff member, for example, is a form of recognition and a sign of confidence. Deferring to subordinates at meetings by asking them to explain procedures and solve problems accomplishes this as well.

Keeping and being on time for appointments with subordinates, notifying them well in advance if an appointment cannot be kept, and generally respecting the employee's time are signs of respect. Giving employees sufficient time to understand a particular procedure or set of directions, rather than leaving them feeling confused and insignificant, also adds to their perceptions of the supervisor's regard for them.

Motivation Through Setting Goals

Too often, subordinates believe that they are pleasing their supervisors only to learn that what they were doing was not what was desired or expected. When giving instructions, the manager should select language that is specific in meaning. Telling an employee to "work hard," to "be sincere," to "be confident," to "be conscientious," to "show cooperation," or to "maintain an open-minded point of view" are examples of vague instructions that could confuse employees and cause them to fail. Telling an employee to "type a letter," "interview a patient," "conduct a performance appraisal," "investigate an accident," "ask questions," or "come to work on time" are examples of specific instructions that encourage success by allowing the employees to know exactly what is being asked of them (42).

One of the most damaging on-the-job sources of stress is the absence or delay of feedback on one's performance (42, 51). Setting goals with subordinates as well as following up with subsequent periodic reviews provides feedback and promotes improved performance. Telling an employee, "Do your best," is useless. To the employee, who is faced with numerous alternatives for ways to spend his "working" time, this instruction can mean dozens of things. Setting goals complements the theories of Maslow and Herzberg. An effective way to assist others who wish to increase their esteem, growth, development, realization, and achievement is to teach them to be proactive in planning specific ways to accomplish more or to improve quality by setting goals.

The effect of setting goals on individual performance has been demonstrated. Theory and experiments support the proposition that supervisors should play an active role in setting goals with subordinates. Goals should be specific, clearly stated, and measurable. When they fulfill these conditions, they provide a criterion for feedback, accountability, and evaluation. An individual can be highly motivated by knowing the objective and working on a plan with the dietetics manager to accomplish it. The three identifiable elements in goal setting are (a) an action verb, (b) a measurable result, and (c) the cost and/or date by which the objective will be accomplished. It is essential for both the employee and manager to agree on their mutual expectations, to clarify the difference, for example, between "I want you to get your work done soon," and "I want to see an increase of 10% by June 16th." Perhaps the single most significant advance in the field of management has been the growth of participative management. A major advantage of goal setting, a form of participative management, is that it directs work activities toward organizational goals and forces planning (52).

Individuals who have specific and challenging goals tend to perform best. Goals seen as "sure things" may discourage motivation as much as those that are believed to be impossible. The best goals—the ones that inspire quality performance—are those that are perceived as difficult and challenging but attainable. A major proposition, supported experimentally, is that employees who set or accept harder goals perform at levels superior to those who set or accept easier goals (53, 54).

Regardless of whether the goal is actually set by the manager or the employee, the two parties need to agree. When staff members feel that they are actively participating in setting their own goals, even if the goals are originally proposed by the supervisor, they are more solidly motivated to perform with distinction than if they feel that they are merely being told what to do (55). For the process to work, however, employees must trust their supervisors. When employees feel used, or when they feel that the goals are a means of exploiting them, they tend to resist the goals.

Motivation Through Reinforcement

Reinforcement, or knowing how to encourage desirable behavior and to discourage undesirable behavior, is related to motivation. One way to increase the likelihood that a performance or behavior will recur is to follow the performance with a positive event. A positively reinforced response has a greater probability of recurring simply because it pays off. Most of the suggestions in the previous sections on motivation through enhancement of self-esteem and recognition are examples of positive reinforcement.

Another type of reinforcement is the removal of something negative after the performance. In this case, the persons are likely to repeat the behavior because something they dislike is taken away as a consequence of the behavior. This removal or elimination of adverse conditions is referred to as negative reinforcement. A hospital dishwasher, for example, who is constantly being checked by the manager and who has been able to decrease dish breakage by 30% from the previous month, will be motivated to continue improving if the manager checks this employee less often during the following week. The manager, then, can encourage the desired ac-

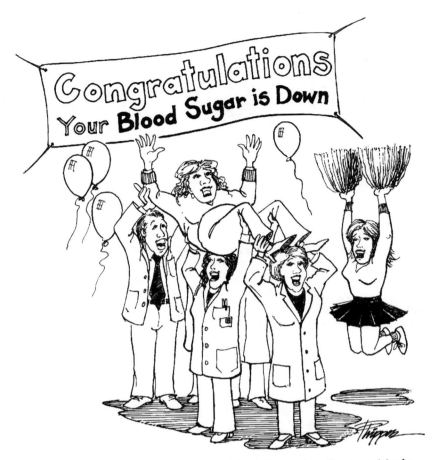

FIGURE 9.7. The counselor should reinforce the client positively.

tion by removing an unfavorable condition, the frequent inspections.

Two strategies that may discourage a given behavior are punishment and extinction. Reprimanding an employee for being late is an example of formal punishment. Although punishment is often used to eliminate undesirable behavior, its value is questionable because of its negative side effects. Punishment can make an employee hostile and prone to retaliation. If the punishment is perceived as unwarranted by the employees, they may resume the undesirable behavior as soon as punishment stops. The way to overcome the employee's feelings of resentment when punished is to provide frequent constructive feedback each time an infraction occurs. In that way, when formal punitive action is taken, it is perceived by the employee as warranted and rational.

The other basic technique for decreasing the likelihood of a behavior is extinction. With extinction, the undesirable performance is neither punished nor rewarded; it is simply ignored. Ignored behaviors tend to diminish, and ultimately to become extinguished, as a result of a consistent lack of reinforcement. For example, a manager who never acknowledges an employee's suggestions is actually encouraging the employee to stop sending them. Although its use may be unintentional, extinction is an effective technique for terminating behavior. A manager should be aware of the potentially negative consequences of ignoring desired behavior. Motivated performances can be unintentionally extinguished by managers through carelessness.

Summary of Recommendations. Managers should give recognition to the employees in the presence of their peers. Recognition provides positive feedback and builds a worker's confidence and self-esteem. Organizations can benefit from involving their employees in the decision-making process. The more employees are involved, the higher the level of their performance and satisfaction. Employees who participate in making decisions feel a sense of ownership and commitment.

Administrators at all levels lessen stress and increase efficiency and motivation when they provide employees with clearly defined goals and objectives. The more employees understand what they are expected to do, the more highly motivated they become. Supervisors should give respect and dignity to their staff. The more they respect the rights and privileges of employees, the better the employees feel about themselves and the more they produce. Managers must become familiar with reinforcement techniques, training themselves to recognize and comment on good work in order to reinforce it. Ignoring

CASE STUDY

Joan Stivers, RD, has been invited to present a class on nutrition to mothers of elementary school children. Her presentation will be about an hour long. She assumes that some degree of motivation toward the subject exists, but is concerned to enhance motivation toward healthy food choices for all family members.

1. What can she do to encourage a positive attitude toward the learning situation?
2. What can be done to satisfy individual needs?
3. How can the learning activities be structured to increase the mothers' feeling of competence?

good work may lead to extinction of desired behavior. Top management needs to instill in lower-level management an appreciation of the human resources of the organization, supporting the development of increased self-esteem, recognition, and growth among all staff.

This chapter has emphasized the complexity of motivation and has discussed its behavior implications for dietetics professionals. Practitioners are involved daily with motivation of both staff and clients. Understanding motivational concepts and being able to employ the strategies and techniques associated with them can add immeasurably to the professional's effectiveness.

REVIEW AND DISCUSSION QUESTIONS

1. What processes is the word "motivation" used to describe?

2. Give an example of positive external factors that enhance motivation.

3. Explain intrinsic motivation.

4. Why should clients be told to expect problems?

5. Why is it impossible for teachers to motivate learners directly?

6. What are the critical periods of motivation?

7. What are the factors within each period?

8. List Maslow's need-priority model.

SUGGESTED ACTIVITIES

1. List the factors that motivate you to go to work or to continue with your present job. Explain your reactions in terms of the Maslow and Herzberg models.

2. Interview someone who is on a diet, and determine the positive and negative influences for motivation that have resulted from adherence to it. Discuss your interview and data using the variables motivating change in food choices and health behavior model presented in the chapter (see Fig. 9.1).

3. Examine the forces that motivate you to learn something new. Are they related to your desire to remain physically well, secure, well-liked and respected, or are they related to your desire to prepare yourself for taking on additional responsibility, having more control, and achieving realization and actualization?

4. Indicate why the following statements would have a negative impact on an employee's motivation and how they might be amended so that they maintain the employee's self-esteem.
   A. That job has been done incorrectly! What do I have to do to get you to understand?
   B. I'm tired of listening to you complain. Just keep still and do your job.
   C. You will probably make a mess of this, but there isn't anyone else to do it.
   D. If you would listen, you would understand.
   E. You can't be serious about that suggestion.

5. For each of the following examples, list the reinforcement technique used and the feelings it might produce in the employee.
   A. Employee: Mrs. Jones, since you told us to be on the lookout for problems with equipment, we have discovered two more.
      Dietetics professional: Yes, but I'm looking for Helen now. Have you seen her?
   B. Employee: Mrs. Jones, I've finished all the work in the kitchen and have begun to rearrange the cabinets.
      Dietetics professional: You mean it took you all this time just to do that?
   C. Dietetics professional: Mary, I am putting you on suspension for 3 days.
   D. Dietetics professional: Mary, I want you to know that I appreciate how effectively you work with others. Several people have told me how thorough you are in using the new procedures.

REFERENCES

1. Wlodkowski RJ. Strategies to enhance adult motivation to learn. In: Galbraith MW, ed. Adult learning methods. Malabar, FL: Krieger Publishing Co, 1990.
2. Wlodkowski RJ. Motivation and teaching. Washington, DC: Nat Educ Assoc, 1986.
3. Hoban JD, Cariaga LL, Bennett BB, et al. Incentives for teaching. Acad Med 1996;71:106.
4. Misener TR, Haddock KS, Gleaton JU, et al. Toward an international measure of job satisfaction. Nurs Res 1996; 45:87.
5. Lima-Basto M. Implementing change in nurses' professional behaviors: limitations of the cognitive approach. J Adv Nurs 1995;22:480.

6. Santurno PJ. Training health professionals to implement quality improvement activities. Int J Qual Health Care (England) 1996;7:119.

7. Armstrong ML, Clark DW, Stuppy DJ. Motivational orientations of urban and rural based RNs. J Nurs Staff Dev 1996;11:131.

8. Borgio JP. Motivation. J Emerg Med Serv 1995;20:74.

9. McConnell TR. Motivating your staff. Leadership Health Serv (Canada) 1996;4:25.

10. Peckos PS. Stimulating the patient in self-motivation. J Am Diet Assoc 1972;61:423.

11. Harris P, Hewitt C, Jones NH. Motivating staff; the pain free week. Am J Nurs 1996;96:23.

12. Burnstein JC, Gollwitzer PM. Effects of failure on subsequent performance: the importance of self-defining goals. J Personal Soc Psychol 1996;70:395.

13. Proch ML. Creating a climate to promote internal motivation in employees. J Nurs Admin 1996;25:5.

14. Krondl M, Lau D. Social determinants in human food selection. In: Baker LM, ed. The psychobiology of human food selection. Westport, CT: AVI Publishing Co, 1982.

15. Gilbert DT, Silvera DH. Overhelping. J Personal Soc Psychol 1996;70:678.

16. Hochbaum GM. Behavior and education. In: Levy R, Rifkind B, Dennis B, et al., eds. Nutrition, lipids, and coronary heart disease. New York: Raven Press, 1979.

17. Hochbaum GM. Strategies and their rationale for changing people's eating habits. J Nutr Educ 1981;13:S59.

18. Johnson DW, Johnson RT. Nutrition education's theoretical foundation. J Nutr Educ 1985;17:S8.

19. Kachroo R. Motivational theory in the work environment. Hosp Cost Mgmt Account 1996;7:1.

20. Owen AV. Management for doctors: getting the best from people. Br Med J (England) 1996;310:648.

21. Maslow AH. Motivation and personality. New York: Harper and Bros, 1954.

22. Clark K. Simply motivate. Industr Soc 1989;22:26.

23. Herzberg F. Work and the nature of man. Cleveland: World Publishing Co, 1966.

24. Kivimaki M, Voutilainen P, Koskinen P. Job enrichment, work motivation, and job satisfaction in hospital wards. J Nurs Mgmt (England) 1996;3:87.

25. Herzberg F. Innovation: where is the relish. J Creative Behav 1987;21:179.

26. McClelland DC. The achieving society. New York: Van Nostrand Reinhold, 1961.

27. McClelland DC. Power; the inner experience. New York: Irvington, 1975.

28. McClelland DC, Winter DG. Motivating economic achievement. New York: Free Press, 1969.

29. McClelland DC. Toward a theory of motive acquisition. Am Psychol 1965;10:321.

30. Robbins SP. Organizational behavior, 7th ed. Englewood Cliffs, NJ: Prentice Hall, 1996.

31. Vecchio RP. Models of psychological inequity. Organizat Behav Hum Perform 1984;10:266.

32. Vroom VH. Work and motivation. New York: Wiley, 1964.

33. Heneman HG, Schwab DP. Evaluation of research on expectancy theory prediction of employee performance. Psychol Bull 1979;12:1.

34. Wendling W. Responses to a changing work force. Personnel Admin 1988;33:50.

35. Sandroff R. What managers need to know about the hiring crisis of the '90's. Work Wom 1989;14:92.

36. Little K. The baby boom generation: confronting reduced opportunities. Employ Relat Today 1989;16:57.

37. Modic S. Motivating without promotions. Indust Week 1989;238:24.

38. Karp H. Supervising the plateaued worker. Supervis Mgmt 1989;34:35.

39. Mills D, Cannon M. Managing baby boomers. Mgmt Rev 1989;78:38.

40. Blanchard M. Motivating people to top performance. Exec Excell 1989;6:11.

41. Welter T. New-collar workers. Indust Week 1988;237:36.

42. Rosenbaum BL. How to motivate today's workers. New York: McGraw-Hill, 1982.

43. Wiegand R. The care and nurture of the company yuppie. Bus Horiz 1988;31:62.

44. Ahmadian A. Motivation: in search of a better way. J Human Behav Learn 1987;4:17.

45. Kiechel W. The workaholic generation. Fortune 1989;119:50.

46. Knippen J, Green TB. Building self-confidence. Supervis Mgmt 1989;34:22.

47. Penzer E. How to motivate a small staff. Incentive 1989;163:186.

48. Pierce JL, Gardner DG, Cummings LL, et al. Organization-based self-esteem: construct definition, measurement, and validation. Acad Mgmt J 1989;32:622.

49. Rosenthal R, Jacobson L. Pygmalion in the classroom. New York: Rinehart and Winston, 1968.

50. Richardson HL. Communicate through listening. Transport Distr 1989;30:32.

51. Larson JR, Jr. The dynamic interplay between employees' feedback-seeking strategies and supervisors' delivery of performance feedback. Acad Mgmt Rev 1989;14:408.

52. Boissoneau R. New approaches to managing people at work. Health Care Superv 1989;7:67.

53. Sherman A, Bohlander G, Snell S. Managing human resources, 10th ed. Cincinnati: South-Western Publ, 1996.

54. Quick TL. The best-kept secret for increasing productivity. Sales Market Mgmt 1989;141:34.

55. Mia L. The impact of participation in budgeting and job difficulty on managerial performance and work motivation: a research note. Account Organizat Soc 1989;14:347.

ten

PRINCIPLES AND THEORIES OF LEARNING

How do people learn? How do they retain what they learn? The field of educational psychology studies questions about learning, learners, and teaching. Its major focus is on the processes by which knowledge, skills, attitudes, and values are transmitted from teachers to learners. The social and behavioral sciences provide most of the health education theories and principles. Dietetics practitioners are concerned with discovering the most effective methods of teaching to influence the dietary behaviors of clients and the work behaviors of employees. Although theory alone does not guarantee effective education, applying theories to planning and implementing feasible interventions does.

What is learning? Learning is defined as a change in an individual as a result of experience (1). Changes may be in knowledge, skills, attitudes, values, and behaviors, and they are relatively permanent outcomes of learning brought about by some experience. As you experience reading this chapter, for example, you are learning something. Other than learning by reading, the practitioner's problem is how to present people with the right stimuli and experiences on which to focus their attention and mental effort so that they acquire new knowledge, skills, attitudes, and behaviors.

LEARNING THEORIES

There is no single theory to explain human learning, and theories often overlap. To explain how people learn, psychologists have developed two principle types of learning theories: behavioral or stimulus-response theories and cognitive theories. Behavioral learning theories are explanations of learning that are limited almost exclusively to observable changes in behavior, emphasizing the effects of external events on the individual (2). Theorists are interested in the way pleasurable or painful consequences of behavior may change the person's behavior over time. It is an approach based on the belief that what we learn has readily identifiable parts and that identifiable rewards and punishments can be given to produce the learning (3). The teachers' role is to arrange the external environment to elicit the desired response (4). The social

learning theory represents an expansion of the behaviorist view.

Rather than observable changes brought about by external events, cognitive learning theories are explanations of learning that focus on internal, unobservable mental processes that individuals use to learn and remember new knowledge or skills (2). Learning processes that are less visible, such as thinking, perceiving, remembering, creating, concept formation, and problem solving, are the domain of cognitive learning. The teacher's role is to structure the content of the learning experiences (4). The boundaries between the two theories, however, have become less distinct over time with a shift toward learning based on cognitive theories. Each theory and the implications for dietetics practitioners are described in this chapter as well as social learning theory, theories of adult learning, and learning styles. There is little doubt that one's preference for a theory will greatly influence how one plans and implements learning for clients and employees.

Behavioral Learning Theories

Most educational interventions to reduce the risk of chronic diseases incorporate behavioral change strategies based on social learning theory and behavioral self-management (5). Behavioral learning theories evolved from the research of several individuals including Ivan Pavlov on classical conditioning, Edward Thorndike who noted that the connections between stimuli and subsequent responses or behaviors are strengthened or weakened by the consequences of behavior, and B.F. Skinner on operant conditioning (2, 6). Other information on their research may be found in the chapter on ''Behavior Modification.''

Skinner's work focused on the relationship between the behavior and its consequences. The use of pleasant and unpleasant consequences following a particular behavior is often referred to as operant conditioning (2, 6). Skinner's work with rats and pigeons established a set of learning principles that have been confirmed with human beings. In the following sections, four consequences following a behavior are discussed: positive reinforcement, negative reinforcement or escape, punishers, and extinction. In addition, shaping, the timing of reinforcement, and social learning theory are examined.

Positive Reinforcers. One of the most important principles of behavioral learning theory is that behavior changes according to its immediate consequences. Pleasurable consequences are called "positive reinforcers" and may be defined as consequences that strengthen and increase the frequency of a behavior that one wants an individual to do again (2). The term "reward" is used also; examples are praise for a job well done, grades one receives in school, money in the form of a salary increase, and token reinforcers, such as stars or smiley face stickers on a chart. When behaviors persist or increase over time, one may assume that the consequences are positively reinforcing them (2). The pleasure associated with eating, for example, is a positive reinforcer.

These reinforcers are highly personal, however, and none can be assumed to be effective at all times. For an employee who has a poor relationship with a superior, for example, the supervisor's praise may not affect his or her behavior. And the professional's praise of a client who has followed a dietary regimen may not matter to that specific individual. The person must value the reinforcer in order for it to increase the frequency of a desired behavior. The professional needs to explore with individuals the things that are considered as positive reinforcers and to help arrange the reinforcement in the person's environment. Knowledge of results is also an effective secondary positive reinforcer. Clients and employees should know their stage of progress. If they know they are doing something properly, that knowledge reinforces the response.

The way the praise is given is also important, and the person doing the praising must be believable (2). The praise should recognize a specific behavior, so the person clearly understands what he or she is being recognized for. "Good job" as a praise is not as effective as saying specifically, "Thanks for completing the extra project on time. I appreciate it."

Negative Reinforcers/Escapes. Reinforcers that are "escapes" from unpleasant situations are called "negative reinforcers." These also strengthen behaviors because they withdraw unpleasant situations (2). Overeating may be reinforcing if the individual "escapes," for example, feelings of loneliness, unhappiness, fatigue, and the like. Or an employee may "escape" the supervisor's wrath by behaving correctly. If some action allows you to stop, avoid, or escape something aversive, you are likely to repeat that action again when faced with a similar situation.

Punishers. Negative reinforcers, which strengthen behaviors, should not be confused with punishers that weaken behaviors. Unpleasant consequences, called "punishers," decrease the frequency of or suppress a behavior (2). Punishment may take one of two different forms. One type is to remove positive reinforcers the person already has, such as removing a privilege. A second form includes the use of unpleasant or aversive consequences as when one is scolded for improper behavior. Punishment can make an individual avoid the situation in the future, so scolding a client who has not lost any weight is not appropriate. Learning theorists disagree about the use of punishers, and some believe that they should be tried only as a last resort when positive reinforcement has been attempted and failed (1).

Extinction. What happens when reinforcers are withdrawn? A behavior will weaken and eventually disappear. This process is called "extinction" of a behavior (2). If an individual starts an exercise program, for example,

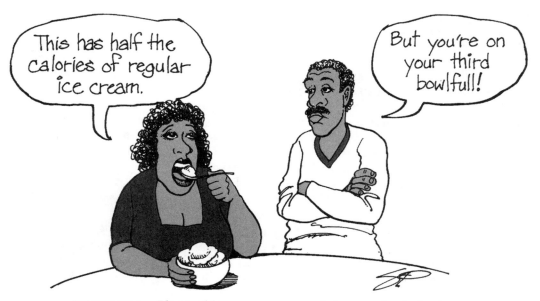

FIGURE 10.1.   Pleasurable consequences reinforce eating behaviors.

and there are no continuous positive reinforcers, the person may exercise less and less and eventually not at all.

When behaviors are undesirable and the reinforcers for it can be identified and removed, the behavior also may become extinct. An employee's boisterous behavior, for example, may change if the supervisor and other employees ignore the individual and do not give him the attention he is seeking. Instead, the supervisor will want to positively reinforce nonboisterous behavior in this individual.

Shaping. The decision of what and when to reinforce with a client or employee is also important. Does one wait until the desired behavior is perfect? No! Most people need reinforcement along the way to something new. Reinforcing each step along the way to successful behavior is called "shaping," or successive approximations (2). It involves reinforcing progress rather than waiting for perfection. When client or employee goals can be broken down into a series of identified steps or subskills, positive feedback may be given as each step or subskill is mastered or accomplished.

Timing Reinforcement. An important principle is that positive consequences that are immediate are more effective than those that are delayed. Then the connection between the behavior and the consequences is better understood in the person's mind. As a result, the dietetics professional needs to identify with the client or employee not only what is positively reinforcing to that individual, but also a time schedule for dispensing that reinforcement for proper behaviors. This concept also explains why it is difficult for people to change their eating behaviors. Usually the positive consequences of the change, such as weight loss or better health, are in the future, while eating disallowed foods is positively reinforcing immediately. It tastes good or hunger is reduced. Eating is intrinsically reinforcing, i.e., a behavior that is pleasurable in itself.

The frequency of reinforcement has also been studied. In the early part of a behavior change, continuous reinforcement after every correct response helps learning. Later on, a variable or intermittent schedule of reinforcement is preferable. When rewards are overused, they lose their effect, so that after an individual has had some rewarded successes, rewards should be given less frequently. Table 10.1 summarizes some of the implications of the theories discussed in the chapter.

Modeling/Social Learning Theory

Behavioral psychologists found that operant conditioning offered too limited an explanation of learning and overlooked important social influences (2). Albert Bandura's work on social learning theory is an outgrowth of behavioral theory. Bandura believed that the observation of and imitation of other people's behavior, vicariously learning from another's successes and failures, had been ignored. He felt that people learned not only from external factors,

TABLE 10.1.

Implications of Learning Theories and Models

THEORY/MODEL	IMPLICATIONS
Behavioral theory	Find out what reinforcers are valued
	Tell the person their stage of progress
	Use positive reinforcement
	Praise specific, not general, behaviors
	Reinforce progress on the way to mastery
	Use continuous reinforcement, then intermittent
	Ignore undesirable behaviors
	Avoid punishment
Social learning	Be a good role model
	Provide other good role models
	Avoid negative models
	Have new skills demonstrated and practiced
Cognitive theory	Explore prior knowledge
	Gain and maintain attention
	Ask questions
	Use goal setting
	Use repetition and review
	Make information meaningful
	Organize information
	Link new information to the memory network
Learning styles	Identify preferences for styles
	Offer several methods/ techniques of learning
Adult learning	Adults are self-directed
	Prior experience should be recognized
	Use participatory methods
	Orient learning to problems and projects
	Use goal setting

but also from observing models or "modeling." People who focus their attention on watching others are constructing mental images, analyzing, evaluating, remembering, and making decisions that affect learning (2). Professionals need to be aware of this and be good role models themselves. If we do not eat nutritiously and exercise regularly, for example, how can we expect others to do so?

When Oprah Winfrey lost weight the first time, many of her viewers started on the same diet to model after her success. It is preferable, of course, if the model is an attractive, successful, admired, and well-known individual. Then people will imitate the behavior, hoping to capture some of the same success.

In group learning situations, clients and employees can learn from good models. In demonstrating the operation of kitchen equipment to a new employee, part of the learning comes from watching the trainer. Then the employee imitates what he or she has seen. In group classes for individuals making dietary modifications due to heart disease, for example, people may be influenced to make dietary changes by modeling after the success stories of others in the group.

We also learn vicariously from watching negative models. When we see that something does not work, or we disagree with it, we decide not to imitate it. Seeing an obese person can trigger this type of reaction in some people. "I'll never be like that" may be a response. People judge behaviors against their own standards and decide which models to follow. Sometimes employees model after others who take short cuts and do not follow proper procedures. And if the supervisor takes extra long breaks and lunches, employees may conclude that this behavior is permissible.

When the professional wants people to model knowledge or skills they are acquiring, it is important to have them practice and demonstrate the skill, not just rehearse it mentally. This shows whether or not they are modeling correctly. The practitioner may want a client learning a new modified diet to plan several menus in order to model the new knowledge and skill, for example. A new employee who can demonstrate the proper use of equipment is modeling correctly. If they are correct, feedback and positive reinforcement, such as praise, should be given. Self-efficacy and motivation are then enhanced. If they are partially correct, using "shaping," one may give positive reinforcement for the correct portion and then assist in altering the rest. Mentoring another individual is another example of using these principles as the mentor models and guides new roles and behaviors.

Cognitive Theories

Which is easier to learn—the formulas for the essential amino acids or the Food Guide Pyramid? Which is easier to remember—a phone number used yesterday for the first time or what was eaten for dinner last evening? The difference is between rote learning, which requires memorizing facts not linked to a cognitive structure, and learning and remembering more meaningful information without deliberately memorizing it. Both, of course, are necessary.

The cognitive view sees learning as an active mental process of acquiring, remembering, and using knowledge instead of the passive process influenced by external environmental stimuli of the behaviorists (2). Individuals pursue goals, seek information, solve problems, and reorganize information and knowledge in their memories. In pondering a problem, the solution may come as a flash of insight as people reorganize what they know. The focus is more on internal mental processes.

The cognitive approach suggests that an important influence on learning is what the individual brings to the learning situation, i.e., what he or she already knows (2). Prior knowledge is an important influence on what we learn, remember, and forget. The cognitive view sees reinforcement as feedback about what is likely to happen if behaviors are repeated (2). Remembering and forgetting are other topics in cognitive psychology. There is however, no single cognitive model or theory of learning (2). Table 10.2 compares the theories discussed in this chapter.

Discovery learning is an example of a cognitive instructional model. When people learn through their own active involvement, they discover things for themselves. This approach, using experimentation and problem solving, helps people to analyze and absorb information rather than merely memorize it (2). The professional can provide problem situations that stimulate the client to question, explore, and experiment. Examples of questions are: What can you eat for breakfast? In a restaurant? On trips? The individual has to discover the answers.

MEMORY

There are a number of theories of memory to explain how the mind takes in information, processes it, stores it, retains it, and retrieves it for use. The dietetics professional not only wants people to acquire information, skills, and attitudes, but also to remember them and use them. As individuals are bombarded with information all day long from family, friends, coworkers, supervisors, newspapers, magazines, television, radio, how do they remember it all? They don't. Much is, of course, immediately discarded.

Some information enters short-term memory until it is used, such as the time of an appointment, and then it is forgotten. Of course, nothing even enters short-term memory until the person pays attention to it, i.e., focuses on certain stimuli and screens out all others (2). So the dietetics professional needs to think of obtaining and then maintaining a client's or employee's attention. Otherwise, the individual may be thinking about something else.

There are various ways to gain attention, such as by using media or bright colors, by raising or lowering one's

TABLE 10.2.

Learning Theories and Strategies

	BEHAVIORAL THEORY	SOCIAL LEARNING THEORY	COGNITIVE THEORY	ANDRAGOGY
Teacher's role	Arrange environment to get desired response Arrange reinforcement	Serve as role model Arrange for other role models	Structure content or problems with essential features Organize knowledge	Facilitator Plan, implement, evaluate jointly Provide resources
Management	Teacher centered	Learner centered	Learner centered	Learner centered
Learner participation	Passive/active	Active Imitate models	Active Test hypotheses	Active
Motivation	Rewards motivate External	Both external and internal	Internal Use goal setting	Internal
View of learning	Rote learning Subject matter approach Practice in varied contexts	Observation of others	Insight learning Understanding	Performing tasks Solving problems Goal oriented
Strategies	Stimulus-response Behavioral objectives Task analysis Competency based Computer-assisted learning	Social roles Discussion Mentoring Role playing	Inquiry learning Discovery learning Simulation Learning how to learn	Oriented to problem solving and task performance

voice, by gestures, by starting a discussion with a question, by explaining a purpose, by repeating information more than once, and by saying, "This is important." Gaining someone's interest in a topic at hand and explaining its importance to him as well as putting it in the context of what he already knows will help. One should try to indicate how it will be useful or important (2).

Asking questions arouses curiosity and interest. Ask a new employee, "What do you know about the meat slicer?" or a new client with heart disease, "What do you know about saturated fats?" Ask why they think that learning this information is important to them. This will force the person to focus attention (2).

Short-term memory. The human mind may be likened to a computer. It receives information, performs operations on it to change its form and content, stores it, and retrieves it when needed (2). Not all information or stimuli are selected for further processing, but some is organized in short-term memory.

After the person attends to something new, it enters short-term memory. There are limits, however, to the amount of new information that can be retained at one time and on the length of time it will be retained, probably less than a minute. Repeating something new over and over again, such as the name of a person one has just met, helps to keep information longer in short-term memory. But if one meets five new people all at once, this can be too much new information to handle at one time. Besides repetition, one may attempt to associate new information with information currently in long-term memory. Because of memory limits, it is helpful to give not only oral information, but also a written dietary regimen to a client, or a written task analysis to an employee, since details are forgotten quickly.

Long-Term Memory. On a computer one takes the input and "saves" it onto a disk or hard drive so that it can be retrieved later. To move new information from short-term memory to long-term memory, one tries to organize it and integrate it with information already stored there. Here the professional needs to make clear to clients and employees what is important and probably repeat it more than once. It takes time and effort to reflect, to grasp the implications, to interpret and experience, and to guide an internal representation of new knowledge in the brain (2).

Individuals need to remember what they learn. How do they make sense mentally of the world? One's ability to recall rote information is limited while meaningful information is retained more easily. The implication for planning educational sessions for clients and employees is to make the information meaningful to the individual, present it in a clear and organized manner, and relate it to what the individual already knows. The person can then connect it to other known information and apply it if necessary.

Which is easier to store and later retrieve—something one hears, something one sees, or something one both sees and hears? As noted in the chapter on media, visual plus verbal images are retained better. Some people use imagery to aid retention by picturing something in the mind (2, 6). Can you picture the food guide pyramid, for example?

There are various strategies to help people to remember. The professional can summarize in the middle and at the end of a presentation. Repetition and review are good. One may put an outline on an overhead transparency as organized information is helpful. Get people involved with active, not passive, situations. Present information in a clear, organized fashion, not as isolated bits of information. Which of the following is easier to remember, for example?

361542

or

36 15 42

People also remember stories, metaphors, and examples better than isolated facts. In teaching employees about food sanitation, for example, one may use stories of actual outbreaks of foodborne illness. The story of British sailors and scurvy is often related in teaching about vitamin C. When teaching about modified diets, examples of actual client cases are used. In discussion of fiber with a client, examples of whole grain breads and cereals, fruits, and vegetables may be discussed. Learning requires people to make "sense out of information," to sort it "in our minds until it fits in a neat and orderly way," and to use "old information to help assimilate new information" (1).

Long-term memory requires connections of new knowledge to known information. Information is probably stored in networks of connected facts and concepts. New information that fits well into an individual's existing memory network is "more easily understood, learned and retained" than that which does not fit as well (1).

Following is an example of a partial knowledge network on water-soluble vitamins:

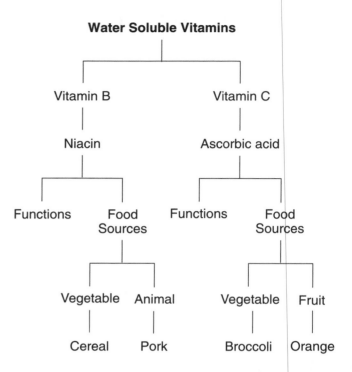

If one already has the above network and learns something new about vitamin C, for example, such as that raw cabbage is a good food source of vitamin C, it is easy to file it into the existing network. If, however, one knew nothing about vitamin C, it would be much more difficult to file the new information into long-term memory.

Following is a knowledge network on food sanitation:

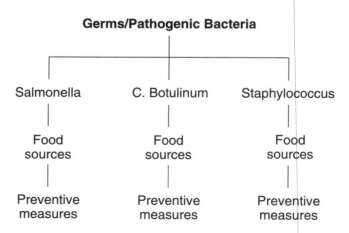

For food service workers, the term "germs" may be more meaningful to them than "pathogenic bacteria." Probably they have not heard the term pathogenic bacteria. One wants to add new information to their existing network. If the above is their network, one can more easily add to it a new "germ" they have not heard of before, such as *E. coli* or hepatitis A.

Dietetics professionals should spend time finding out

what people already know, what words they use, and what topics are in their knowledge networks; they should ask a lot of questions and then help the individual to link new information into the existing network by organizing it accordingly. Material that is organized well is much easier to learn and remember than material that is poorly organized (1). Our motivation to learn is intrinsic or internal as we seek to make sense of what is happening in our world (3).

Organizing around concepts also helps the learner to organize vast amounts of information into meaningful units. Following is an example of organizing around the concept of meals:

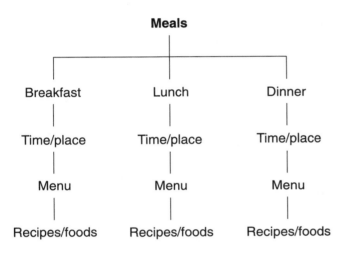

Meals

Breakfast   Lunch   Dinner

Time/place   Time/place   Time/place

Menu   Menu   Menu

Recipes/foods   Recipes/foods   Recipes/foods

Using questions from time to time helps people learn by asking them to assess their understanding of what they are hearing or reading.

When teaching about concepts, one needs to use a lot of examples (1). What mental picture or ideas does the client or employee have if the professional discusses "cholesterol," "saturated fatty acids," "blood glucose," "microorganisms," "grams" as a weight, "ounces" of meat, "quality assurance," and the like. Finding out the words they use in the current content of their knowledge network will help in using examples with them.

Transfer of learning. In human resource management, as well as in other situations, the question frequently asked is "Did the training transfer?" In other words, can an individual take the knowledge, skills, attitudes, and abilities learned in the training situation, remember them, and apply them effectively on the job in a new situation or in a dissimilar one (2). Transfer of learning cannot be assumed. It depends partly on "the degree of similarity between the situation in which the skill or concept was learned and the situation to which it is applied" (1). The implication is that one should teach people to handle the range of situations that they are likely to encounter most frequently at work (employees) or at home (clients). The practitioner needs to give many different examples from the range of problems the per-

son may encounter in using the knowledge or skills learned (7). When people do use their new knowledge and skills to solve problems, transfer of training is indicated.

For a client on a modified diet, for example, it is not enough to teach which foods to eat and avoid, but also how to transfer that information into planning menus, reading food labels, adapting current or using new recipes, eating in restaurants or while traveling, and the like. Using knowledge or skills to solve problems, such as what to do in a restaurant, helps people to apply what they learned. Can a person with diabetes, for example, calculate what one-half of an exchange of fruit is if one exchange of orange juice is one-half a cup? Can you? In school, one would multiply $\frac{1}{2} \times \frac{1}{2} = \frac{1}{4}$.

The professional cannot assume that learning transfers. For employees, it is best to teach them in the actual situation they will encounter. Cashiers, for example, need to be trained on the actual equipment they will be using, as well as how to handle all types of transactions. When training does not transfer to the job, possible reasons are that trainees found the training irrelevant, that they did not retain it, or that the work environment or supervisor does not support the newly learned behavior (7).

Since most individuals consider that it is "bad" to be wrong, and "good" to be right, some people may avoid answering questions or solving problems for fear of being wrong, with the psychological discomfort this brings. The implication is that one should handle incorrect answers carefully, with every effort to preserve the person's self-image and avoid making the person feel dumb. If the answer is partially correct, concentrate on that part. If totally wrong, one may say, for example, "Perhaps I did not phrase my question well" and then rephrase it. A relaxed atmosphere and a noncritical professional are important.

LEARNING STYLES/TEACHING STYLES
Learning Styles
Many factors affect how well an individual learns. One's learning style plays an important role in how effectively people deal with new information. Each of us has a unique learning style and teaching style. Think for a minute about the ways you learn best, or how you process and remember new information. If you remember your own school experiences, you preferred some teaching methods to others, and processed and retained material presented in a preferred manner for a longer time than material delivered in another way.

A unique learning style differentiates individuals in terms of preferences for content, methods of delivery, learning environment, and teaching techniques. Learning-style preferences are defined as "preferred ways of studying and learning, such as using pictures instead of text, working with other people versus alone, learning in structured or in unstructured situations, and so on"

(2). Emphasis is placed on the learner and the learning environment.

Different styles of learning reflect the fact that learners differ in their preferences for and ability to process the content of various instructional messages. Brilliant individuals who do well learning principles and theories from reading or watching (visual learners), for example, may be all thumbs in a hands-on experience enjoyed by others (tactile learners). Those who prefer a quiet environment may be annoyed by those who learn while listening to music. While some learn well by listening to lectures (auditory learners), those who do not enjoy this method may like learning in a group discussion. Their own discussion may enhance remembering. These preferences influence how easy or difficult learning is for the individual and therefore, have important implications for educators.

Components of style that influence learning include cognitive, affective, and environmental factors. Cognitive factors include the person's preferences in thinking and problem solving. Those who think through an experience tend more to abstract dimensions of reality. They reason and analyze what is happening. Schools tend to value these analytical learners. Others who sense and feel (affective) tend to prefer learning by way of more concrete, actual, hands-on experiences and are more intuitive. While some learn best by thinking through ideas, others learn best by testing theories and through self-discovery, or by listening and sharing ideas.

In addition to perceiving differently, people process information in different ways. Some are reflective, watching what is happening and thinking about it. Others are doers who prefer to jump right in and try things. In learning to use a computer, for example, some read the directions first and others just try different things. In a study environment, some require absolute silence to process information, some can block out sound, and others prefer sound and turn on a radio or stereo when studying and learning.

The learner's style preference may vary from situation to situation, affected by the subject matter or skill to be learned. People may learn both by thinking and feeling, and by reflecting and doing.

One's instruction can be improved and learners should perform better if the professional identifies the learner's preferred learning style and makes the instructional environment compatible. To measure learning styles, researchers have developed a variety of inventories. Though perhaps helpful, they have been criticized for lacking reliability and validity (2). Learning preferences may be too complicated for a simple test or inventory (8).

The instructor can attempt to diagnose learning style by observing how people learn or by asking them questions about their preferences, such as: "Do you prefer to read, to view, to listen, or to have actual experiences?" "Do you prefer to learn alone or in groups?" People are different and it is a good idea to accommodate styles.

Whether training employees or designing adult nutrition education programs, professionals should offer new information in a variety of ways, since people learn in different ways—by thinking through ideas reflectively, by hands-on experiences, by solving problems, by experimentation, by trial-and-error, by viewing material, and by self-discovery. The next chapter discusses various methods in more detail. Since preferred style varies with the situation, offering alternative techniques and methods that reflect the variety of ways that individuals acquire knowledge and skills allows the learners to learn in their preferred mode at least some of the time.

Teaching Style

In addition to learning style, teaching style is a related matter that affects learning significantly. Teaching style refers to the sum of what one does as a teacher—the preferred instructional methods, activities, organization of material, interactions with learners, and the like. People may be categorized as either teacher-centered or learner-centered (9). The teacher-centered approach is more associated with Skinner, and it assumes that learners are passive and that they respond to stimuli in the environment. In the learner-centered approach, individuals are assumed to be proactive and to take responsibility for their actions. Subject matter is presented in a manner conducive to the person's needs. Some evidence suggests that teachers tend to select learning activities based on how they themselves prefer to learn when they should be focusing on the learner's preferred style. Good teachers seek to improve their styles and search for better ways to adapt to the styles of the learners (8).

ADULT LEARNING THEORY

Besides behavioral and cognitive theories of learning, others have explored the differences between adults and children as learners. If one could explain how adults learn, one should be able to arrange for it to happen. When the dietetics professional accepts responsibility for teaching a client, patient, or employee, it is natural to think back to one's own past experiences, or how we were taught in school and college. Most educational experiences were the result of pedagogy, which may be defined as the art and science of teaching children (10, 11). The teacher was an authority figure, and students were dependents who complied with assignments.

Adult education has challenged some of the basic ideas and approaches of pedagogy. Knowles has focused attention on beliefs about educating adults and instead of "pedagogy," uses the term "andragogy." He maintains that the basic assumptions regarding adult learners differ from those regarding child learners. He focuses on learner characteristics, life situations, and the desired outcomes of learning more than on the learning process (4). His five major assumptions for adult learners involve the following (10–12):

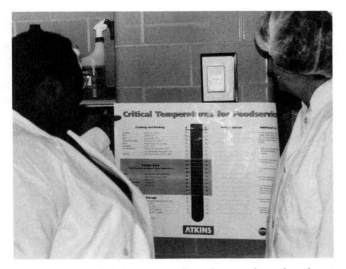

FIGURE 10.2. Adults are ready to learn when they have a need for learning.

1. In adulthood, the self-concept changes from being a dependent to being a self-directed learner.

2. Expanding experiences are a growing resource for learning.

3. Readiness to learn is based on the developmental tasks of social roles.

4. Orientation to learning shifts from subject matter in young people to problem solving in adults and from a future-oriented to a present-oriented focus.

5. Motivation to learn comes more from internal than external sources.

Self-Concept

Childhood is a period of dependency. As a person matures, the self-concept changes, and the individual becomes increasingly independent and self-directed. People make their own decisions and manage their lives (10). Once individuals become self-directed adults, they prefer to be independent and self-directing in learning experiences. Any educational experience in which one is treated as a dependent child is a threat to the self-concept. Negative feelings may result, and resentment, resistance, or anxiety will interfere with learning.

Experience

As compared with children, adults have more experiences and different kinds of experiences that they bring to new learning situations. This background is a resource for learning. Ignoring the adult's quantity and quality of experiences may be misinterpreted as a sign of rejection. A client who has had diabetes for 5 years, for example, has a wealth of experience that should be recognized when the dietetics professional discusses the diabetic diet. To ignore this prior experience and start from the beginning may annoy, bore, or possibly antagonize the

client, and may place obstacles in the way of the learning process. Teaching methods such as lectures are de-emphasized in adult education in favor of more participatory methods that tap a person's wealth of experience, such as group discussion, problem-solving activities, role playing, simulation, and the like.

Practical applications that apply learning to the individual's day-to-day life are appropriate. Focus group members planning a worksite cholesterol education program, for example, were "adamant about the importance of activities that allowed them to participate actively" (13). They wanted programs on snack ideas, easy breakfasts, dining out, fast foods, brown-bag lunches, easy recipe substitutions, and evaluating cholesterol information. A review of over 200 nutrition education interventions found that the educational process requires active participation and decision making on the part of the learner, not only in activities, such as food tasting, but also in analyzing one's diet and setting goals (5).

Readiness to Learn

Readiness to learn differs between children and adults. Children are assumed to be ready to learn because there are subjects they ought to know about, and there are academic pressures from teachers and parents to perform. Adults have no such pressures and are assumed to be ready to learn things required for performing their social roles in life—as spouses, employees, parents, and the like, or in order to cope more effectively in some aspect of their lives. Education of adults should be appropriate to the individual's readiness or need to know something, and the timing of learning experiences needs to coincide with readiness. People seek information and are ready to learn when they are confronted by problems that they must solve. For example, new employees may be ready to learn about their job responsibilities, but not necessarily about the history of the company. Clients may not be ready to learn about their modified diets until they have accepted the fact that their medical conditions and future health require it.

Orientation to Learning

A child's learning is oriented toward subjects, while an adult's learning is oriented toward performing tasks and solving problems. These different approaches involve different time perspectives. Because children learn about things that they will use some time in the future, the subject matter approach may be appropriate. Adults approach learning when they have an immediate need to learn because of a problem to solve, or a task to perform. The implication is that learning should be applied to problems or projects that the individual is currently dealing with. Adults learn what they want to learn when they want to learn it, regardless of what others want them to learn.

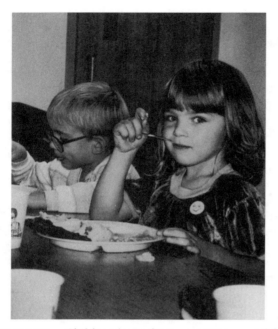

FIGURE 10.3. Children learn from experience and from the example set by adults.

Motivation

Children are motivated primarily by external pressures from parents, teachers, competition for grades, and the like. The more potent motivators for adults are internal ones, such as recognition, self-esteem, the desire for a better quality of life, and the like.

From an examination of various educational theories, Knowles described the appropriate conditions for learning to take place (10, 11). He suggested that learners should feel the need to learn something and should perceive the goals of any learning experience as their own personal goals. Before undertaking new learning, adults need to know why they need to learn it. Adults should participate actively in planning, implementing, and evaluating learning experiences to increase their commitment to learning, and the process should make use of the person's life experiences. The physical and psychological environment needs to be comfortable, as discussed in the next chapter. The relationship between the professional and learner should be characterized by mutual trust, respect, and helpfulness, and the environment should encourage freedom of expression and the acceptance of differences (10).

The professional who accepts the assumptions of "andragogy" becomes a facilitator of learning or a change agent rather than a teacher. The practitioner involves the learner in the process of learning and provides resources for assisting learners to acquire knowledge, information, and skills, while maintaining a supportive climate for learning.

In summary, there is no one educational theory or model for dietetics practitioners to use to facilitate learn-

ing and behavioral change. However, the theory that one prefers will undoubtedly influence the way one teaches and the relationship one has with clients and employees. Table 10.2 summarizes the learning theories and strategies. Individuals and groups are more likely to be motivated if the information presented emphasizes the personal consequences of behaviors as mentioned in the Health Belief Model and is appropriate to the individual's Stage of Change discussed in Chapter 1. Positive reinforcement appropriate to the needs and interests of the individual should be arranged (5). Other chapters covered the influence of cognitions, self-efficacy, relapse prevention, goal setting, social support, and behavioral self-management, which are important to explore with clients.

ADOPTION OF INNOVATIONS

The Cooperative Extension Service of the U.S. Department of Agriculture and other groups have used a model to promote the adoption of innovations (14). The process by which adults adopt new ideas and practices, such as healthy eating patterns, involves five stages:

1. **Awareness.** A person becomes aware of a new idea, practice, or procedure.

2. **Interest.** A person is concerned enough to seek further information about something, is aware of his current behavior, and is willing to discuss it. The individual sees possibilities for the use of something new.

3. **Evaluation.** A person mentally weighs the advantages and disadvantages of the new idea. The individual asks, "Can I do it?"

4. **Trial.** A person tries or tests the usefulness of the new idea or practice on a small scale once or twice. It is still a low priority.

5. **Adoption (or rejection).** A person performs consistently as a habitual procedure indicating that something is accepted, highly valued, and found satisfying.

The nutrition labeling on foods, for example, or the food guide pyramid, require a series of steps from awareness of its existence, to interest in it as a source of information, knowledge of its meaning and use, trying to understand and apply it, and adopting or rejecting its use. Nutrition education and employee education are incomplete until stage five is reached. People learn only what they want to learn, and adopt new behaviors to satisfy the basic needs of survival or to achieve some personal goal.

The characteristics of the innovation influence whether or not it is adopted. Innovations are more readily adopted if they offer sufficient advantage over current practices or products, if they are compatible with current beliefs, values, habits, and practices, if they are simple to understand and to use, if they can be divided into

CASE STUDY

"I am about ready to give up on this batch of new trainees," said Ross to his boss in frustration.

"I thought you liked training the entry-level employees, Ross," replied Bob, the Department Director.

"I do, but it seems like this latest batch of trainees just is not retaining the information," Ross said. "Now they get two additional days of classroom training before going on-the-job for a total of five days of instruction. Before I changed the program they only got three days of classroom training and then two days on-the-job. They have two extra days of lecture now. I just don't understand what is wrong with these people."

1. Where is the problem? With the trainees, the trainer, or the training program?
2. What impact did changing the training schedule have on the trainees?
3. How should a training program be designed in order to provide more effective results?

smaller units for trial, and if their benefits are clearly and quickly demonstrated before a total commitment is required. Nutrition education rates poorly on some of these criteria (15). Research findings suggest that reaching the level of adoption requires considerable communication and a lengthy time span. It may be unrealistic to expect new behaviors to be adopted from short-term educational endeavors. A dietary regimen with the achievement of one or two goals for change instead of total change may not be what the professional considers best, but limited benefits may be preferable to total abandonment of the dietary regimen.

REVIEW AND DISCUSSION QUESTIONS

1. Compare and contrast the behavioral and cognitive theories of learning in terms of what is learned, the role of reinforcement, and the like.
2. Explain the four types of consequences and their effect on behaviors.
3. What effect does the timing of reinforcement have?
4. How can you encourage persistence in a client's or employee's behavior?
5. What is modeling?
6. How can you reinforce yourself after reading this chapter?
7. What information that you learned yesterday do you remember today?
8. What makes information easy for you to learn and remember?
9. What strategies enhance long-term memory?
10. How do adults differ from children as learners?
11. What steps are involved in adopting innovations?
12. What are learning styles and teaching styles?

SUGGESTED ACTIVITIES

1. Match these types of consequences with the examples A through C following them:

   _____ positive reinforcement

   _____ negative reinforcement

   _____ punishment

   A. "With the diet you are on, you should know better than to eat fried chicken and French fries."
   B. "Employees who learn the new procedures this afternoon will not have to take any work home to study this evening."
   C. "Congratulations on your success. I'm proud of you."

2. Extinction occurs as a result of which of the following?
   A. Not rewarding a response.
   B. Punishing a response.

3. According to cognitive learning theory, which of the following statements is true?
   A. Learning involves associations that are arbitrary.
   B. Learning involves specific information being organized into more generalized categories.
   C. Learning involves observing and modeling after others.

4. Cognitive educators believe that
   A. New information and knowledge should be presented in an organized fashion considering prior knowledge.
   B. New knowledge and information should be presented separately from prior knowledge.
   C. It does not matter how new knowledge is presented as long as rewards are given.

5. Discuss in small groups each person's examples of experiences with positive reinforcement, negative reinforcement, punishment, and extinction.

6. Discuss in groups the techniques or methods individuals use in enhancing their memories of new information.

7. Discuss in groups the individuals' learning styles and environments preferred for learning.

REFERENCES

1. Slavin RE. Educational psychology: theory into practice. 4th ed. Boston: Allyn and Bacon, 1993.
2. Woolfolk AE. Educational psychology. 6th ed. Boston: Allyn and Bacon, 1995.

3. Caine RN, Caine G. Teaching and the human brain. Alexandria, VA: Assoc for Supervision and Curriculum Development, 1991.

4. Merriam SB, Caffarella RS. Learning in adulthood: a comprehensive guide. San Francisco: Jossey-Bass, 1991.

5. Contento I, Balch GI, Bronner YL, et al. Nutrition education for adults. J Nutr Educ 1995;27:312.

6. Elliott SN, Kratochwill TR, Littlefield J, et al. Educational psychology. 2nd ed. Madison: Brown & Benchmark, 1996.

7. Garavaglia PL. How to ensure transfer of training. Train Dev 1993;47:63.

8. Apps JW. Mastering the teaching of adults. Malabar, FL: Krieger Publ Co, 1991.

9. Conti GJ. Identifying your teaching style. In: Galbraith MW, ed. Adult learning methods. A guide for effective instruction. Malabar, FL: Krieger Publishing, 1990.

10. Knowles MS. The adult learner: a neglected species. 4th ed. Houston: Gulf Publishing, 1990.

11. Knowles MS. The modern practice of adult education. New York: Association Press, 1970.

12. Knowles MS. Andragogy in action. San Francisco: Jossey-Bass, 1984.

13. McCarthy PR, Lansing D, Hartman TJ, et al. What works best for worksite cholesterol education? Answers from targeted focus groups. J Am Diet Assoc 1992;92:978.

14. Nestor J, Glotzer J. Teaching nutrition. Cambridge, MA: Abt Books, 1981.

15. Yarbrough P. Communication theory and nutrition education research. J Nutr Educ 1981;13:S16.

eleven

PLANNING LEARNING

Teaching is one of the major job responsibilities of all dietitians and dietetic technicians, whether they specialize in clinical, community, or administrative practice. In the health care setting, practitioners are responsible for assisting patients and clients in the management and control of their diseases and medical problems. Health care facilities approved by the Joint Commission on Accreditation of Healthcare Organizations (JCAHO) are required to provide the patient, family, and/or significant others with education specific to their needs and to document the education given in the medical record (1). Administrative professionals and managers teach and train their staff.

Dietetics practitioners must be skilled in providing appropriate learning opportunities to patients, clients, and employees to facilitate their acquisition of knowledge, attitudes, skills, and new behaviors. Most professionals are experts in the content that they teach. Since they spend substantial amounts of time teaching, they are also expected to be effective teachers. Chambers noted that "a well-informed and well-intentioned dietitian who lacks the communication skills necessary for effective nutrition instruction is not competent" (2).

Dietetics professionals in clinical and community practice educate clients and patients about normal nutrition and about dietary modifications necessitated by such medical problems as cardiovascular disease and diabetes. The practitioner may one day be teaching a 50-year-old man about fatty acids and cholesterol in foods and the next day be teaching an 18-year-old pregnant woman about prenatal nutrition. A study of Army dietitians reported that the time dedicated to nutrition education varied from 13 hours weekly for chiefs of nutrition care divisions to 36 hours for chiefs of clinical dietetics (3). A wide variety of group and individual interventions was offered including weight control, prenatal nutrition, well-baby clinic, basic nutrition, alcohol rehabilitation, diabetic, low sodium, fat controlled instructions, fitness, wellness, and drug, alcohol, and cardiac rehabilitation programs.

Nutrition education has been defined as (4):

... the teaching of validated, correct nutrition knowledge in ways that promote the development and maintenance of positive attitudes toward and actual behavioral habits of eating nutritious foods (within budgetary and cultural constraints) that contribute to the maintenance of personal health, well-being, and productivity.

Nutrition education has also been defined as "any set of learning experiences designed to facilitate the voluntary adoption of eating and other nutrition-related behaviors conducive to health and well-being" (5). Recently patient education has focused more on "self-management" training and education that promote independent living. The professional assists people in the development of the knowledge, skills, and motivation in making appropriate decisions about food choices throughout life to promote optimum health. The practitioner wants the individual not only to know what to do, but also to change current dietary behaviors, adopt and practice new ones, and manage their environments.

The purpose of nutrition education is to change or reinforce eating practices. The goal is the improvement of dietary behaviors either related to reducing the risk of chronic diseases or improving nutritional adequacy and health (5). The changes sound simple: to avoid or decrease consumption of certain foods (such as fats), to increase consumption of others (fruits and vegetables), to shop for different foods (reduced in fat), to read food labels (for fat, calories, sodium, fiber, etc.), to change cooking methods (bake instead of fry), to order different foods at a restaurant (baked potato instead of French fries), and the like. But they are not simple to accomplish. They are complex.

The internal and external forces that have shaped people's eating habits are of long-standing, and create barriers to successful, long-term change. Nevertheless, the ultimate criterion for effectiveness of nutrition education is behavioral change in food and health habits (5). The dietetics professional must be a facilitator of positive behavioral change in an ongoing educational process (6). Studies have found that interventions that used educational methods directed at goals of behavioral change

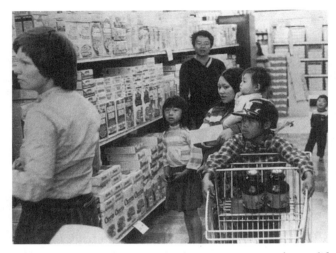

FIGURE 11.1. Cultural and ethnic groups may have different needs for learning.

were more successful than those directed at disseminating information with the assumption that the information would lead to changes in behaviors and attitudes (5).

Many practitioners are responsible for the supervision of employees. Orientation, training, and development programs (human resource development) are necessary for these subordinates. An employee's on-the-job performance must meet standards acceptable to the organization, and it is the responsibility of the supervisor to ensure that training needs are recognized and met. The goal of training is to have employees know their job responsibilities and, when necessary, learn and substitute new practices for current ones. The fact that an employee knows proper procedures but may not always follow them is an indication of the difficulty involved in getting a person to change.

Frequently, the terms "teaching" and "learning" are confused. Some people have the mistaken notion that if they teach something, the audience or individual learns automatically and will transfer the learning to appropriate situations. One may teach a pregnant woman about the food guide pyramid, for example, tell her why it is important to use it in menu planning, and give her printed handouts. A passive learner who has not participated actively in the learning may not make any connection between what was taught and her own food selection or menu planning. To change behavior, education should endeavor to further the adoption of better practices. Although knowledge is a prerequisite for change, knowledge in itself does not necessarily lead to a different behavior. In a study of the consumption of foods high in fat, nutrition knowledge was not found to relate to attitudes or to food consumption behaviors (7). Research has shown that knowledge accounts for "4 to 8% of the variance in eating behavior, leaving 92 to 96% of the behavior to be accounted for by other influences" (8). Motivation and intention are vital for change. A person may

be knowledgeable about a healthy diet but lack perseverance. A client may be familiar with the sodium-restricted diet, for example, but still may consume salted pretzels.

Teaching factual information should not be mistaken for education. Education may be defined as the process of imparting or acquiring knowledge or skills in the context of the person's total matrix of living. Education should assist people in coping with their problems as they adapt to circumstances. The term "teaching" suggests the educator's assessment of the need for knowledge and the utilization of techniques to transfer knowledge to another individual.

The term "learning" refers to the cognitive process through which the individual acquires and stores the knowledge or skill and changes his behavior due to an interaction with, or experiences in, an educational environment. The change in behavior may be related to knowledge, attitudes, values, or skills.

Achterberg describes the nutrition educator as a person who "deliberately seeks to progressively empower learners to act on food and nutrition-related issues such that the learner is gradually freed from the intervention and the materials" (9). She suggests that there is a planned effort, that the effort is a step-by-step process, that people are enabled to act on their nutrition knowledge, and that eventually people can act on their own, making positive changes in their behavior and practicing self-care and self-management. Self-management education is described as the cornerstone of training for all individuals with diabetes (10).

This chapter examines the educational environment for learning and examines a model or framework for planning, implementing, and evaluating learning. The first three steps, which are preassessment of the learner or needs assessment, planning performance objectives, and determination of the content, are examined along with information on grouping people together for learning. Discussion of the additional steps in the learning process follows in the next chapter. The question of motivation is examined in another chapter.

ENVIRONMENT

An educational environment has two components, the psychological environment and the physical environment. Both are important to enhancing teaching and learning (11).

Psychological Environment

The psychological climate for learning is important, and it is determined by the approach of the dietetics professional. A supportive and friendly environment with a tolerance for mistakes and with a respect for individual and cultural differences makes people feel secure and welcome. Openness and encouragement of questions create an informal atmosphere. Individuals should be known by their names, and respect for their opinions should be demonstrated.

In group teaching of clients or employees, participants should be encouraged to introduce themselves and to get to know one another at the first session. Collaboration and mutual assistance rather than competition should be promoted, and initial feelings of anxiety should be reduced so they do not inhibit learning. The professional who creates this informal, supportive, and caring environment for adult learners can obtain better results than one who creates a formal, authoritative environment. Since some learners have negative memories of their early experiences in school, for example, if clients or employees were dismissed from high school, a physical or psychological climate that reminds them of their past unpleasant experiences will create barriers to learning.

Physical Environment

One considers not only the psychological climate, but also the physical environment. Comfort should be provided with appropriate temperature, good lighting, ventilation, and comfortable chairs to create conditions that promote learning rather than inhibit it. Noise from a radio, television, telephone, or people talking may be distracting and interfere with a client's, patient's, or employee's attention. Individuals should be able both to see and to hear. Interaction is facilitated by seating groups of people in a circle or around a table where everyone has eye contact, as opposed to seating people in row upon row of chairs.

STEPS TO EDUCATION

Successful educational efforts that meet the needs of the adult learner include a number of interactive steps. The framework and components are as follows:

1. Assessment of the needs of the individual or group.

2. Planning of performance objectives that are measurable, feasible, and able to be accomplished in a stated period of time.

3. Determination of the content based on the preassessment and the objectives.

4. Selection of methods, techniques, materials, and resources appropriate to the objectives and the individual or group.

5. Implementation of the learning experiences to provide opportunities for the person to practice new information.

6. Evaluation of progress performed continuously and at stated intervals, including rediagnosis of learning needs.

7. Documentation of the results of education.

NEEDS ASSESSMENT

The first step in education is to conduct a preassessment or needs assessment with the client or employee. Preassessment is a diagnostic evaluation performed prior to instruction for the purpose of placement, or for establish-

ing a starting point, and it serves to classify people regarding their current knowledge, skills, abilities, aptitudes, interests, personality, educational backgrounds, age, culture, lifestyle, disease process, and psychological readiness to learn. Each individual is unique.

A need for learning may be defined as a gap between what people should know and what they do know now, or the difference between how employees should perform and their actual performance.

Desired knowledge, skill, performance, or results	−	Current knowledge, skill, performance, or result	=	Need for learning

If preassessment determines that an individual already has some prior knowledge and experience, such as a client with long-term diabetes who knows how to count carbohydrates, more advanced material is indicated. One determines in advance how much the individual already knows, since it would be a waste of everyone's time to repeat known information, and could lead to boredom or lack of attention on the part of the learner. Does the client have the intellectual capabilities to understand the instruction? Some people are unable to read, and such limitations require that the instruction be planned at the client's level. Educational planning should be based on the dietetics professional's preassessment of the client's or employee's knowledge, skills, ability, and lifestyle factors.

In determining what the person already knows, preassessment may be handled by oral interviewing. One may inquire: "Have you been on a diet before?" "Can you tell me what foods are good sources of potassium?" "Can you explain the relationship between your diet and your health?" In general, the line of questioning should be based on what the person needs to know or would like to know. Interviewing may be used with employees as well. "Have you ever used a meat slicer before?" "Can you show me how you set tables at the restaurant where you worked previously?"

Psychological preassessment is also necessary since the dietetics professional must understand the attitudes that influence the client's or employee's behavior. Attitudes are thought to be predispositions for action. Problems in learning may not be cognitive, or caused by deficits in knowledge; the cause and solution may be found in the affective domain, or in attitudes, values, and beliefs. Nutrition behaviors are the result of many motivations, and having nutrition information does not necessarily mean that it will be applied (4). For example, the hospitalized patient who has just learned of a confirmed diagnosis of chronic illness is unlikely to learn much about a prescribed dietary treatment at that moment. The patient may be thinking: "Why me?" "What did I do to deserve this?" "How will this affect my job? my lifestyle? my marriage?'' A new employee may feel high levels of anxiety, which may interfere with learning for the first few days on the job. Anxiety may arise whenever a superior trains a subordinate. "What does the superior think about me?'' "I will appear to be dumb if I don't understand, so I had better pretend I do understand." These feelings are barriers to learning that must be recognized, reduced, or eliminated prior to teaching.

In more formal situations, a preassessment questionnaire or test may be developed and administered. The purpose of a test is to evaluate the individual's knowledge and capabilities before instruction begins and to identify what the individual already knows. Pretest results may be compared later with posttest results after instruction has been completed. Preassessment is most necessary when the dietetics professional is unfamiliar with the knowledge, ability, and values of the client, patient, or employee. At the community level, a survey questionnaire, a focus group, or a telephone interview survey may be used. The focus group interview technique was useful, for example, in developing a nutrition education intervention for rural seniors (12).

In business, training and development programs are planned to meet current and future goals and objectives of the organization. Training provides specific skills, under the guidance of established personnel so that employees meet quality standards acceptable to the organization. Training is needed, for example, by new employees and by current employees accepting new assignments, such as after a promotion or transfer. A need for training is described as the difference between a person's actual and desired knowledge, skill, or performance or the gap between current and desired results (13). Training needs assessment may be handled in a number of ways, for example, by discussing needs and problems with supervisors or subordinates; by directly observing the work; by structured interviewing of employees; by seeing what is done correctly and especially what is not; by examining reports of accidents, incidents, grievances, turnover, productivity, and quality control and assurance; and by administering employee attitude surveys (14–16). One may ask: "What are the knowledge, skills, abilities, and attitudes that employees need in order to perform their jobs successfully?" This assessment deals with ends, not the means to the ends, which are selected later (13).

PERFORMANCE OBJECTIVES

Developing precise statements of goals can help to organize one's thinking regarding the purpose of instruction, i.e., what is to be learned. The professional needs to decide what is to be learned prior to selecting the methods and techniques to accomplish it. References to goal statements are found in the literature under the terms "behavioral objectives" and "measurable objectives." Because the term "behavioral objectives" may be erroneously confused with behaviorism, the term "performance objectives" is used in this chapter. Written performance objectives are helpful tools in planning, implementing, and evaluating learning.

A well-stated performance objective communicates the practitioner's instructional intent for the patient, client, employee, or audience. It specifies the person's behavior or degree of competence after instruction is complete. Writing performance objectives has many advantages. It results in less ambiguity regarding what is to be learned. Also, clear performance objectives make it possible to assess or evaluate the degree to which the objectives have been achieved. Both the practitioner and the individual benefit from clearer instructions. When people know what they are supposed to learn, it does not come as a surprise. They should not be kept guessing about what should be learned or about what is important. This is a waste of their time. Performance objectives have been criticized for focusing on increasingly smaller behaviors (17). More broad-scope objectives may also be written for a whole program.

Thus, initial effort is devoted to delineating the intended results of instruction for the individual, rather than to the methods or processes of learning. One first defines the ends and then explores the means to the ends. Instruction must benefit the learner, not the professional, so one must focus initially on the result in the individual. If clear objectives are not written, the professional cannot select content or materials for instruction. One cannot select an educational video, for example, without knowing what it is to accomplish. As pointed out by Mager, "If you're not sure where you're going, you're liable to end up someplace else" (18).

Objectives should focus on the person learning, not on the health educator. The following objective is poorly stated: "The dietetics professional will teach the client about his diet." Note that this statement focuses on what the practitioner will do, and not on what the client or

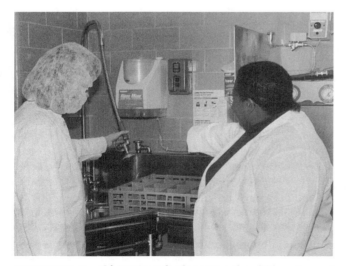

FIGURE 11.2. Objectives for learning should be planned around what the employee needs to know.

learner will do. The following is preferred because it focuses on the client: "After instruction, the client will be able to plan appropriate menus using the sodium-restricted diet as a reference."

One of the most useful guides to writing performance objectives was written by Robert Mager (18). A key to writing measurable performance objectives is the selection of the verb that describes the desired outcome. Some verbs are vague and subject to misinterpretation, as in the following objectives:

To know (is able to know which foods contain potassium).

To understand (is able to understand that foods high in potassium should be consumed daily when certain medications are prescribed).

To appreciate (is able to appreciate the importance of following the practitioner's instructions).

In the written objective for "to know," it is not clear whether "knowing" means that the client will purchase foods high in potassium, be able to tell a friend which foods are high in potassium, or recognize them on a list. "Understanding" could mean being able to recall reasons, being able to read an article about it, or being able to apply knowledge to one's own situation. The meanings of knowing, understanding, and appreciating are vague and unclear.

Instead, one should select verbs that describe what the person is able to do after learning has taken place. Note that the phrase "after learning, the individual is able to" is understood to precede the phrase, since one is describing what the person will be capable of doing. Another method involves starting with the action verb. The first two examples are rewritten from the unsatisfactory objectives in the previous list. Better verbs to use are summarized in Table 11.1 and include the following:

To recall (is able to recite five good food sources of potassium).

To explain (is able to explain why foods high in potassium should be consumed).

To write (is able to list the groups in the food pyramid).

To compare (is able to compare the nutrient needs of an adult woman with those of a pregnant woman).

To identify (is able to identify on the menu those foods that are permitted).

To solve or use (is able to plan menus using a diet instruction sheet).

To demonstrate (is able to demonstrate the use of the mixer).

To operate (is able to slice meat on the meat slicer).

Mager noted that three characteristics improve written objectives: *(a)* performance, *(b)* conditions, and *(c)* criterion (18). The "performance" tells what the learner will be able to do after instruction has been given. The second characteristic describes under what "conditions"

TABLE 11.1.
Verbs Describing Performance

Verbs to use		
analyze	discuss	prepare
apply	distinguish	produce
assemble	evaluate	recall
calculate	explain	recite
cite	identify	recognize
classify	illustrate	recommend
compare	interpret	repair
complete	list	select
construct	measure	solve
contrast	name	state
define	operate	summarize
demonstrate	plan	use
describe	practice	write
Verbs to avoid		
appreciate	feel	learn
believe	grasp	like
comprehend	hope	realize
discern	know	understand

the performance is to occur. Finally, a "criterion" tells how good the individual's performance must be to be acceptable. Table 11.2 summarizes the three-part system for writing objectives. Conditions and criterion may not be included in all objectives. In general, the more that can be specified, the better the objective and the more likely that the patient, client, or employee will learn what the dietetics professional intends.

Performance

The performance component of an objective describes the activity in which the individual will be engaged. The performance may be visible or heard, such as listing, reciting, explaining, or operating equipment, or invisible, such as identifying or solving a problem. While overt or visible performance may be seen or heard directly, invisible or covert performance requires that the individual be asked to do something visible to determine whether or not the objective is satisfied and learning has taken place. In invisible performance, one adds an "indicator" behavior to the objective, for example:

Is able to identify the parts of the meat slicer (on a diagram or verbally).

Identifying is invisible until the learner is asked to identify the parts on a diagram or to recite them verbally, which are indicator behaviors. The major intent or performance should be stated using an active verb, and an indicator should be added if the performance cannot be seen or heard.

TABLE 11.2.

Mager's Three-part System for Objectives Client and Employee Examples

PART	QUESTION	CLIENT EXAMPLE
Learner behavior	Do what?	Plans a menu for a day
Conditions	Under what conditions?	Given a list of permitted foods
Criterion	How well?	With no errors

PART	QUESTION	EMPLOYEE EXAMPLE
Learner behavior	Do what?	Measures sanitizer in a bucket
Conditions	Under what conditions?	When cleaning the work area
Criterion	How well?	Using the exact concentration recommended

Conditions

Once the performance has been clearly stated, one may ask whether or not there are specific circumstances or conditions under which the performance will be observed. The conditions describe the setting, equipment, or cues associated with the behavior. With what resources will the individual be provided? What will be withheld? Conditions are in parentheses in the following examples:

(Given the disassembled parts of a meat slicer) is able to reassemble the parts in correct sequence.

(Using the diabetic diet menu for tomorrow) is able to select the proper foods in the correct quantities.

(Given a list of foods including both good and poor sources of potassium) is able to identify the good sources.

(Given a copy of a sodium-restricted diet) is able to plan a menu for a complete day.

(Without looking at the diet instruction form) is able to describe an appropriate dinner menu.

(Without the assistance of the practitioner) is able to explain the foods a pregnant woman should eat on a daily basis.

These objectives give a more accurate and complete picture of the exact performance expected of an individual. While every objective may not have conditions, there

should be enough information to make clear exactly what performance is expected.

Criterion

Once the end performance has been described and the conditions, if any, under which it will be observed, a criterion may or may not be added. The criterion describes a level of achievement, that is, how well the individual should be able to perform. It is a standard with which to measure performance. Possible standards include speed, accuracy, quality, and percentage of correct answers (18).

A time limit can be used to describe the speed criterion. This is necessary only when speed is important, and if it is, it should be included in the objective. The following are examples:

Is able to type (50 words per minute).

Is able to reassemble the meat slicer (in 5 minutes or less).

Is able to complete a diet history (in 20 minutes).

For objectives that require the development of skill over a period of time, one must determine how much time is reasonable in the initial learning period as opposed to the time when the skill is well developed. A new employee cannot be expected to perform a task as rapidly as an experienced person.

While speed is one type of standard, a second is accuracy. Accuracy should communicate how well the individual needs to perform for his or her performance to be considered competent. Examples include:

Is able to type 50 words per minute (with 5 errors or less).

Is able to identify good sources of potassium (with 80% accuracy), when given a list of foods including both good and poor sources.

Is able to plan a menu for a complete day (with no errors) when given a copy of a sodium-restricted diet.

Is able to calculate the carbohydrates in the diabetic diet (within 5 grams).

If the individual is expected to perform with a degree of accuracy, this should be included in the objective.

After considering whether speed and accuracy are important, one should examine the quality to assess what constitutes an acceptable performance. It is easier to communicate quality when objective standards are available to both the individual and the practitioner. Any acceptable deviation from the standards can then be determined. Examples of such standards are as follows:

Is able to reassemble the meat slicer (according to the steps in the task analysis).

Is able to measure the amount of sanitizer (according to the directions on the label).

Is able to substitute foods on a diabetic menu (using carbohydrate counting).

In these examples, the quality of performance has been stated according to a known standard.

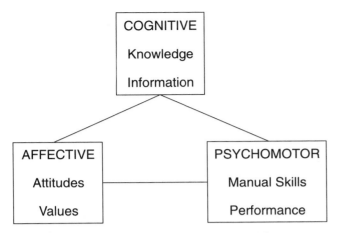

FIGURE 11.3. The interrelationships of objectives.

Domains of Learning

After developing skill in writing measurable performance objectives, one should consider the range of objectives that may be written. Objectives have been organized into taxonomies or classification systems to focus on precision in writing, and one may examine the range of possible outcomes desired from instruction. There are three basic types of objectives: *(a)* cognitive, *(b)* affective, and *(c)* psychomotor. Each is a hierarchy from simple to complex. Figure 11.3 shows their interrelationship.

COGNITIVE DOMAIN

A taxonomy of educational objectives in the cognitive domain was published by Bloom and others (19). The cognitive domain involves the acquisition and use of knowledge or information and the development of intellectual skills and abilities. According to Bloom and coauthors, the cognitive domain has six major levels or categories and a number of subcategories as shown in the following (19):

1.0 KNOWLEDGE
   1.1 Knowledge of specifics
   1.2 Knowledge of ways and means of dealing with specifics
   1.3 Knowledge of the universals and abstractions in a field
2.0 COMPREHENSION
   2.1 Translation
   2.2 Interpretation
   2.3 Extrapolation
3.0 APPLICATION
4.0 ANALYSIS
   4.1 Analysis of elements
   4.2 Analysis of relationships
   4.3 Analysis of organizational principles

5.0 SYNTHESIS
   5.1 Production of a unique communication
   5.2 Production of a plan, or proposed set of operations
   5.3 Derivation of a set of abstract relations
6.0 EVALUATION
   6.1 Judgments in terms of internal evidence
   6.2 Judgments in terms of external criteria

The classes are arranged from simple to complex, from concrete to more abstract. The objectives in any one class are likely to be built on the behaviors in the previous class. The subcategories help to define the major headings further and make them more specific.

The dietetics professional needs to think beyond the simplest levels of knowledge and also to write objectives at higher, more complex levels. Without examining the possibility of writing higher-level objectives, one may tend to think only in terms of knowledge and comprehension, which are the easiest objectives to write. The client or employee may then be denied the opportunity of applying knowledge or using it in problem solving and will be reduced to memorizing facts. In nutrition education, for example, knowing facts is necessary, but the client also needs the ability to analyze food labels, to synthesize all information learned so that she may tell others about it, and to evaluate nutritional information in making wise food choices. In the following discussion of the six levels in the taxonomy, examples of objectives are given.

Knowledge. At the lowest levels in the cognitive domain, knowledge involves the remembering and recall of information without necessarily understanding it. This includes the recall of specific bits of information, terminology, and facts, such as dates, events, and places, chronological sequences, methods of inquiry, trends over time, processes, classification systems criteria, principles, and theories. Table 11.3 suggests verbs describing performance in the cognitive domain.

Example: Is able to list foods high in sodium.

Comprehension. The second level, comprehension, is the lowest level of understanding. It involves knowing what is communicated by another person and being able to use the information communicated. The use of information may include translation, restatement or paraphrase, interpretation, summarization or rearrangement of the information, and extrapolation or extension of the given information to determine implications or consequences.

Example: Is able to explain (verbally or in writing) why certain foods are excluded on the diabetic diet.

Application. At the level of application, one is able to use information, principles, concepts, or ideas in concrete situations. Knowledge is understood sufficiently to be able to apply it to solve a problem.

Example: Is able to plan a sodium-restricted menu for the day.

TABLE 11.3.

Verbs Describing Performance—Cognitive

LEVEL	VERBS TO USE
Knowledge	cites, defines, describes, identifies, labels, lists, matches, memorizes, names, outlines, recalls, recites, repeats, reproduces, selects, states
Comprehension	converts, defends, discusses, distinguishes, estimates, explains, generalizes, gives examples, paraphrases, predicts, recognizes, rewrites, selects, summarizes
Application	applies, assembles, calculates, changes, computes, demonstrates, designs, manipulates, modifies, operates, plans, practices, prepares, produces, shows, solves, uses
Analysis	analyzes, compares, differentiates, discriminates, distinguishes, identifies, illustrates, interprets, investigates, outlines, relates, researches, separates, solves, studies
Synthesis	assembles, categorizes, classifies, combines, compiles, composes, creates, designs, explains, formulates, generates, organizes, plans, recommends, revises, rewrites, summarizes, writes
Evaluation	assesses, appraises, compares, concludes, contrasts, criticizes, discriminates, evaluates, judges, justifies

Analysis. This level entails the breakdown of information into its parts to identify the elements, the interaction between elements, and the organizing principles or structure. Relationships may be made among ideas.

Example: Is able to analyze the nutrition labeling on a food product.

Synthesis. Synthesis requires the reassembling of elements or parts to form something new. One may assemble a unique verbal or written communication, a plan of operation, or a set of abstract relations to explain data.

Example: Is able to explain the low cholesterol diet accurately to a friend.

Evaluation. At the highest level in the cognitive taxonomy, evaluation is the ability to judge the value of materials or methods in a particular situation. Such judgment requires the use of criteria, which may be internal criteria, such as logical accuracy or consistency, or external criteria, such as external standards.

Example: Is able to evaluate a nutrition article from the daily newspaper.

AFFECTIVE DOMAIN

The affective domain deals with changes in attitudes, values, beliefs, appreciation, and interests. Often, one wants a client or employee not only to comprehend what to do, but also to value it, accept it, and find it important. Attitudes and beliefs about food are widely recognized as important determinants of an individual's food habits. According to Johnson and Johnson, the purpose of nutrition education is "to create informed consumers who value good nutrition and consume nutritious foods throughout their lives" (4). When imparting information fails to bring about behavior change, the common response is to redouble efforts to teach facts and explain why something should be done. Instead, the examination of attitudes and values should be considered.

The affective domain involves a process of internalization from least committed to most committed. It categorizes the inner growth that occurs as people become aware of, and later adopt, the attitudes and principles that assist in forming the value judgments that guide conduct. For the client learning about prenatal nutrition, the dietetics professional may desire the person not only to be knowledgeable (cognitive domain) about the proper foods to eat during pregnancy, but also to value the knowledge so much (affective domain) that she eats nutritious foods and practices good nutrition. Note that an objective in one domain may have a component in another. Cognitive objectives may have an affective component, and affective objectives may have a cognitive one.

Affective objectives are more nebulous and resist precise definition; therefore, evaluation of their achievement is more difficult. The practitioner may find it a formidable task to describe affective behaviors involving internal feelings and emotions, but they are as important as overt behaviors. Because affective objectives are more difficult to express, most written objectives express cognitive behaviors.

Krathwohl and others published a taxonomy of educational objectives in the affective domain (20). It includes five categories and a number of subcategories:

1.0 RECEIVING (ATTENDING)

    1.1   Awareness

    1.2   Willingness to receive

    1.3   Controlled or selected attention

2.0 RESPONDING

    2.1   Acquiescence in responding

    2.2   Willingness to respond

    2.3   Satisfaction in response

3.0 VALUING

    3.1   Acceptance of a value

    3.2   Preference for a value

    3.3   Commitment

4.0 ORGANIZATION

    4.1   Conceptualization of a value

    4.2   Organization of a value system

5.0 CHARACTERIZATION BY A VALUE OR VALUE COMPLEX

    5.1   Generalized set

    5.2   Characterization

The ordering of classes describes a process by which a value progresses from a level of mere awareness or perception to levels of greater complexity until it becomes an internal part of one's outlook on life that guides or controls behavior. This internalization may occur in varying degrees, and may involve conformity and high commitment or nonconformity. At higher levels, behavior may be so ingrained that it is unconscious rather than a conscious response, and responses may be produced consistently in the absence of external authorities, and in spite of barriers. Thus, a client may eventually select a proper diet or an employee may wash his hands without thinking about it at the conscious level. Table 11.4 suggests verbs describing performance in the affective domain.

Receiving. At the lowest level of the affective domain, the learner is willing to receive certain phenomena or stimuli. Receiving represents a willingness to attend to what the professional is presenting. The individual may move from a passive level of awareness or consciousness, to a neutral willingness to tolerate the situation rather than to avoid it, and then to an active level of controlled or selected attention despite distractions.

Example: Is able to focus attention on instructions on a diabetic diet.

Responding. The second level, responding, indicates a desire on the part of the individual to become involved in, or committed to, a subject or activity. At the lowest level of responding, the client or employee may passively acquiesce, or at least comply, in response to the practi-

TABLE 11.4.

Verbs Describing Performance—Affective

LEVEL	VERBS TO USE
Receiving	asks, attends, chooses, describes, follows, gives, identifies, listens, replies, selects, uses
Responding	answers, assists, complies, conforms, cooperates, discusses, helps, participates, performs, practices, presents, reads, recites, reports, responds, selects, tells, writes
Valuing	completes, describes, differentiates, explains, follows, imitates, joins, justifies, proposes, reads, selects, shares
Organization	accepts, adheres, alters, arranges, combines, compares, defends, discusses, explains, generalizes, identifies, integrates, modifies, organizes, prefers, relates, synthesizes
Characterization	acts, advocates, communicates, discriminates, displays, exemplifies, influences, listens, performs, practices, proposes, questions, selects, serves, supports, uses, verifies

tioner. At a higher level, a willingness to respond or voluntarily make a commitment to a chosen response is evident. Finally, a feeling of satisfaction or pleasure in response involves an internalization on the part of the individual.

Example: Is able to read diet materials with interest and ask questions.

Valuing. At the third level, valuing, the individual believes that the information or behavior has worth. The individual values it based on a personal assessment. When the value has been slowly internalized or accepted, the client or employee displays a behavior consistent with the value. When something is valued, motivation is not based on external authorities or the desire to obey, but on an internal commitment. The individual may demonstrate acceptance of a value, preference for a value, or commitment and conviction.

Example: Is able to select a nutritious meal from the cafeteria line.

Organization. At this level, the individual discovers situations in which more than one value is appropriate. Individual values are incorporated into a total network of values, and at the level of conceptualization, an individual relates new values to those he already holds. New values must be organized into an ordered relationship with the current value system. Perhaps a client has valued eating whatever he wants, for example. If the dietetics professional is teaching a client a new diet, he has to learn a new value (different foods) and change an old one (some of his current eating patterns).

Example: Is able to discuss plans for following a new dietary regimen.

Characterization. The highest level, characterization, indicates that the values have been internalized for a sufficient time to control behavior, and the individual acts consistently over time. A generalized set is a predisposition to act or perceive events in a certain way. At the highest level of internalization, beliefs or ideas are integrated with internal consistency.

Example: Is able to select only those foods permitted on the diet at almost all times.

Behavioral change in the affective domain takes place gradually over a period of time, whereas cognitive change may occur more rapidly. Affective change may take days, weeks, or months at the higher levels.

PSYCHOMOTOR DOMAIN

The psychomotor domain involves the development of physical abilities and skills. Knowledge and attitudes are interrelated and may be necessary to perform these skills. For example, one could not drive a car or operate a meat slicer, tasks requiring manual skills, without some basic knowledge of the equipment. The authors who developed the cognitive and affective domains did not develop a taxonomy for the psychomotor domain, but more than one has been published (21, 22). Table 11.5 suggests verbs describing performance at the various levels of the psychomotor domain. The performance of physical ability proceeds to increasingly complex steps. Simpson's seven levels and subcategories are as follows (21):

1.00   PERCEPTION

    1.10   Sensory stimulation

        1.11   Auditory

        1.12   Visual

        1.13   Tactile

        1.14   Taste

        1.15   Smell

        1.16   Kinesthetic

    1.20   Cue Selection

    1.30   Translation

2.00   SET

    2.10   Mental set

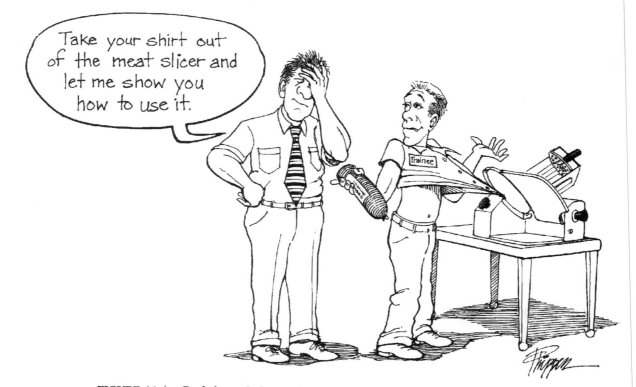

FIGURE 11.4. Both knowledge and skills are needed in operating equipment.

TABLE 11.5.
Verbs Describing Performance—Psychomotor

LEVEL	VERBS TO USE
Perception	attends, observes, perceives, recognizes, watches
Set	demonstrates, positions, prepares, senses, touches, uses
Guided response	calculates, computes, cuts, imitates, performs, practices, repeats, replicates, tries
Mechanism	assembles, disassembles, operates, performs, practices, repairs, uses
Complex overt response	demonstrates, masters, performs
Adaptation	adapts, changes, develops, modifies, organizes, produces, solves
Origination	operates, originates, uses

2.20   Physical set

2.30   Emotional set

3.00   GUIDED RESPONSE

    3.10   Imitation

    3.20   Trial and error

4.00   MECHANISM

5.00   COMPLEX OVERT RESPONSE

    5.10   Resolution of uncertainty

    5.20   Automatic performance

6.00   ADAPTATION

7.00   ORIGINATION

Perception. The lowest level of the psychomotor domain is perception. It involves becoming aware of objects by means of the senses—hearing, seeing, touching, tasting, and smelling—and by muscle sensations or activation. The individual must select which cues to respond to in order to perform a task. The individual then must mentally translate the cues received for action.

Example: Is able to recognize a need to learn how to use the meat slicer.

Set. The second level, set, suggests a readiness for performing a task. In addition to being ready mentally, the employee must be ready physically by correct positioning of the body, and emotionally, by having a favorable attitude or willingness to learn the task.

Example: Is able to demonstrate readiness to learn to use the meat slicer.

Guided Response. The third level is guided response. The professional or trainer guides the employee during the activity, emphasizing the individual components of a more complex skill. The subcategories include imitation of the practitioner and trial and error until the task can be performed accurately. Performance at this level may initially be crude and imperfect.

Example: Is able to practice the steps in using the meat slicer under supervision.

Mechanism. Mechanism, the fourth level, refers to habitual response. At this stage of learning, the employee demonstrates an initial degree of proficiency in performing the task, which results from some practice.

Example: Is able to use the meat slicer properly.

Complex Overt Response. The fifth level of complex overt response suggests that a level of skill has been attained over time in performing the task. Work is performed smoothly and efficiently without error. Two subcategories are resolution of uncertainty, in which a task is performed without hesitation, and automatic performance. Performance is characterized by accuracy, control, and speed.

Example: Is able to demonstrate considerable skill in using the meat slicer.

Adaptation/Origination. Adaptation requires altering manual skills in new but similar situations, such as in adapting slicing procedures to a variety of different foods on the meat slicer. The final level, origination, refers to the creation of a new physical act, such as slicing something that has not been done before.

In understanding the psychomotor domain, it may be helpful to recall the process of learning to drive an automobile, responding to the physical and visual stimulation, feeling mentally and emotionally ready to drive, learning parallel parking by trial and error under the guidance of an instructor, developing a degree of skill, and finally starting the car and driving without having to think of the steps. With time, sufficient skill is developed so that the person can adapt quickly in new situations on the road and create new responses automatically.

Using the taxonomies ensures that the objectives of learning are not limited to the lowest levels, that is, to the recall of facts, or to the cognitive domain only. The taxonomies assist the dietetics professional in thinking of higher levels of knowledge, which may be more appropriate behaviors for the learner. They also serve to remind the practitioner that there are interrelationships among

CASE STUDY

Joan is the dietetics professional responsible for employee education at a worksite. She moderated a focus group interview consisting of 10 employees. The purpose was to determine the employees' concerns about nutrition and health. At the top of the list of concerns was the relationship of diet and cholesterol to heart disease.

1. The follow-up focus group will determine more precisely what the employees' needs and interests are related to the topic. What questions would you ask the focus group?

2. What objectives could you write for an educational presentation to employees on the relationship of diet and cholesterol to heart disease?

the three domains. The professional should be concerned not only that clients can plan menus using their diets, but also that they think that the diet is important enough to their health to follow it. Employees need not only to know proper sanitation procedures, for example, but also to value them if they are going to practice optimum sanitary procedures regularly.

DETERMINING THE CONTENT

A close examination of the objectives helps to identify the content of the instruction. The objective states what the patient, client, or employee will be able to do when instruction is complete and directs attention to the appropriate content. The preassessment may have eliminated certain objectives as unnecessary, and those that remain should be examined in planning content. Some individuals may need to start at the lowest level in the taxonomy, while those who have already mastered the lower level objectives are ready for those at higher levels.

ORGANIZING TRAINING GROUPS

Learning may take place individually or in groups. Groups are advantageous in that they save time and money and provide opportunities for people to share experiences. Those who are successful in making dietary changes can model behaviors and discuss information with those who have been unsuccessful in coping. The more complex the information to be learned, the greater the need to discuss it in groups.

Even when one individual is involved, the dietetics professional should consider whether or not others should be present. In nutrition counseling and education, the individual responsible for purchasing the food and preparing the meals should be present. When a child is placed on a modified diet, such as a diabetic diet, for example, usually the mother requires instruction as well, since her cooperation is essential to the child's successful adherence to the diet and management of the disease.

Training sessions for employees may be organized in several ways. Frequently, all new employees are grouped together for initial orientation and training. Although current employees may be grouped by age, educational level, amount of experience, or job title, the best grouping probably occurs when employees with similar learning needs are together. Waitresses, for example, may re-

quire sessions on sanitary dish and utensil handling while cooks may need classes on sanitary food handling. The learning needs of employees differ according to their job content and level of current knowledge. The preassessment should show differences in knowledge levels and should assist in making grouping decisions.

Another question is whether supervisors should be grouped in the same classes as their employees. One disadvantage of such a grouping is that the employees may be reluctant to participate by asking questions when the superior is present. The final decision rests on the size of the group. There is more opportunity for individual participation in small groups of 10 to 15 than in groups of 30 to 50 or more.

This chapter has explored the initial steps in planning learning. After needs assessment has been completed, performance objectives should be written in the cognitive, affective, and psychomotor domains. Either individual or group instruction may be organized. The content of instruction may be determined from an examination of the objectives. The next chapter explores the remaining steps in the framework for education.

REVIEW AND DISCUSSION QUESTIONS

1. What is the difference between teaching and learning?

2. What are the 3 parts of Mager's learning objectives? What question does each answer?

3. What are the 3 domains of learning objectives? What are the levels in each domain?

4. How are the objectives in the 3 domains interrelated?

5. What in-service topics would be appropriate for food-service employees in the 3 domains? For clients?

6. How should the physical and psychological environments be arranged?

7. What are the steps to education?

8. What are the reasons for conducting a preassessment or needs assessment?

SUGGESTED ACTIVITIES

1. Make a list of questions you would ask in the preas-

sessment of knowledge of some subject with which you are familiar.

2. Write three performance objectives using active verbs to describe behavior.

3. Write examples of performance objectives containing conditions and a criterion.

4. Write examples of objectives in various levels of the cognitive, affective, and psychomotor domain. Note overlap from one domain to another.

5. Decide which of the following performance objectives are measurable as opposed to nonmeasurable.
   A. Presented with a menu, the patient will be able to circle appropriate food selections according to his diet.
   B. At the close of the series of classes, the clients will be more positively disposed toward following their diets.
   C. After counseling, the patient will know which foods he should eat and which he should not.
   D. The patient will be able to explain the diabetic diet to her husband.

6. Examine the following objectives and decide whether each concerns primarily the cognitive, affective, or psychomotor domain.
   A. All clerical staff should be able to type 50 words per minute without errors.
   B. Given a series of objectives, the student will be able to classify them according to the taxonomies in the chapter.
   C. At the end of the session, clients will request more weight control classes.

REFERENCES

1. Hartman TJ, McCarthy PR, Park RJ, et al. Focus group responses of potential participants in a nutrition education program for individuals with limited literacy skills. J Am Diet Assoc 1994;94:744.

2. Chambers DW, Gilmore CJ, Maillet JO, et al. Another look at competency-based education in dietetics. J Am Diet Assoc 1996;96:614.

3. Johnson KD, Rinke WJ. Nutrition education: a review of results and a report provided by Army dietitians. J Am Diet Assoc 1988;88:1582.

4. Johnson DW, Johnson RT. Nutrition education: a model for effectiveness, a synthesis of research. J Nutr Educ 1985;17:S1.

5. Contento I, Balch GI, Bronner YL, et al. Executive summary. J Nutr Educ 1995;27:279.

6. Franz MJ. Diabetes and nutrition: state of the science and the art. Top Clin Nutr 1988;3:1.

7. Sepherd R, Stockley L. Nutrition knowledge, attitudes, and fat consumption. J Am Diet Assoc 1987;87:615.

8. Fleming PL. Nutrition education and counseling. In: Paige DM, ed. Clinical nutrition. 2nd ed. St. Louis: Mosby, 1988.

9. Achterberg C. A perspective on nutrition education research and practice. J Nutr Educ 1988;20:240.

10. National standards for diabetes self-management education programs. Diabetes Educ 1994;21:189.

11. Galbraith MW. Attributes and skills of an adult educator. In: Galbraith MW, ed. Adult learning methods: a guide for effective instruction. Malabar, FL: Krieger Publishing, 1990.

12. Crockett SJ, Heller KE, Peterson JM. Assessing beliefs of older rural Americans about nutrition education: use of the focus group approach. J Am Diet Assoc 1990;90:563.

13. Kaufman R. Needs assessment and analysis. In: Tracey WR, ed. Human resources management and development handbook. 2nd ed. New York: American Management Assoc, 1994.

14. Laird D. Approaches to training and development. 2nd ed. Reading, MA: Addison-Wesley, 1985.

15. Rose JC. Handbook for health care food service management. Rockville, MD: Aspen Publishing, 1984.

16. Kaufman R. A needs assessment primer. Train Dev J 1987;41:78.

17. Popham WJ. Educational evaluation. 3rd ed. Boston: Allyn and Bacon, 1993.

18. Mager RF. Preparing instructional objectives. 2nd ed. Belmont, CA: Lake, 1984.

19. Bloom BS, Engelhart M, Furst E, et al. Taxonomy of educational objectives, handbook I: cognitive domain. New York: David McKay, 1956.

20. Krathwohl D, Bloom BS, Masia B. Taxonomy of educational objectives, handbook II: affective domain. New York: David McKay, 1964.

21. Simpson E. The classification of educational objectives in the psychomotor domain. Illinois Teacher of Home Econ 1966;10:110.

22. Harrow A. A taxonomy of the psychomotor domain. New York: David McKay, 1972.

twelve

IMPLEMENTING AND EVALUATING LEARNING

The initial steps in planning learning, discussed in the previous chapter, include a preassessment of the learner's current knowledge and competencies, the development of performance objectives in the cognitive, affective, and psychomotor domains, and the determination of the content to be learned. This chapter discusses the selection and implementation of appropriate learning activities for the cognitive, affective, and psychomotor domains. In addition, plans for the evaluation of the results of learning and for documentation are also discussed, as these steps are necessary to complete the educational process.

SELECTING AND IMPLEMENTING LEARNING ACTIVITIES

Various methods and techniques of educational presentation are available to turn the objectives of learning into action. Techniques are the ways the instructor presents information to learners to influence the internal processes of learning (1). They establish a relationship between the teacher and the learner, and between the learner and what he or she is learning. They include lectures, discussions, simulations, demonstrations, and the like. All are not equally effective in facilitating learning, and each has its advantages and disadvantages, its uses and limitations, which are summarized in Table 12.1. In deciding which one will be most effective, the dietetics professional may be guided by several factors, including the educational purpose they serve, learner preference, needs, or style, group size, facilities available, time available, cost, and one's previous experience or the degree of success with the techniques (2). In addition, an examination of the performance objectives may suggest which approach is most appropriate, as methods and techniques may differ for the cognitive, affective, and psychomotor domains. All factors being equal, one should select the technique that requires the most active participation of the leaner. As Confucius said:

I hear and I forget,
I see and I remember,
I do and I understand.

The dietetics professional must also be concerned that clients and employees remember and retain what they learn. Studies show that the more actively one is involved in the learning process, the better the retention. See Fig. 12.1, which shows that reading and hearing information is not as productive as both seeing and hearing or, better yet, discussing it or doing something with it.

Lecture

The lecture is the presentation technique most familiar to people. It has been used for years as a method of informing and transferring knowledge—the lowest level in the cognitive domain—from the teacher to the learner. It is especially useful in situations where there are large numbers of learners, a great deal of information to be communicated, and a limited amount of time is available. Examples are a class on sanitation for food service employees or on cholesterol and fat in relation to heart disease for work-site employees or hospital clients.

In spite of the advantages of efficiency, a major drawback is that there is no guarantee that the material is learned and remembered since the individual is a passive participant whose learning depends on listening skills. This may be the least effective technique for use with adults. A review of over 200 nutrition education interventions found that often there was a mismatch between stated goals related to dietary change and a didactic, information-based educational methodology used (3) (Fig. 12.2).

While many educated people may respond positively to lectures because of long experience with this mode, people with less education may learn better with other methods. Their attention may wane quickly as they tune out, especially if the lecturer is not an effective speaker or if the lecture is dull, and new information may be rapidly forgotten. A focus group of clients with limited literacy skills considered lectures an ineffective way to obtain nutrition information and preferred more hands-on activities where they could share ideas and experiences (4). Furthermore, lectures do not meet the requirements of adult education, or "andragogy," for self-directed learning and problem-solving approaches as discussed in an earlier chapter. When lectures are

TABLE 12.1.

Strengths and Weaknesses of Teaching Methods

	STRENGTHS	WEAKNESSES
Lecture	Easy and efficient Conveys most information Reaches large numbers Minimum threat to learner Maximum control by instructor	Learner is passive Learning by listening Formal atmosphere May be dull, boring Not suited for higher level learning in cognitive domain Not suited for manual learning

Discussion
  Panel
  Debate
  Case study
	More interesting, thus motivating
	Active participation
	Informal atmosphere
	Broadens perspectives
	We remember what we discuss
	Good for higher level cognitive, affective objectives
		Learner may be unprepared
		Shy people may not discuss
		May get sidetracked
		More time-consuming
		Size of group limited

Projects	More motivating Active participation Good for higher level cognitive objectives	
Laboratory experiments	Learn by experience Hands-on method Active participation Good for higher level cognitive objectives	Requires space, time Group size limited

Simulation
  Scenarios
  In-basket
  Role playing
  Critical incidents
	Active participation
	Requires critical thinking
	Develops problem-solving skills
	Connects theory and practice
	More interesting
	Good for higher level cognitive and affective objectives
		Time-consuming
		Group size limited

Demonstration	Realistic Appeals to several senses Can show a large group Good for psychomotor domain	Requires equipment Requires time Learner is passive, unless can practice

employed, it is advisable to limit the number of concepts presented, use examples frequently, add visual aids, and provide ample time for a question-and-answer or discussion period.

Discussion

In discussion techniques, whether on a one-to-one basis or in groups, individuals are active participants as they examine their own thinking and internalize the knowledge through their verbal responses. Discussion may be guided by the dietetics professional's raising open-ended questions, problems, or key issues so that clients or employees make comparisons or work to draw conclusions, or it may be more group-centered if individuals are fairly well acquainted. With a series of classes on weight reduction, for example, clients could discuss what they have done to change their food habits, recipes, and shopping habits. Debates and panel discussions, in which several people of notable competence and specific knowledge of a topic informally discuss or debate the topic in front

10%
What they read

20%
What they hear

30%
What they see

50%
What they both see and hear

70%
What they say

90%
What they both say and do

FIGURE 12.1. What people remember.

of a larger group, are other approaches. The basis for discussion may be common experiences, problem solving, topics that were preannounced so that the group has prepared, or case studies or real-life situations, which are developed.

For best results, seating should be arranged in a circle so that everyone can see and hear one another, and so that the practitioner can participate as a member of the group. Smaller group sizes of 10 to 15 offer more opportunity for participation as learners explore their thoughts, values, and experiences, think critically, and influence others.

While it is more time-consuming than lecture, discussion may be more interesting for learners, and thus more motivating, especially with higher-level cognitive objectives and with affective objectives. Discussion and oral summarization facilitate and promote the individual's acquisition and retention of information since we remember what we say out loud. When people study alone, or are passive listeners, some cognitive processing may not take place.

Simulation

Simulation of real-life situations may also be considered in developing learner knowledge, skills, and competencies. Several means of representation may be used, such as scenarios, in-basket exercises, critical incidents, and role-playing. These methods involve learning by "doing" something or "experiential learning" rather than learning by "listening." Active learner involvement is necessary for optimum transfer of learning.

Simulation may be based on scenarios or models of real-life problem situations. Clients on sodium-restricted diets, for example, could take restaurant menus and determine what they should order. Learners use a process of inquiry in exploring the problem.

In-basket exercises test the person's ability to handle day-to-day challenges. The techniques have been used, for example, to simulate a supervisor's decision-making ability in handling problems that arrive in the in-basket on the desk each day. Written memos, notes, requests, or reports are given to an individual and require a decision.

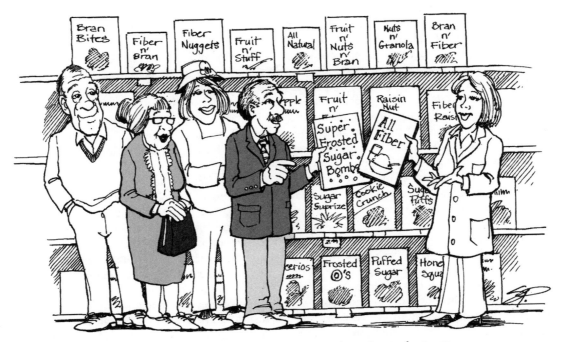

FIGURE 12.2. People prefer hands-on learning to lectures.

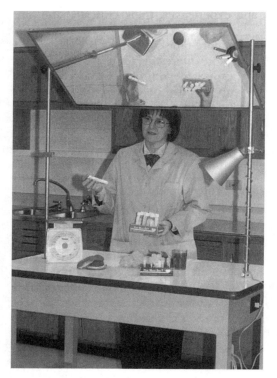

FIGURE 12.3. A demonstration is one approach to presentations.

Critical incidents also require the learner's responses to specific situations. Emergencies, such as fires or electrical blackouts, or unusual incidents are used, and the learner has to provide a solution in handling the situation or problem.

The use of role-playing, in which two or more persons dramatize assigned parts or roles simulating real-life situations, is another possibility. Role playing allows learners to try or practice new behaviors in relatively safe environments, and it can be used to work through real problems (5). This is followed by discussion of the problem, ideas, feelings, and emotional reactions, as, for example, role-playing of handling an employee disciplinary problem or clients learning to say ''no'' when offered disallowed foods. While time-consuming, simulations may be helpful in providing opportunities for individuals to make a connection between theory and practice, to engage in critical thinking as active participants, and to develop problem-solving and coping skills. Simulation may be used with both cognitive and affective objectives.

Demonstration

A demonstration may be used to show how something is done, or to explore processes, techniques, ideas, or attitudes. Learning to prepare low-fat recipes or how to use a meat slicer are examples of times when demonstration is appropriate. Usually, the client or employee observes as the dietetics professional makes the presentation, although a participant volunteer may do it. The

demonstration may be a dramatic learning experience if the individual's attention is held and may be appropriate for any type of learning objective. If skills are demonstrated, the individual will need an opportunity to practice the task or skill soon after and evaluate the performance. Job Instruction Training (JIT) discussed later in this chapter is an example of the use of demonstration to achieve mastery. Sometimes, duplicate work operations are set up independent of the work site and are used for training.

Audiovisual Aids

According to an old Chinese proverb, ''one picture is worth more than 1000 words.'' An effective media presentation can enhance learning by providing variety and improving memory through visual stimulation. The appropriateness of such material to the learning situation, and to the individual or group, should be considered. A videotape of one's own setting, for example, would probably foster better learning among employees than one that is purchased. Such materials are an adjunct to learning and should not be considered the total learning experience. Another chapter discusses this in more detail.

Other techniques to promote learning by individuals rather than by groups include coaching, programmed instruction, and computer-based training, which is used by more than half of U.S. organizations with 50 or more employees. Laboratory experiences, apprenticeship, job rotation, job enlargement, personal reading, and interactive video instruction are other approaches (6, 7). A WIC program used client-directed, interactive, multimedia software to deliver nutrition education to a high-risk, low-income population. Positive changes in knowledge, attitudes, or behavioral intentions, and a high level of client acceptance were found (8).

Techniques for Different Domains

For learning in the cognitive domain, most of the above techniques may be effective. There are additional factors to consider in fostering learning in the affective and psychomotor domains. In reviewing 80 studies of nutrition education interventions, there appeared to be some advantage to using mixed methods rather than only one (3, 9).

In the affective domain the dietetics professional seeks to influence the learner's interests, attitudes, and values. This cannot be accomplished in an hour or a day, but requires ongoing contacts. At the lowest level in the affective domain, receiving and awareness, the professional may gain the learner's attention through the use of audiovisual materials or guided discussion. At higher levels where the adoption of new attitudes and values is important, the individual must participate more fully. Attitudes are acquired through interpersonal influences, and commitments that are made public are more likely to be adopted than those that are private (10).

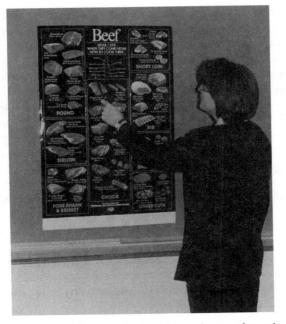

FIGURE 12.4. The professional needs to plan visuals along with her presentation.

Discussion in a group or where experiences are shared, discussion of case studies or critical incidents, and role-playing may be effective, They may lead to higher self-awareness and public commitment. People may perceive that all members of the group support the new attitudes and behaviors. Active oral summarization following discussion is recommended because it leads to more elaborate thinking and integration into the person's conceptual framework.

Effective instructional strategies that influence deeper-level learning of nutrition and the modification of attitudes and dietary behaviors have been recommended. Strategies promoting the active involvement of participants and interpersonal interaction in a group, which are related to the social context, help to achieve deeper-level learning, attitude modification, and behavioral change. The strategies suggested to accomplish this include *(a)* cooperative learning, *(b)* inquiry learning, *(c)* nutrition experiments and experiences, *(d)* out-of-class experiences, and *(e)* academic controversies (10). Competitive and individual learning are not as effective.

In cooperative learning, individuals work together to achieve goals for learning that are mutually held. They collaborate, effectively share information and analyses, and teach and assist each other. In the process of teaching others, people enhance their own learning.

A second strategy, inquiry learning, requires use of the problem-solving process, in which the dietetics professional presents a puzzling situation or problem. The professional could ask people, for example, to figure their daily fat allowance from food labels. Individuals identify and clarify the problem, form hypotheses, gather

data, analyze and interpret data, select possible solutions, test solutions, and finally draw conclusions and select the best solution to the problem. People learn how to solve problems, evaluate possible solutions, and think critically. Clients can be guided through this process so that they learn to solve their own nutrition problems.

Experiments, such as with modifying recipes for fat or sodium, and hands-on activities, such as planning nutritious menus and preparing varieties of new foods for a diet, are a third approach. An example of experiences outside of the classroom as a means of instruction is to require individuals to shop for and evaluate certain foods.

In using academic controversies, participants take opposing sides of an issue, explore their differences, and try to come to consensus. These five types of experiences promote more elaborate cognitive processing, higher-level reasoning, problem solving, decision making, positive attitudes, and motivation. They can lead to group decisions in which members commit themselves publicly to better food habits (10).

Modeling is also a method of influencing behavior (10, 11). People learn by imitating others in unfamiliar or new situations. The dietetics professional should behave as the client or employee is expected to behave, modeling the desirable attitude or behavior. People are more likely to accept new behaviors when they meet and have discussions with people who have successfully adopted them. This technique is appropriate for nutrition education.

Focus group research was used to plan diabetes nutrition education for a hard-to-reach, low-income, African-American community. Members wanted positive sessions rather than "don'ts," the demonstration of alternatives in preparing food, and not too many words. The resulting program "Learn, Taste, and Share" de-emphasized lecture for more participatory methods that included games, food prizes, a cooking demonstration, and cooking participation. Activities included ranking boxes of cereal from low to high fiber, guessing the amount of fat in foods, finding whole-grain crackers at a grocery store, experiments with recipes, and preparing a dinner (12).

Skills in the psychomotor domain are learned with direct experience and practice over time. The professional may begin with a demonstration, but then the individual needs to practice the skill under supervision. Coaching is a term that describes the assistance given to someone learning a new skill, and it can apply to an educational experience as well as a sport. It suggests a one-on-one, continuous, supportive relationship from which an individual learns over time. It is perhaps the best method of on-the-job training of employees. The trainer can give encouragement, confidence, and guidance as the trainee performs the task (12). Coaching takes into consideration different learning abilities and needs, allows actual practice, and provides people with immediate feedback regarding their performance.

TASK ANALYSIS

In instruction that requires the individual to develop a skill, a task analysis is helpful. Employees need to learn the skills related to their jobs, and clients may need to develop skills in menu planning and food preparation using a new dietary regimen. Regardless of the kind of skill involved, the learner needs to be able to perform the skill initially and then to improve the skill through continued practice. After grasping the basics of tennis, driving a car, or baking a cake, for example, an individual requires repeated experience to develop a skill.

Instruction involving the initial development of a skill requires examination of what the job or task entails, the conditions under which it is performed, and the proper method of performance. The task should be broken down into its elements and key points and put into writing.

If available, a job description may be used as a starting point in determining job content, but job descriptions do not give specific enough information for determining the content of training (13). All of the tasks included in a job should be listed individually. If the job description is unavailable or incomplete, it may be necessary to interview employees or observe their work to determine the job content. Wait-staff, for example, complete a number of tasks during the day, such as greeting customers, taking their orders, placing orders in the kitchen, serving the courses of the meal, busing dishes, setting tables, receiving payment for services, and maintaining good public relations. Each is a separate task making up the total job, and each task or set of actions can be defined.

The next step is to complete a written task analysis or series of task analyses for each different task of the job. A task analysis, sometimes referred to as a job breakdown, is a sequential list of the steps involved in performing any task from beginning to end. Usually, the major steps are numbered, and each step describes what to do (13). Many job-related tasks involve the psychomotor domain; thus actions are listed in the analysis. It is often necessary, however, to have some background knowledge from the cognitive domain in performing the task. Balancing a checkbook, for example, is both a manual and intellectual skill, as is operating a cash register.

After the sequential steps are listed, each one should be examined to see whether there are explanations from the cognitive domain that need to be added. If step one, for example, is to plug in the meat slicer, a key point is to have dry hands to avoid the danger of electrical shock. If a final step in the wait-staff's task analysis for busing dirty dishes includes washing hands, an explanation may be added regarding the transfer of microorganisms to clean food and utensils. In food service, sanitation and safety statements are frequently needed. Other explanations of reasons why a step is necessary or notes on materials or equipment may be important to add. There are a number of different ways to complete a task analysis (13–16).

Once written, the task analysis should be used both by the professional and by the individual. The practitioner or trainer may examine the task analysis in order to construct learning objectives, which describe the behavior expected at the end of training. In assessing the person's need for instruction, the professional should consider the difference between the skill described in the task analysis and the individual's current skill to define the gap in knowledge or skill that must be addressed. The person doing the training should demonstrate to the individual what to do, and then allow him or her to perform the task. The individual may use the task analysis as a reference since it describes what to do in sequence. Using the task analysis in coaching or in supervised on-the-job training facilitates the learning of skills.

After mastering the basic skill involved and being able to recognize the correct sequence of procedures, the individual needs repeated practice to improve the skill. With time and practice, improvements in speed and quality of work should develop.

JOB INSTRUCTION TRAINING (JIT)

A great deal of employee training takes place not in the classroom, but on the job. New employees require orientation and training with either an experienced worker or a supervisor. Current employees may need retraining periodically, may be assigned new tasks, or may receive promotions that require the development of new skills and abilities. A four-step process entitled Job Instruction Training (JIT) was delineated for rapid training of new employees. It may be used to teach skills and is based on performance rather than subject matter. The four steps are *(a)* preparation, *(b)* presentation, *(c)* learner performance, and *(d)* follow-up. This is similar to Tell/Show/Do/Review. Before instruction, a task analysis should be completed, and the work area arranged with the necessary supplies and materials that the employee is expected to maintain (17, 18). Table 12.2 summarizes the main points.

Preparation. Part I of JIT prepares the employee psychologically and intellectually for learning. Since a superior may be the trainer, any tension, nervousness, or apprehension in the subordinate employee must be overcome, since it may interfere with learning. A friendly, smiling trainer puts the person at ease by creating an informal atmosphere for learning, where mistakes are expected and tolerated. The trainer states the job to be learned and asks specific questions to determine what the individual already knows about it. When employees become interested in their jobs, their motivation for learning increases. Finally, the trainer should be sure that the employee can physically see what is being demonstrated.

Presentation. In Part II, the trainer presents and explains the operation as the employee is expected to perform it. The trainer shows, tells, and illustrates the opera-

TABLE 12.2.

How to Instruct

Part I: Prepare the learner.
          Put the learner at ease.
          State the job.
          Find out what the individual knows about
              the job.
          Develop interest.
          Correct the person's position.

Part II: Present the operation.
          Tell, show, and illustrate.
          Explain one important step at a time.
          Stress key points.
          Instruct clearly, completely, and patiently,
              but no more than the learner can
              master.
          Summarize the operation in a second run-
              through.

Part III: Try out performance.
          Have the learner do the job.
          Have the learner explain key points while
              performing the job again.
          Make sure that the learner understands.
          Continue until you know that the person
              knows the job.

Part IV: Follow-up.
          Put learner on his own.
          Designate where to obtain help.
          Encourage questions.
          Taper off.
          Continue with normal supervision.

tion one step at a time using a prepared task analysis. Key points should be stressed. The instruction should be carried out clearly, completely, and patiently, with the trainer remembering the employee's abilities and attitudes. Since the ability to absorb new information is limited, the trainer needs to determine how much the learner can master at a time. It may be 5 to 10 steps with key points, or it may be more. It may be 15 minutes or 1 hour of instruction. Overloading anyone with information is ineffectual since the information will be forgotten. After this initial instruction, the operation or task should be summarized and performed a second time.

Performance. Part III tests how much the employee has retained as he or she tries out the operation using the written task analysis as a reference. The individual does the job while the trainer or coach stands by to assist. This is a form of behavior modeling. Accuracy, not speed, is stressed initially. As the individual completes the task a second time, the trainer should ask the employee to state the key points. To be sure of understanding, the trainer should ask such questions as "What would happen if . . . ?" "What else do you do . . . ?" and "What next . . . ?" Employees may need to repeat the operation 5 times, 10 times, or however many times are needed until they know what to do. The trainer continues coaching and giving positive feedback, encouragement, and reassurance until the employee learns the operation.

Follow-up. Follow-up occurs in Part IV as supervision tapers off. At first, the employee is left alone to complete the task. The individual should always know, however, where to obtain assistance if it is needed. Any additional questions should be encouraged in case problems arise. Normal supervision continues to ensure that the task is done as instructed, since fellow workers may suggest undesirable shortcuts.

Mager pointed out that when the learner's experience is followed by positive consequences, the individual will be stimulated to approach the situation, but that when aversive consequences follow, the learner will avoid the situation (11). A positive consequence may be any pleasant event, praise, a successful experience, an increase in self-esteem, improvement in self-image, or an increase in confidence. Aversive conditions are events or emotions that cause physical or mental discomfort, or that lead to loss of self-respect. They include fear, anxiety, frustration, humiliation, embarrassment, and boredom. In influencing learners in the affective domain, as well as the other domains, the dietetics professional should positively reinforce learner responses.

SEQUENCE OF INSTRUCTION

Since there is a great deal to learn, instruction requires some type of organized sequence. Sequence of instruction is characterized by the progressive development of knowledge, attitudes, and skills. Learning takes place over time, and the process should be organized into smaller units. Since the ultimate outcome is able performance, it is important to consider how meaningful the sequence is to the individual, not the teacher or trainer, and whether or not it promotes learning. Mager provides several recommendations for sequencing. Instruction may be arranged from the general to the specific, from the specific to the general, from the simple to the complex, or according to interest, logic, or frequency of use of the knowledge or skill (2, 15).

In moving from the general to the specific, an overview or large picture should be presented first, and then the details and specifics are presented. For example, an overview of the reasons for the diabetic diet and the general principles of the diet should be presented prior to the details. With a new employee, a general explanation of the job should precede the specifics. Once the individual has digested some information, it is possible to consider a specific to general sequence.

Material may be organized from the simple (terms, facts, procedures) to the complex (concepts, processes, theories, analyses, applications) so that the individual handles increasingly difficult material. If the cognitive, affective, and psychomotor taxonomies (see Chapter 11) are used in writing objectives for learning, the hierarchy of the taxonomies provides a simple to complex sequence.

Another possibility is sequencing according to interest, or from the familiar to the unfamiliar. One may begin instruction with whatever is of most interest or concern to the individual. Initial questions from patients, clients, employees, or other audiences suggest such interest and should be dealt with immediately so that they are free to concentrate on later information. "How long will I have to stay on this diet?" "Can I eat my favorite foods?" Information desired by the individual is a good starting point for discussion. Similarly, if the person perceives a problem, the dietetics professional can start with that problem rather than with her preset agenda. As learning proceeds, the individual may develop additional needs for information or goals for learning, which they may then address. Individuals who have assisted in directing their own learning tend to feel more committed to it.

Logic may suggest the sequence. Certain things may need to be said before others. Safety precautions may need to be introduced early, for example, when discussing kitchen equipment. Sanitary utensil handling may be important to discuss with wait-staff prior to discussing how to set a table.

Frequency of use of the knowledge or skill may also dictate sequence. The skill used most frequently should be taught first, followed by the next most frequently used skill. If training time runs out, at least the learner has learned all except the least frequently used skills. The dietetics professional should teach first what people "need to know" rather than the "nice to know" information.

Finally, the practitioner should provide learners with total job practice. While learners may have been practicing individual elements of the job, they also need practice on the total job. This practice may be provided in the actual job situation or through simulation.

EVALUATION OF RESULTS

The step most often overlooked is probably that of evaluation. The literature indicates that evaluation of nutrition programs is frequently omitted (19, 20). Evaluation connotes the determination of the value or worth of something. Everyone makes these judgments daily, both consciously and unconsciously. "Does the food taste good?" "Is she dressed well?" "Was the television show worth watching?" "Did I learn anything?" One's thoughts turn to evaluation automatically.

According to Popham, systematic educational evaluation "consists of a formal appraisal of the quality of educational phenomena," such as programs, products, or goals (21). That it is systematic suggests that advance planning has taken place and that the process will provide data on the quality or worth of the educational endeavor.

One must consider not only what to evaluate, but also when to evaluate and how the evaluation will be done. Evaluation involves a number of steps: defining objectives or outcomes; designing the evaluation based on objectives; choosing what to evaluate; deciding how to collect data; constructing a data collection instrument or method; implementing the data collection; analyzing results; and reporting them.

Although the terms "measurement" and "evaluation" are sometimes interchanged, their meanings are not equivalent. Evaluation is based on measurement (22). Measurement is the process of collecting and quantifying data in terms of numbers on the extent, degree, or capacity of people's achievement in knowledge, attitudes, skills, and performance. Testing is one kind of measurement, for example. Measurement involves determining the degree to which an individual possesses a certain attribute, as when one receives an 85 on a test, but it does not determine quality or worth. Measurement systems require experimental designs, data collection, and statistical analysis of the data (21). Some use the term "educational assessment" instead of measurement.

Evaluation, on the other hand, is based on the measurement of what people know, think, feel, and do (22). Evaluation compares the observed value or quality to a standard or criteria of comparison. Evaluation is the process of forming value judgments about the quality of programs, products, goals, and the like from the data. One may evaluate the success of an educational program, for example, by measuring the degree to which goals or objectives were achieved. Evaluation goes beyond measurement to the formation of value judgments about the data. To be effective, evaluation designs should specify not only what will be evaluated, but also when. Sometimes several measurements are needed, as in pretesting and posttesting.

Purpose of Evaluation

Careful evaluation should be an integral part of all nutrition education programs and employee education programs (3). There are several purposes of evaluation. Program evaluation may be used for planning, improvement, or justification (7). Evaluation is a system of quality control to determine whether the process of education is effective, to identify its strengths and weaknesses, and to determine what changes should be made. To determine accountability, one needs to know whether people are learning, whether dietetics professionals are teaching effectively, whether programs accomplish the desired outcomes, and whether money is well spent. It is important to determine whether the objectives were accomplished, and whether the individual learned what was intended or developed in desired ways (23).

Evaluation helps dietetics professionals to make better decisions and to improve education. Evaluation will be helpful in making decisions concerning teaching, learning, program effectiveness, and the necessity of making modifications in current efforts or even of terminating them. In times of limited financial resources, accountability requires an examination of cost/benefit ratios. Is the program so useful and valuable that costs are justified (23)? Is there concrete evidence that training is changing employee behavior on the job and contributing to the bottom line? Evaluation provides evidence that what one is doing is worthwhile. Plans for evaluation should be made early when one is in the planning stages of an educational endeavor, and not after it has begun or is completed.

With employees, training evaluation should demonstrate improved job performance and financial results. A question asked often is: "Does training transfer?" One needs to determine whether the skills and knowledge taught in training are applied on the job. If they are, this demonstrates the value of the training to the organization, and the effectiveness of the method of training. If not, change is needed (24).

As with other parts of his adult education model, Knowles has suggested that evaluation should be a mutual undertaking between the educator and the learner (25). He recommends less emphasis on the evaluation of learning, and more on the rediagnosis of learning needs, which will suggest immediate or future steps to be taken jointly by the professional and the client or employee. This type of feedback from evaluation becomes more constructive and acceptable to adults. Thus, evaluation may be considered something one should do with people, not to people. If problems are apparent, then solutions may be found jointly by the professional and the individual.

Formative and Summative Evaluation

Formative and summative evaluation are two types of evaluation used to improve any of three processes—curriculum construction, teaching, or learning. Formative evaluation refers to that made early or during the course of education, with the feedback of results modifying the rest of the educational endeavor. Summative evaluation refers to a summary assessment of quality at the conclusion of learning (21).

FORMATIVE

Formative evaluation is a systematic appraisal that occurs before or during a course of instruction or learning activity for the purpose of modifying or improving teaching or learning. It can help to diagnose problems in student learning and in teaching effectiveness. It pinpoints parts that are mastered and those not mastered, and allows for revision of plans, methods, techniques, or materials.

Formative evaluation may be performed at frequent intervals. If the learner appears bored, unsure, anxious, quizzical, or lost, or if one is unsure of the person's abilities, it is appropriate to stop teaching and start the evaluation process. Ask the person to repeat what he has learned. In diabetic education, for example, if formative evaluation shows that the individual does not understand the concept of carbohydrate counting, he will not be able to master more complex behaviors, such as menu planning. Having located the problem that carbohydrate counting is not comprehended, the dietetics professional can change approaches to try to overcome the problem. Perhaps the use of an alternative explanation that is clearer or simpler, or the use of concrete illustrations is indicated. Ideas and concepts may need to be reviewed. Sometimes, in group education, a group member is able to provide an explanation that the person understands better than the professional's explanation.

Before nutrition messages are designed and implemented, formative evaluation or market research activities, such as focus group interviews, are designed and implemented. This type of evaluation helps to learn about individuals' thoughts, ideas, and opinions, and tells whether message recipients are likely to ignore, reject, or misunderstand the message or accept it and act upon it (3, 26, 27). Formative research is essential to tailoring intervention strategies. The moderator of a focus group uses open-ended interviewing strategies with groups of 8 to 15 people (28). The focus group approach has been used to assess consumer preferences, to plan and evaluate nutrition education interventions, and to pretest print materials. This qualitative evaluation may be audiotaped or videotaped for later review and reference.

Failure to learn may not always be related to instructional methods or materials per se, but may derive from problems that are physical, emotional, cultural, or environmental in nature. By performing an evaluation after smaller units of instruction, one can determine whether the pacing of instruction is appropriate for the patient, client, or employee. Frequent feedback is necessary to facilitate learning. It is especially important when a great deal has to be learned. Mastery of smaller units can be a powerful positive reinforcement for the learner, and verbal praise may increase motivation to continue learning. When mistakes are made, they should be corrected quickly by giving the correct information. Avoid saying: "No, that's wrong." "Can't you ever get things right?" "Won't you ever learn?" Positive, not negative, feedback should be given. Approach the problem specifically by saying, for example, "You identified some of the foods that are high in sodium, which is good. Now let's look a second time for others."

SUMMATIVE

Summative evaluation has a different purpose and time frame than formative evaluation. Summative evaluation is considered final, and it is used at the end of a term, course, or learning activity. The purpose of summative evaluation is to appraise quality or worth. It may include grading, certification, or evaluation of progress, and the evaluation distinguishes those who excel from those who do not. Judgment is made about the learner, teacher, program, or curriculum with regard to the effectiveness of learning or instruction. This judgment aspect creates the anxiety and defensiveness often associated with evaluation.

Evaluation should be a continuous process that is pre-planned along with educational sessions. Evaluation pre-assessment determines the individual's abilities before the educational program, and progress should be evaluated continuously during, as well as immediately following, the educational program. Follow-up evaluation at 3 to 6 months may measure the degree to which one has forgotten knowledge or has fallen back to previous behaviors.

Norm-Referenced and Criterion-Referenced Methods

NORM-REFERENCED EVALUATION

Besides formative and summative evaluation, there are norm-referenced and criterion-referenced methods of evaluation. In norm-referenced testing, the group that has taken a test provides the norms for determining the meaning of each individual's score (21, 29). A norm is like the typical performance of a group. One can then see if an individual is above or below the norm. The college entrance examinations are an example.

Some instructors may believe that a test should not be too easy, but the degree of difficulty of a test may not be as important as whether an individual can perform. Or the instructor believes that some of the questions have to be difficult so that a spread of scores is produced, to separate the brightest from the rest, the "A's" from the "B's" and "C's." Some tests are purposely developed so that not everyone is successful, and variation in individual scores is expected. Students are graded in a norm-referenced manner by comparison with other individuals on the same measuring device or with the norm of the group. A norm-referenced instrument indicates, for example, whether the individual's performance falls in the 50th percentile or the 90th in relation to the group norm (21, 30). This method is not as appropriate for affective and psychomotor objectives (29).

CRITERION-REFERENCED EVALUATION

A more important question is whether or not the learner can perform what is stated in the objectives. Another approach to evaluation is the criterion-referenced method. Instead of comparing learners with each other, the instructor compares each individual with a predefined, objective standard of performance of what the learner is expected to know or to be able to perform after instruction is complete. A criterion-referenced measurement ascertains the person's status in respect to a defined objective or standard, and test items, if tests are used, correspond to the objectives. If the learner can perform what is called for in the objective, he has been successful. If not, criterion-referenced testing, which tends to be more diagnostic, will indicate what the learner can and cannot do, and more learning can be planned (21).

No doubt everyone has had the experience of being told to learn one thing and then being tested on another. Instruction should benefit the learners, not the teacher. What is important should be made known to the learners so that their time and effort are not wasted. Well-written performance objectives accomplish this. They should be the basis for assessing the results of instruction. If everyone does well on the evaluation, the instruction has been successful (30). The Registration Examinations for Dietitians and for Dietetic Technicians are examples of criterion-referenced tests.

Formative evaluation is almost always criterion-referenced. The practitioner wants to know who is having trouble learning, not where they rank compared to others. Summative evaluation may be either norm-referenced or criterion-referenced.

Types of Evaluation

After considering the purpose and timing of evaluation, one should resolve the question of what to evaluate. Four types of evaluation have been suggested. These are (a) measures of participant (client, employee) reactions to programs, (b) measures of behavioral change, (c) measures of results in an organization, and (d) evaluation of learning in the cognitive, affective, and psychomotor domains (23, 31). The evaluation of health education is usually focused on one or more of three types: knowledge, attitudes or beliefs, and/or behavior (32).

PARTICIPANT REACTION TO PROGRAMS

The first type of evaluation deals with participant (employee, client) reactions to educational programs. One needs to decide what should be evaluated. Were participants pleased and satisfied with the program, subject matter, content, materials, speakers, room arrangements, and learning activities? When a program, meeting, or class is evaluated, the purpose is to improve decisions concerning its various aspects, to see how the parts fit the whole, or to make program changes (33). These aspects may include structure, arrangements, administration, physical facilities, and personnel. The quality of learning elements, such as objectives, techniques, materials, and learning outcomes may be included also. Hedonistic scales or happiness indexes, such as smiley faces or numerical scales, have been used to determine the degree to which participants "liked" various aspects. Although these judgments are subjective, they are not useless since learners who dislike elements of a program may not be learning (34).

BEHAVIORAL CHANGE

A second type of evaluation is the measurement of behavior. Did employee or client behavior or habits change based on the learning? In measuring behavior, the focus is on what the person does. In employee training, for example, one may assess changes in job behaviors to see whether transfer of training to the job has occurred. Continuous quality improvement has influenced the need for this type of evaluation (34). It is necessary to know what the job performance was prior to training and to decide who will observe or assess changed performance—the supervisor, peers, or the individual. While the participants' reactions can always be done, this type is more difficult to measure and can be done selectively.

The ultimate criterion for effectiveness of nutrition education is not merely the improvement in knowledge of what to eat, but also changes in dietary behaviors and practices as the individual develops better food habits (3, 35, 36). Is the person consuming more fruits and vegetables, for example. These changes are difficult to confirm and often depend on direct observation, which is time-consuming, on self-reports, and on indirect outcome measures, such as weight gained or lost by a person on a weight reduction diet, reduction in blood pressure in hypertensive individuals, or better control of blood sugars in diabetes mellitus (32).

ORGANIZATIONAL RESULTS

Professionals involved with employee training gather a third type of evaluative data to justify the time and expense to the organization. Management may want to know how training will positively benefit the organization in relation to the cost. Results in terms of the following aspects may be attributed, at least in part, to training: improved morale, improved efficiency or productivity, improved quality of work, more customer satisfaction, less employee turnover, less frequent accidents or worker's compensation claims, less absenteeism/better attendance records, dollar savings, number of employee errors, number of grievances, amount of overtime, and the like. Did changing employee's behavior on the job improve business results? If not, it is not useful.

LEARNING

Whether learning has taken place is a separate question, even if the program rated highly on entertainment value. The learning of principles, facts, attitudes, values, and skills should be evaluated on an objective basis, and this task is more complex. If the learning objectives are written in terms of measurable performance, they serve as the source of the evaluation. To what degree were the objectives achieved by the learner?

Whether one has succeeded in learning can be determined by developing situations, or test items, based on the objectives of instruction. It is important for the test items to match the objectives in performance and conditions. If they do not match the objectives, it is not possible to assess whether instruction was successful, i.e., whether the learner learned what was intended.

Mager pointed out that several obstacles must be over-

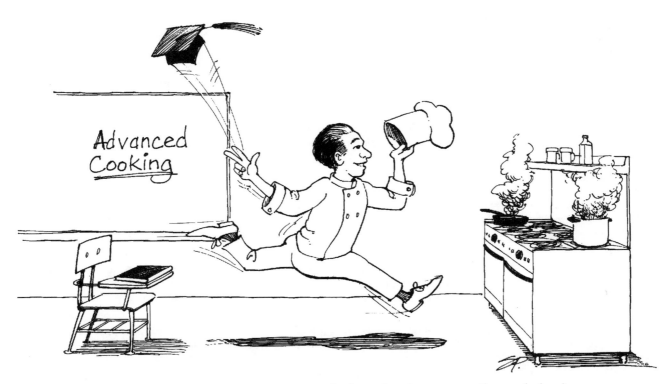

FIGURE 12.5.   Does the training transfer from the classroom to the workplace?

come to assess the results of instruction successfully. Some obstacles are caused by the objectives, while others result from attitudes and beliefs on the part of instructors (30).

One of the problems in evaluation results from inadequately written objectives. If the performance is not stated, if conditions are omitted, and if the criterion is missing, it will be difficult to create a test situation. If these deficiencies are discovered, the first step is to rewrite the objective.

Mager suggested a series of steps to select appropriate test items (30):

1. Match the performance and conditions of the test item to those of the objective.

2. Check whether the performance is a main intent or an indicator.

3. If the performance is an indicator, note the main intent. Note whether the performance is covert or overt.

4. Test for the indicator in objectives which contain one.

The first step is to see whether the performance specified in the test item is the same as that specified in the objective. If they do not match, the test item must be revised, since it will not indicate whether the objective has been accomplished. If the objective states that the performance is "to plan menus," or "to operate the dishwashing machine," the test should involve planning menus or operating the dishwashing machine. It would be inappropriate to ask the learner to discuss the principles of writing menus or to label the parts of the dishwashing machine on a diagram.

In addition to matching performance, the test should use the same specific circumstances or conditions that are specified in the objective.

Example: (Given the disassembled parts of the meat slicer), is able to reassemble the parts in correct sequence.

The conditions are "given the disassembled parts of the meat slicer." The practitioner should provide a disassembled machine and ask the employee to reassemble it. An inappropriate test would be to ask the learner to list the steps in reassembling the meat slicer, or to discuss the safety precautions to be taken.

If the individual must perform under a range of conditions, it may be necessary to test performance using the entire range. If a client eats at home and in restaurants, the dietetics professional must determine whether the individual is capable of following the dietary regimen in both environments. If students are learning to take a diet history, they should be taught to handle the range of conditions, including people of different age, socioeconomic, and ethnic groups. Not every condition will be taught and tested, but the common conditions that the individual will encounter should be included in the objectives and in testing.

The main intent of an objective may be stated clearly or it may be implied. The main intent is the performance, while an indicator is an activity through which the main intent is inferred.

Example: (Given a copy of a sodium-restricted diet), is able to plan a menu for a complete day.

In the above example, the main intent is to discriminate between foods permitted and omitted on the diet, and the indicator is the ability to plan menus. One infers that the client knows what is permitted and what is not if accurate sodium-restricted menus are planned. One should test for the indicator in objectives which contain one.

Some performances are overt while others are covert. Overt actions are visible or audible, such as writing, verbally describing, and assembling. If the performance is overt, determine whether the test item matches the objective.

Example: Is able to reassemble the parts of the meat slicer.

The employee should be provided with the parts of the meat slicer and asked to reassemble them. Performance tests are appropriate when skills are taught. If the employee is being taught to use equipment, the evaluation should be to have him demonstrate its operation. If a student is learning interviewing skills, an interview session is indicated as the evaluation.

Covert actions are not visible, but are internal or mental activities, such as solving problems or identifying. If the performance is covert, an indicator should have been added to the objective as explained in the previous chapter, and the indicator should be tested.

Example: Is able to identify the parts of the slicer (on a diagram or verbally).

For this example the employee should be provided with the indicator, a diagram of a meat slicer, and asked to identify the parts.

The discussion to this point has used examples of objectives in the cognitive and psychomotor domains. Affective objectives describe values, interests, and attitudes. While the cognitive and psychomotor domains are concerned with what an individual can do, the affective domain deals with what he is willing to do. These changes are covert or internal, and may develop more slowly over time. Evaluation of their achievement is more difficult and needs to take different forms. In measuring attitudes, the person needs the opportunity to express agreement rather than deciding on "right" or "wrong" answers.

To assess whether the individual has been influenced by education, the professional may conduct a discussion and listen to what the individual says or observe what he does, since both saying and doing are overt behaviors. To evaluate change in the person's behavior, the practitioner attempts to secure data that permit an inference to be made regarding the individual's future disposition in similar situations. In the affective domain, this is a more difficult task.

It is conceivable that the individual may display a desirable overt behavior only in the presence of the practitioner. The attitude toward following a diabetic diet or an employee work procedure may differ depending on the dietetics professional's presence or absence. Since time is required for change in the affective domain, evaluation may have to be repeated at designated intervals. To determine realistically how the person is disposed to act, the measurement approach needs to evaluate volitional rather than coerced responses.

The criterion of nutrition education program effectiveness has generally been improvement in knowledge and awareness, and in dietary behaviors and/or physiologic parameters (3). Other outcomes of nutrition education may be measures of nutrition and health status, such as body mass index or weight loss; decreased blood pressure; change in clinical or biochemical indices, such as serum cholesterol level in cardiovascular disease, hemoglobin level in pregnancy, and glycosylated hemoglobin level in diabetes; or reduction in risk factors for disease and improved health, both long-term goals. Care must be taken in interpreting some of these results since they may reflect other variables besides education. For example, stress can affect one's blood sugar even when the diabetic diet is followed.

Data Collection Techniques

There are a number of techniques for collecting evaluation data. They include paper-and-pencil tests, questionnaires, interviews, visual observation, job sample or performance tests, simulation, rating forms or checklists, individual and group performance measures, individual and group behavior measures, and self-reports (23, 31). As measurement devices that will be analyzed statistically, they require the use of specific experimental designs. Regardless of the particular instrument or technique used, it should be pretested with a smaller group prior to actual use. Since comparisons are desired, it is usually necessary to collect preliminary data on current performance or behaviors.

TESTS

Tests, especially written tests, are probably the most common devices for measuring learning. Tests sample what one knows. Schools depend heavily on them, and as a result, they are familiar to everyone. Multiple-choice, true-false, short-answer, completion, matching, and essay questions are used to measure learning in the cognitive domain. These tests have been used when several people are expected to learn the same content or material. Sometimes, both a pretest and a posttest are used to measure learning. This method assists in controlling variables, but one should be careful not to attribute all of the changes noted on the posttest to the learning experiences, since other factors may have been involved (21). In a child's

school experiences, the teacher assigned grades based on tests. With adults, the dietetics practitioner should avoid evoking childhood memories associated with the authoritarian teacher, the dependent child, or the assigned degree of success and failure based on right or wrong answers. In one-on-one situations, the practitioner may ask the individual to state verbally what she has learned as though she were telling it to a spouse or friend.

QUESTIONNAIRES

Questionnaires may be preplanned and are often used to assess attitudes and values, which do not involve correct answers. Questions may be open-ended, multiple-choice, ranking, checklist, or alternate-response, such as yes/no or agree/disagree. In evaluating behavioral change on the job, trainees and supervisors can both complete a questionnaire.

INTERVIEWS

Interviews conducted on a one-to-one basis are another form of evaluation. They are the oral equivalent to written questionnaires used to measure cognitive and affective objectives. Before the interview, the dietetics professional should draw up a list of questions that will indicate whether learning has taken place. After instruction, evaluation may consist of asking the client or employee to repeat important facts. An advantage of an interview is that the evaluator can put the person at ease and immediately correct any errors. Another advantage is that the interviewer can probe for additional information. Although this method is time-consuming, it is appropriate for the illiterate or less educated. Focus group interviews, mentioned earlier, are an example of a qualitative, formative evaluation.

OBSERVATION

In many cases, visual observation is an appropriate method of evaluating learning. The behaviors to be observed should be defined, and an observation checklist may be helpful. When employees are under direct supervision, systematic ongoing observation for a period of time is a basis for evaluating learning. The supervisor can observe and report whether the employee is operating equipment correctly or following established procedures properly. If the employee has been taught sanitary procedures, for example, the professional can see whether or not they are incorporated into the employee's work. One should evaluate the performance, using what was taught as a standard. If discrepancies are found, further learning may be indicated.

PERFORMANCE TESTS

Where direct observation is not possible or would be too time-consuming and costly, a simulated situation or performance test can be observed. Performance tests are appropriate in the cognitive and psychomotor domains. One could ask wait-staff to set a table, a cook to demonstrate the meat slicer, or a client to indicate what to select from a restaurant menu. The patient could be given a list of foods, some of which are permitted on the diet and some of which are not, and asked to differentiate them. Audiotape or videotape may be used to record the simulation, so that the instructor and learner may discuss the results together and plan further learning to correct any deficiencies. The learner should give permission in advance if taping is to be used. The observer needs to delineate which behaviors are being observed and what is to be acceptable behavior.

RATING SCALES/CHECKLISTS

Rating scales or checklists have been used to evaluate learner performance and teacher effectiveness. Categories or attributes, such as knowledge level or dependability, are listed, and these should be defined in detail to avoid ambiguity. Emphasis should be placed on attributes that can be confirmed objectively rather than judged subjectively. A five- or seven-point scale is used, allowing a midpoint, and the ratings should be defined, e.g., from "excellent" to "poor" or from "extremely acceptable" to "very unacceptable." The list should include as a possible response, "No opportunity to observe."

Rating scales are subject to a number of errors. Two evaluators may judge the same individual differently. To avoid error, definition of the terms and training of evaluators are essential. The ratings may suffer from personal biases. In addition, some raters have the tendency to be too lenient. Error may result if the rater is a perfectionist. Some evaluators tend to rate most people as average, believing that few people rank at the highest levels. Another possible error is the "halo" error, in which an evaluator is so positively or negatively impressed with one aspect of an individual that he judges all other qualities according to this one impressive aspect.

PERFORMANCE MEASURES

In employee training programs, individual and group performance measures, such as work quality and quantity, and number of errors, may be assessed. Individual and group behavioral measures, such as amount of absenteeism, number of grievances, and other types of problems that affect work performance, may be noted.

SELF-REPORTS

Self-reports, self-evaluation, and self-monitoring are another approach to evaluation. In the affective domain, written questions or statements are presented, and the individual supplies responses. Responses may be distorted if the individual can ascertain the socially acceptable answer. Role-playing, simulation, and attitudinal scales have also been used. Self-reports, such as a 3-day food record, have been used to measure behavioral change. In the Multiple Risk Factor Intervention Trial (MRFIT), a food score was developed, permitting participants to score their own food choices (37). A cholesterol-

saturated fat index (CSI) scorecard was developed for self-monitoring in order to facilitate the adoption and maintenance of a cholesterol-lowering dietary pattern (38). Studies have shown that self-evaluation or self-assessment of dietary status and behaviors enhanced motivation in older children, adults, pregnant women, and older adults (3).

All methods of evaluation have advantages and limitations, which need to be considered. While evaluation may not provide proof that treatment and education worked, it does produce a great deal of evidence (34). Evaluation of nutrition education programs is complex and federal food assistance programs often have limited budgets to undertake evaluation (39). In assessing adult learning, the dietetics professional should be careful to protect the individual's self-concept and to treat errors as indicators for additional instruction.

Reliability/Validity

VALIDITY

The concepts of reliability and validity are important to the measurement of learning. Validity indicates whether a test measures what it is intended to measure (40). There are different types of validity, such as content, construct, concurrent, and predictive validity, all of which help to "defend" the validity of the instrument. Content validity, which is the simplest and probably the most important for criterion-referenced testing, refers to whether the test items correspond to the content of instruction or to the knowledge, skills, or objectives they are supposed to measure.

RELIABILITY

Reliability refers to the consistency and accuracy with which a test or device measures something in the same way in each situation (40). For example, if a test is given twice to the same students to sample the same abilities, the students should place in the same relative position to others each time if the test is reliable. Methods for determining the reliability and validity of tests may be found in the educational literature (21). In all cases, one must keep in mind that the test or measuring device should assess whether the learner has attained the requisite knowledge, skill, or competence needed. If the learner has not attained the intended knowledge or skill, additional learning may be indicated.

Once the data from evaluation have been collected, they should be compiled and analyzed. The statistical analysis of data that is required is a lengthy subject of its own beyond the scope of this book. Future plans or programs may be modified based on the results of the evaluation. Results should be communicated through evaluation reports to others, such as participants, management staff, decision makers, and future learners.

LESSON PLANS/PROGRAM PLANS

A lesson plan is a written summary of information about a unit of instruction. It is prepared and used by the instructor and may be submitted to an administrator. Various formats for lesson plans are available, but the content is essentially the same.

A lesson plan is a blueprint that describes all aspects of instruction. It includes the following (15):

Preassessment or needs assessment.

The performance objectives identified.

The content outline.

How the content will be sequenced.

A description of the activities learners will engage in to reach the objectives.

Instructional procedures.

Resource materials, teaching aids, media, and equipment.

Amount of time allotted or scheduled.

Facilities to be used.

Method of evaluating whether the learner reached the objectives, outcomes, or other results measured.

Once written, a lesson plan is a flexible guide to instruction that can be used with many different individuals or groups.

A series of lesson plans or activities may be grouped into a larger unit of instruction covering a longer time frame, such as a whole day or several days. The term program planning is also used. A plan for a longer program would include essentially the same components as a lesson plan with the addition of the names of speakers or those responsible and cost considerations. Sample lesson plans are found in Tables 12.3 and 12.4.

DOCUMENTATION

Dietetics professionals are accountable for the nutrition care they provide in all settings, including in consulting and private practice and at the work site. Accepted standards of practice for quality control and accreditation agencies, such as the Joint Commission on Accreditation of Healthcare Organizations (JCAHO), mandate that dietetic services be documented and communicated to other health professionals providing care (41). Patient records also provide evidence in malpractice suits and are important to the denial of liability (42).

Documentation has been described as "the method by which others are made aware of specific approaches to client problems and outcomes," and it provides a "developmental history" of nutrition services to clients (20). What takes place between the dietetics professional and the patient or client should be recorded, including such data as nutritional assessment, nutrition care plans with timetables, goals, means of achieving goals and their outcomes, meal intakes and tolerance problems, nutrition counseling and education provided to the patient and/or significant other, patient's or client's reactions, progress notes including adherence to recommendations, actual outcomes, and behavioral changes, as well as where efforts should be directed in the future. The information

---

TABLE 12.3.

Sample Lesson Plan on Sanitary Dish Handling

I. Target audience: New wait-staff.

II. Objective: When setting tables, wait-staff will be able to handle dishes and utensils in a sanitary manner.

III. Time allotted: 15 minutes.

IV. Preassessment: Question new employees to determine what they already know about sanitary dish and utensil handling.

V. Content and sequence:
1. Handling of flatware by the handles.
2. Handling of cups by the base or handle and glassware by the base.
3. Handling plates and bowls on the edge without touching the food.
4. Use a tray.
5. The hands and skin as major sources of disease causing bacteria and their transmission to food and utensils.
6. Proper busing of dishes to avoid contamination of the hands.
7. Hand washing.

VI. Learning activities:
Demonstration and discussion of proper handling of dishes and utensils when setting tables, servicing food, and busing tables.
Discussion of hand washing.
Actual practice by new wait-staff.

VII. Materials: Dishes, utensils, tray, handout of important points to remember.

VIII. Evaluation: Whether or not dishes and utensils were handled properly during the actual practice; continued observation of the employee's performance on the job.

---

communicated demonstrates what the dietetics professionals contribute to health care delivery and that their services provide the patient or client with a specific benefit that will offset the cost of the service.

The usual place for documentation is in the medical or client's record. Although several formats are available, frequently, the professional makes notes on the patient's medical record using the SOAP procedure (41). The acro-

TABLE 12.4.

Sample Lesson Plan on Calcium in Pregnancy

I. Target audience: Pregnant women.

II. Objective: To be able to identify foods and quantities of foods that will meet the daily calcium needs for pregnancy and plan menus using these foods.

III. Time allotted: 30 minutes.

IV. Preassessment: Question audience about what foods contain calcium and how much of these foods should be eaten daily during pregnancy. Determine any previous pregnancies and what was eaten.

V. Content and sequence:
1. Total daily calcium needs with the important functions of calcium during pregnancy.
2. Dairy foods as a source of calcium with quantities of calcium in each.
3. Other foods as good sources of calcium with quantities of calcium in each.
4. Calcium sources for lactose-intolerant individuals.
5. Have audience suggest a breakfast, lunch, dinner, and snacks that meet the need for calcium.
6. Questions from the audience.
7. Have each individual plan her own menu for tomorrow.

VI. Learning activities: Group discussion of food sources of calcium. Show actual foods and food models for portion sizes. Group planning of a day's menu followed by each individual planning something appropriate for herself for the next day's menu.

VII. Materials: Actual food samples, food models, paper and pencils for menu planning, chalkboard or flip-chart for writing menus, handout with good sources of calcium and the amount of calcium in each including the RDA for pregnancy, and a sample menu.

VIII. Evaluation: The menu planned by each individual. Discussion with individuals during their follow-up prenatal visits.

nym SOAP stands for Subjective data, Objective data, Assessment, and Plan. Subjective data, obtained primarily through an interview, includes the patient's or client's perception and thoughts about the nutrition problem and his or her food intake. Objective data are the results of laboratory tests, such as serum albumin, or physical findings, such as weight and height. Assessment is the practitioner's analysis of the person's problem based on the subjective and objective data. The plan tells what the professional recommends or intends to do to solve a particular problem, such as plans for patient counseling, education, referral, or other follow-up practices.

Documentation of employee education and training programs is also essential. Records should be kept of all information included in employee orientation. The use of an orientation checklist is helpful in ensuring that everything the employee needs to know has been communicated to him. Records should be kept on file showing the date and content of ongoing training sessions such as in-service programs, and off-the-job experiences, such as continuing education.

This chapter has examined the selection and implementation of learning activities in the cognitive, affective, and psychomotor domains. The use of a task analysis and job instruction training have been explained. The final step in planning learning is evaluation, in which data are collected and analyzed to determine the success of educational endeavors.

The dietetics professional seeks to change people's eating practices, and in training employees, seeks to change the employee's job performance. Techniques and strategies that influence the acquisition of knowledge, the development of appropriate attitudes, and behavioral change were discussed. The relationship of knowledge and attitudes to behaviors is complex, however, since behavior is subject to many motivations all operating at the same time. The fact that clients and employees are informed does not mean that they will always act appropriately. Motives may be conflicting, and information may be disregarded or altered to serve one's own purposes (10). If time is limited, for example, little thought may be given to food choices. Instructional techniques that promote interpersonal interaction and reflect the social context are important influences in nutrition education.

REVIEW AND DISCUSSION QUESTIONS

1. What are the advantages and disadvantages of the various educational methods and techniques?

2. What methods and techniques are appropriate for objectives in the cognitive domain? The affective domain? The psychomotor domain?

3. Explain how a task analysis would be used with Job Instruction Training (JIT).

4. In what ways may educational instruction be organized or sequenced?

5. What are the purposes of evaluation?

CASE STUDY

Susan Grey, RD, has decided that there is a need for prenatal nutrition classes in the outpatient clinic. Many of the patients are teenagers with limited incomes who are on suboptimum diets. The nurse is also interested in cooperating with Susan to reduce the time she spends in individual counseling with patients.

1. Develop a lesson plan for a prenatal nutrition class.
2. What audiovisual materials would you suggest?
3. What handout materials would you recommend?
4. How long should the presentation be?

6. Differentiate between the following: formative and summative evaluation; reliability and validity; criterion-referenced and norm-referenced evaluation.

7. What are the four major types or levels of evaluation? If you had to describe each to someone desiring to evaluate employee training, what major elements of each would you emphasize?

8. What are the parts of a lesson plan or program plan?

9. What should be documented in the medical record?

SUGGESTED ACTIVITIES

1. Complete a task analysis for using a procedure or a piece of equipment (coffee urn, meat slicer, dishwashing machine, mixer, oven, grill, broiler, etc.), listing the sequential steps and key points.

2. Using the Job Instruction Training sequence and a task analysis, teach someone to use an unfamiliar piece of equipment.

3. Plan learning using one of the techniques in the chapter (other than lecture), such as discussion, simulation, or a demonstration. Carry out the plan.

4. Develop one or two performance objectives on a topic of interest for a target audience defined by age, sex, socioeconomic status, and educational level. The audience may be pregnant women, mothers, school children, adolescents, adult men or women, elderly, employees, executives, sports figures, or a person with a chronic disease. Plan the preassessment, content, techniques for presentation, teaching aids and handouts, and evaluation methods. Carry out the educational plan.

5. Develop one or two visual aids to use in teaching.

6. Give a pretest of knowledge on a subject. Instruct the learner on the subject. Follow up with a posttest to examine results.

7. List three ways in which one might evaluate whether an employee learned from a training program. List three ways in which one might evaluate whether a patient comprehended instruction regarding a diabetic diet.

8. Identify which of the following is a norm-referenced test and which is a criterion-referenced test.

A. Learners are given a national test of knowledge and individual scores are reported and compared.

B. Learners are given a test prepared by the teacher based on the learning objectives.

REFERENCES

1. Gagne RM, Briggs LJ, Wager WW. Principles of instructional design. 4th ed. Fort Worth: Harcourt Brace Jovanovich, 1992.
2. Tracey WR. Selecting a delivery system. In: Tracey WR, ed. Human resources management and development handbook. 2nd ed. New York: American Management Assoc, 1994.
3. Contento I, Balch GI, Bronner YL, et al. Executive summary. J Nutr Educ 1995;27:279.
4. Hartman TJ, McCarthy PR, Park RJ, et al. Focus group responses of potential participants in a nutrition education program for individuals with limited literacy skills. J Am Diet Assoc 1994;94:744.
5. Pfeiffer JW, Ballew AC. Using role plays in human resource development. San Diego: University Associates, 1988.
6. Holste P. High tech—hot talk. Computer-based training. Special report. Training Magazine, 1988.
7. Knox AB. Helping adults learn. A guide to planning, implementing, and conducting programs. San Francisco: Jossey-Bass, 1986.
8. Carroll JM, Stein C, Byron M, et al. Using interactive multimedia to deliver nutrition education to Maine's WIC clients. J Nutr Educ 1996;28:19.
9. Contento I, Balch GI, Bronner YL, et al. Nutrition education for adults. J Nutr Educ 1995;27:312.
10. Johnson DW, Johnson RT. Nutrition education: a model for effectiveness, a synthesis of research. J Nutr Educ 1985;17:S1.
11. Mager RF. Developing attitudes toward learning. 2nd ed. Belmont, CA: Lake, 1984.
12. Hahn J. How do you provide diabetes education to hard-to-reach, at-risk populations. J Am Diet Assoc 1996;96:1136.
13. Wexley K, Latham G. Identifying training needs. In: Baird L, Schneier CE, Laird D, eds. The training and development sourcebook. Amherst, MA: Human Resource Development Pr, 1983.
14. Nolan M. Job training. In: Craig RL, ed. The ASTD training and development handbook. 4th ed. New York: McGraw-Hill, 1996.

15. Mager RF, Beach KM. Developing vocational instruction. Belmont, CA: Fearon, 1967.

16. Laird D, House R. Training today's employees. Boston: CBI, 1983.

17. Brinbrauer H. Skills/technical training. In: Tracey WR, ed. Human resources management and development handbook. 2nd ed. New York: American Management Assoc, 1994.

18. Leatherman RW. Conducting one-on-one training. In: Tracey WR, ed. Human resources management and development handbook. 2nd ed. New York: American Management Assoc, 1994.

19. Hornik RC. Development communication: information, agriculture, and nutrition in the third world. New York: Longman, 1988.

20. Wills BB. Documentation: the missing link in evaluation. J Am Diet Assoc 1985;85:225.

21. Popham WJ. Educational evaluation. 3rd ed. Boston: Allyn and Bacon, 1993.

22. Dignan MB. Evaluation of health education. 3rd ed. Springfield: CC Thomas, 1995.

23. Phillips JJ. Handbook of training evaluation and measurement methods. 2nd ed. Houston: Gulf, 1991.

24. Garavaglia PL. How to ensure transfer of training. Training Dev 1993;47:63.

25. Knowles MS. The adult learner: a neglected species. 4th ed. Houston: Gulf, 1990.

26. DiLima SN, Schust CS. Community health: education and promotion manual. Rockville, MD: Aspen, 1996.

27. Betts NM, Baranowski T, Hoerr S. Recommendations for planning and reporting focus group research. J Nutr Educ 1996;28:279.

28. Navaie M, Glik D, Saluja K. Communication effectiveness of postnatal nutrition education in a WIC program. J Nutr Educ 1994;26:211.

29. Woolfolk AE. Educational psychology. 6th ed. Boston: Allyn and Bacon, 1995.

30. Mager RF. Measuring instructional results. Belmont, CA: Lake, 1984.

31. Kirkpatrick DL. Evaluation. In: Craig RL, ed. Training and development handbook. 4th ed. New York: McGraw-Hill, 1996.

32. Dignan MB. Measurement and evaluation of health education. 3rd ed. Springfield: Charles C Thomas, 1995.

33. Edwards PK, Mullis RM, Clarke B. A comprehensive model for evaluating innovative nutrition education programs. J Nutr Educ 1986;18:10.

34. Gerber B. Does training make a difference? Prove it. Training 1995;32:27.

35. Lewis M, Brun J, Talmage H, et al. Teenagers and food choices. The impact of nutrition education. J Nutr Educ 1988;20:336.

36. Franz MJ. Diabetes and nutrition: state of the science and the art. Top Clin Nutr 1988;3:1.

37. Remmell PS, Gorder DD, Hall Y, et al. Assessing dietary adherence in the Multiple Risk Factor Intervention Trial (MRFIT). J Am Diet Assoc 1980;76:351.

38. Mitchell DT, Korslund MK, Brewer BK, et al. Development and validation of the cholesterol-saturated fat index (CSI) scorecard: a dietary self-monitoring tool. J Am Diet Assoc 1996;96:132.

39. Sims LS, Volchick J. Our perspective: nutrition education enhances food assistance programs. J Nutr Educ 1996;28:83.

40. Monsen E. Research: successful approaches. Chicago: American Dietetic Assoc, 1992.

41. Grace-Fargaglia P, Rosow P. Automating clinical dietetics documentation. J Am Diet Assoc 1995;95:687.

42. Cross AJ. Legal requirement of private practice medical records. J Am Diet Assoc 1988;88:1272.

thirteen

GROUP DYNAMICS, LEADERSHIP, AND FACILITATION

When people gather together in groups, they do not act in the same way as when they are alone or with one other person. The "behavior" that is observed when people come together is often discussed under the topic of "Group Dynamics." Each group develops its own pattern of interaction as it goes through various phases and as members become comfortable in the group, learning to know and trust one another. Individuals promoted into management are often expected to convert their behavior from performing a task to managing a staff without being given the necessary training to exercise the required new skills. Activities such as conducting performance appraisals, counseling, disciplining staff, facilitating group meetings, team building, enhancing morale through the building of group cohesiveness among staff, and initiating change and managing any accompanying resistance all require well-honed communication skills.

When people are advanced into management without adequate training in these areas, the chances of their succeeding are hindered. In the 21st century dietetics practitioners who manage need not only an extensive understanding of the applications of computer science and technology to assist them in decision making but also the knowledge and ability of how to harness the power of their employee and client groups (1, 2).

This chapter provides the practitioner with a general overview of the dynamics inherent in groups and the variables that influence their direction, growth, and development. These process variables refer to how the group functions internally, how the members relate to one another, how they communicate among themselves, and how they do their work as a group (3). The following topics are discussed: contemporary leadership, team building and management, change in groups, cohesiveness in groups, informal work groups, facilitator preparation, group facilitation skills, facilitator/participant functions, synergy, guidelines for managing meetings effectively, and groups as a supplement to individual nutrition counseling.

Much of this chapter is devoted to exploring skills re-quired of the group leader and participants. The reader is cautioned, however, that one cannot develop these skills simply from reading a chapter, or even from reading it again and again. To develop these skills, individuals must make a personal commitment to risk feeling unsure and awkward as they attempt to practice them. Individuals need not wait until they are in management positions. In fact, the time to develop group skills is while one is still a student or a subordinate. The skills can be practiced with friends, with family, and in the community. In that way, when one advances to a position of authority, the skills will have become refined from the earlier practice and experience.

Although interpersonal and group interaction skills can be taught, the most effective way for individuals to learn them is through experiencing and observing others whom they admire and view as effective communicators. Communication skills can be effectively "caught" as well as taught, and professionals have an opportunity to develop these skills among staff and clients through their own modeling. Whether or not one intends it, and whether one's behavior is good or bad, the professional is a role model for staff and clients. By learning interpersonal and group skills and then consciously applying them, dietetics practitioners constructively and proactively enhance the development of these skills among staff and clients.

CONTEMPORARY DIETETICS LEADERSHIP

The profession of dietetics is being affected by the new health care technologies and treatments, shifting demographics, the wellness movement, escalating health care costs, and health care reform. These changes are requiring dietetics professionals to develop leadership skills that will allow them to establish a vision and a sense of value for their organizations (4, 5).

Recent literature in the field of dietetics is suggesting that a team-based style of leadership is needed in which the power of ideas is recognized over the power of position (6). The new leadership differs from the former more authoritarian style in that the primary emphasis for leaders is on their ability to communicate a vision to their team and to inspire them to take responsibility for the team's actions and decisions.

During the past few decades most organizations have carefully crafted mission statements. The job of the contemporary team leaders is to communicate to the members of the nutrition team their vision as to how the organization's mission can be actualized within particular departments. Their next step is to develop the specific goals, objectives, and strategic plans to accomplish that mission (6).

Pace distinguishes between the old leadership style and the new and provides a formula for building both teams and leaders in the field of dietetics (6). The traditional style, she points out, is marked by the concentration of power in a single leader; the contemporary new leadership style is marked by power being distributed throughout the team. Formerly the leader was accountable and controlled the organization; however, while the contemporary leaders are still accountable, they surrender control of the organization to teams. In the old style the leader defined the vision, mission, and goals of the organization; in the modern style the leader defines the vision and mission, but the team defines the goals of the organization. Traditionally the leader made all decisions and the employees simply implemented them. Today in the contemporary work groups, each team member has input into the decision-making process. Decisions are arrived at by consensus and agreed to by the whole team. In the old system individuals were recognized for their achievements; in the new system it is the team that is recognized for achievement. Finally, in the past leaders took credit for the end product of the employees' work; today the team takes credit for the end product of the team's work (6).

There are still other ways in which contemporary leaders distinguish themselves. They are concerned with knowing and utilizing sophisticated conflict resolution techniques. They know that in a diverse workplace of mixed generations and ethnic groups, there will always be conflict, and they recognize conflict as a positive, a force to stimulate creative thought when managed carefully. They understand that dictating and demanding compliance from staff is no longer effective and, consequently, are comfortable with managing and facilitating consensus seeking in groups, where they act as the facilitator rather than the "leader." They understand the need to know the "gifts" and talents of their human resources, and attempt in groups to stimulate the involvement of the appropriate persons as resources on an *ad hoc* basis. Finally, they understand the new motivation that supplements the many theories. The professional dietetics practitioners in the 21st century know that providing recognition and building self-esteem among staff will facilitate cooperation, satisfaction, and trust. Their primary responsibility as their teams' directors is to actualize the vision, making it clear and understandable to their staff and to show them the way to accomplishment. They grasp the need to be a model to the others as they enable them to perform optimally, and they comprehend that it is the team who, with a sense of "ownership," will ultimately realize the vision. The team director's job, then, is to articulate the vision, enable the team, show them the way and attend to the team's maintenance functions, allowing them to concentrate on getting the job done right.

Characteristics of an Effectively Operating Team

Wholesale political, economic, and social change is pressuring health care organizations to reinvent themselves as they enter a new area of managed competition. The reengineering of the field is costly and risky. Staff and directors alike live with the anxiety arising from the question of whether or not the belt-tightening efforts, combined with structural changes and strategic alliances, will achieve the necessary improvements in efficiency and help to secure an adequate patient base. It seems reasonable to expect that health care institutions can realize the major gains in quality, productivity, efficiency, and competitive edge that organizations in the manufacturing and service industries have enjoyed for the past several years. It is a logical next step for health care organizations to deploy proven methods, such as work redesign, team-based structures, and an empowered workforce, that have helped to restore competitiveness to many industrial and service firms (7).

There are a spate of studies in health care generally and dietetics specifically examining the values of the team approach. The studies, furthermore, are being done not only within separate disciplines but also across disciplines and among the multidisciplines that are included in health care. Topics such as the efficiency of service and total quality of delivery, overcoming resistance to change within the work units, and the effects of team approaches on stress and burnout of staff are all being considered (8–28).

By and large the studies confirm the superiority of the team approach, albeit directed by an enlightened director/facilitator, rather than the traditional authoritative, individual, and prescriptive approach, widely practiced during most of the 20th century. The studies cited above confirm that the team approach is more cost-effective and efficient, promoting more harmony and less resistance among staff and between the team leader and her work team. The contemporary dietetics professional, therefore, will need to be skilled in the practices of team leadership and development. The most critical of those skills is the operational knowledge of how to create the appropriate "atmosphere" among the team members, a climate that is comfortable, informal, relaxed, and yet encourages the team to perform optimally, free from obvious tensions, working together with interest and involvement.

The team leader must recognize that her role is not to dominate nor unduly defer to the group. In healthy teams leadership often shifts, depending on the circumstances. Different members, because of their special knowledge or experience, may be in positions at various times to act as "resources" for the group. In such teams there is generally little evidence of a struggle for power; the issue is not who controls but how to get the job done.

The team leader also has the responsibility for motivating team members to stay focused on the team's goals and objectives. For example, if two team members are not getting along, she is responsible for bringing the discussion back to the team's goals and away from individual personalities.

The team leader reinforces member behavior that promotes healthy team dynamics. One of her key functions is to teach them to monitor themselves and their work-related responsibilities independently. A well-functioning team processes their progress and attempts to discern what may be interfering with the operation. Whether the problem is an individual whose behavior is interfering with the accomplishment of the group's objectives or a matter of procedure, the preferred method of resolution is open discussion until a solution is found (29, 30).

In an optimal team the members communicate openly and frankly. Although they are cohesive, they are not afraid to disagree or of being rejected by teammates for disagreeing. Conflict is regarded as healthy, and members understand that "managed" disagreement often leads to synergetic solutions. Individuals expect to voice their alternative opinions in order that mutually satisfactory solutions may be found. Criticism is frequent, frank, and given with a minimum of anxiety. When members feel invested in one another, they are freer in expressing their feelings authentically. When all members of the team participate in the problem-solving and decision-making process, team members feel responsible and committed to the successful implementation of the team's decisions and objectives.

CHANGE IN TEAMS/GROUPS

Groups and teams are similar but not the same. All teams are groups, but not all groups are teams. A group is a collection of people who are together because of a common cause, goal, or purpose—they are not just a collection of people. The word "team" implies all of what constitutes a group plus more. Teams ordinarily have structure imposed to facilitate the accomplishment of their agenda, and a team has a director, a coach, or a facilitator whose task it is to act as their catalyst. In order to be such a catalyst, team leaders or facilitators require group skills to manage change with both staff teams and client groups. Ongoing change in organizations is inevitable. When changes are minor, the administrator can simply announce the changes and expect others to follow without resistance; however, other changes may be perceived as threatening by the staff. When changes arouse a sense of fear, ambiguity, and uncertainty, they are resisted. One of the first steps in overcoming this resistance is to facilitate the overt expression of concerns, even when the disclosures may provoke conflict. The profes-

sional needs to learn how to process the conflict that arises in the group in order that it can be managed constructively (31).

There is a direct correlation between the amount of time, consideration, and participation in the proposed change allotted to those affected by the change and the amount of resistance likely to occur. When people are given consideration and an opportunity to voice their anxieties and questions, with their recommendations being incorporated whenever possible, they are less likely to resist the changes and more likely to assist in upholding them among others who may resist. When an entire work group is involved in discussion of problems and potential changes, with their supervisor acting as facilitator, agreement can be reached to employ new methods, procedures, or solutions. Those members of the group who later object are reminded by the others that they had adequate opportunity to make suggestions and express their concerns, and that objecting now is inappropriate (32–35). Subsequent discussion will examine the group phenomena of change and cohesiveness and their effect upon one another.

Communication among work groups is affected by a constellation of variables, each of which is related to every other. Currently no theoretical model exists that takes into account all of the elaborate networks of sender, receiver, and message variables in small groups. In this section the two most salient variables, "change" and "cohesiveness" are explored. It is to the advantage of practitioners not only to understand the power and influence of the two phenomena on organizational life, but also to understand and apply appropriate strategies to use the change and cohesiveness variables for the good of the organization, department, and staff.

COHESIVENESS IN GROUPS

Because employee turnover is constant in most organizations, intense cohesiveness in work groups is rare; however, a knowledgeable manager can enhance the group's level of attraction and support toward one another through an understanding and application of information that behavioral scientists have learned regarding group cohesiveness.

Cohesiveness is an elusive concept; there is no single definition that completely defines it. An eclectic definition is perhaps the best way to discuss the concept. A cohesive group is one which has strong feelings of "we-ness," members talking more in terms of "we" than "I"; one which displays loyalty and congeniality to fellow members; one in which members work together for a common goal with everyone ready to take responsibility for group tasks; one which may endure pain and frustration for the group; and one which defends against criticism and attack. A summary of factors influencing group cohesiveness is found in Table 13.1.

The specific reasons cohesion thrives in some groups, dissipates in others, and fails to emerge at all in still others

TABLE 13.1.

Factors Increasing Group Cohesiveness

1. All members perform worthwhile tasks and feel they are appreciated by the group.

2. Members clearly perceive the group's goals and consider them to be realistic.

3. Members perceive the group as an entity in its own right and refer to it as such, calling it "the group" or "our group."

4. The group develops a history and tradition. All cohesive groups, church, state, family, work, etc., perform traditional rites and rituals, passing on to new members the "secrets" of the past and strengthening the existing ties among the group's veterans.

5. The group has prestige.

6. Members possess knowledge or material needed by the group.

7. There is full and direct member participation in the determination of the group's standards.

8. Members perceive the issues at hand to be of importance.

9. Personal interaction among members is based on equality, with no one exercising much authority over anyone else.

10. There are shared ideals and interests among members, a common enemy outside the group, or a common satisfaction of individual needs for protection, security, and affection.

11. Members are not jealous and competitive with one another.

12. Group size is small rather than large.

13. The group is more homogeneous than heterogeneous.

the esteem they receive from those around them. There is, therefore, always a tendency to go along with the group. Once a group feels itself to be cohesive, it attempts to preserve the state. Cohesiveness, however, is not static. Even highly cohesive organizations change membership, altering the nature of the internal structure and the interaction patterns of members. Over a period of time, therefore, a group may lose its cohesiveness.

Not all teams are cohesive and those that are may not remain so continuously. Cohesiveness relates to the feelings of belonging and acceptance each member feels in the group. Unless the norms of authenticity, openness, and acceptance of differences nonjudgmentally are regularly reinforced among the members, the level of cohesiveness will diminish.

In addition to the increase in self-esteem that generally accompanies members' participation in a cohesive group, other benefits emerge as well: members or individuals can be honest in their dialogue with other members, and they can relax and not be continuously on their guard. Because members feel a stake in the group, they are more likely to disagree and argue about decisions affecting it. When a decision is made, each member feels committed to it and will take responsibility for it. Even if meetings are uninhibited and unruly, the topic is more likely to be fully explored, errors are more likely to be pointed out, and poor reasoning or attempts at manipulation on the part of various individuals are more likely to be exposed in the cohesive group than in the more self-conscious and cautious non-cohesive group. From the dietitian's perspective, maintaining high cohesiveness provides a highly desirable work climate, especially when the manager employs participative decision-making and group problem-solving strategies.

Individuals in non-cohesive groups are likely to argue less, be more polite, and more easily bored. When members disagree, they feel less secure in expressing themselves and often give no overt signs; instead, they may frown, look away, or plead ignorance. Members worried about their own security hesitate to challenge others; therefore, non-cohesive groups frequently stick to irrelevancies, safe topics, or procedures rather than become involved in discussing the real issues. Unlike the members of cohesive groups, they generally do not fully explore the topic, expose manipulation or poor reasoning, argue for what they believe, or take full responsibility for the group's decision. Agreement may be only external for the sake of apparent cohesion, in which case the individual does not feel bound to the group's goals or decisions. Clearly the quality of any group decisions or solutions to work-related problems made in these groups is poorer than that made in more cohesive work groups. It is the manager's responsibility to create a climate in which individuals will dare to differ from the group without fear of expulsion.

It is the newer members who generally are the most easily intimidated because they are more likely to feel

are as elusive as its definition. The most fundamental reason for groups tending to gravitate toward cohesive units stems from a basic tenet of human nature: people like to be liked. This desire to be accepted and liked leads people to engage in actions that will maintain or increase inferior to the established members of the work group. The individual's sense of acceptance in the work group is a highly prized possession, and anything that produces disharmony or conflict of views is likely to disturb it. New members are the most likely to accept and adopt the group's norms because of the pressures of being in a group in which everyone else is acting, talking, or thinking in a certain way. This can occur even without any overt or conscious pressure by group veterans.

In summary, the major advantage of the cohesive group is its tendency toward a greater quality of communication, with the interaction more equally distributed than in the non-cohesive group. Members feel freer to disagree and challenge one another, providing they do not perceive the message as a threat to their own status or security. Messages are usually more fully explored in the cohesive group, and the communicator has a better chance of achieving a shared understanding of the message, which could lead to a favorable attitude change in the entire group. If, however, the group interprets a message as a threat to its cohesiveness, it will reject it more hastily than will the non-cohesive group.

Conforming to norms may stifle the individual's identity and creativity and may restrict, inhibit, and change the values of individual members. It is paradoxical that cohesive teams or groups also provide individuals with opportunities for need fulfillment, personal growth through work satisfaction and camaraderie, and are the most likely to achieve synergy. Developing cohesiveness within the team and then using it to produce superior problem-solving and decision-making skills can only be achieved consistently through the enlightened facilitator's careful monitoring and "fine-tuning" of the group's dynamics. The manager needs to solicit and reinforce authentic reactions from individuals within the group, while at the same time safeguarding the sense of unconditional acceptance among the other team members (36).

The Relationship of Cohesiveness to Change in Groups

A spate of data concerning group influences has been accumulated in recent years, and the evidence of its power and potential force is convincing. The discussion below reviews the relationship of cohesiveness to change in groups.

While group change can be fostered through coercion and intimidation, permanent change promoted in this way is rare. Group change is most easily and optimally developed in meetings and workshops where trust, team building, and open communication are facilitated among members. Change has the best chance for acceptance and permanence when the need for and value of the change arises from within the group. Change occurring under these conditions receives mutual support and reinforcement from the entire group. After all channels of communication are opened and the needs for change explored, the members may experience a short-lived in-crease in hostility, but eventually, after all have shared perceptions and arrived at mutual agreement or compromise, the new norms are enforced.

Although there may be some who disagree with the change and revert to the old behavior, frequently the group pressures and the individuals' perceptions of their own dissonance cause them to abide by the group-accepted behavior. Suggestions for promoting group change are summarized in Table 13.2.

In summary, people's attitudes, beliefs, and values are all rooted in the various groups to which they belong. The more genuinely attached individuals are to their groups and the more attractive these groups become in fulfilling the various needs of group members, the more likely for these members to be in close and continuous contact with their group. Under these conditions group-anchored behaviors and beliefs are extremely resistant to change, with the group being able to exercise firm control over its members. The more attractive a group is to its members, moreover, the greater its power to change them. For the group itself to be used most effectively as an agent of change, it must first be cohesive with a strong sense of oneness existing between those who are to be changed and those who desire change. Attempts at changing individuals must be aimed at either countering the influence of the group or encompassing it in the change. Either way, all attempts at changing individuals must also consider the dynamics of their groups (32, 33) (Table 13.2).

INFORMAL WORK GROUPS

Dietetics professionals need to be aware of the inherent power and influence of the informal work group. Since the 1920s, when the Hawthorne studies were carried out at the Western Electric plant near Chicago, social scientists have been studying the "Hawthorne Effect," which refers to the theory, and its corollaries, that employees perform more efficiently when they believe that they are being given special attention. The theory suggests that the major influences affecting efficiency and production are group social structures, group norms, and group pressures.

Professionals need to be sensitive to the dynamics and influences of the informal work group. They must learn ways to provide a forum where social, task-related, and organizational concerns can be expressed, responses can be offered, and any resistance to change can be overcome. To become conscious of the influence inherent in the informal work group and to tap into the grapevine of informal communication, the manager needs to be aware of the networks of communication that exist within the department as well as those within the organization.

Communication networks are the patterns of message flow, or linkages of who actually speaks to whom (37). In all organizations, there are distinctions between the "permissible" and the actual channels of communication

TABLE 13.2.

Suggestions for Promoting Group Change[a,b]

1. If attitude change is desired, small, open-ended, off-the-record discussion groups where the person feels secure are most effective.

2. When people need to change behaviors, participation in group discussions is 2–10 times more effective than a lecture that presents the reasons and pleas for change.

3. Active discussion by a small group to determine its goals, methods, work, new operations, or to solve other problems is more effective in changing group practices than are separate instructions, supervisor's requests, or the imposition of new practices by an authority. Group involvement brings about better motivation and support for the change and better implementation and productivity of the new practice.

4. Group change is easier to bring about and more permanent than change in the separate individual members of the group. The supposed greater permanence stems from the individual's assumed desire to live up to group norms. It follows that the stronger the group bonds, the more deeply based are the individual's attitudes. Another explanation suggests that the public commitment to carry through the behavior decided on by the group members creates an awareness of the expectations that the members have for each other, thus creating forces on each member to comply.

5. The best way for a teacher or manager to initiate change is to create an atmosphere that will lead to a shared perception by the entire group of the need for change. Then they will call for the change themselves and enforce it. After all facts have been shared with all members and all channels of communication have been opened, there is frequently a sudden but short-lived increase in hostility; however, without this complete sharing among all group members, there can be no real change, only mistrust and subtle hostility.

7. High-status persons have more freedom from group control than do other members. The greater the prestige of individual group members, the greater the influence for change they can exert on the others.

8. The "big brother" or "buddy system" of change, where the change is suggested by a peer, is better than having it demanded by an authority figure.

[a] Modified from Breuer J. Orchestrating culture shock: What happens when companies must change. Inform 1989;3:46.
[b] Modified from Brilhart JK, Galanes GJ. Effective group discussion. 8th ed. Dubuque, IA: William C Brown, 1995.

and network linkages. The permissible channels are the linkages dictated by the organization's structure, which determines the hierarchy of power and influence; the actual channels are the patterns that do, in fact, occur. Often, secretaries are ultimately more influential, because of their connections within the network, than others who are considerably higher on the organizational chart. A later section in the chapter discusses "process meetings" as a way of tapping into the informal group and airing common group concerns.

Although they constitute a minority, some people perform best when under the direction of an authoritarian leader. When persons come from backgrounds where they have not been encouraged to think and have been punished for initiating ideas, it is predictable that in a work situation they will lack the self-confidence to offer suggestions within a group. If treated with patience, however, and given continued positive reinforcement

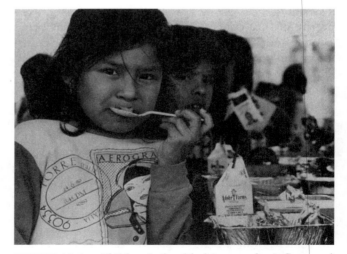

FIGURE 13.1. Children's food habits may be influenced by their peer group.

each time they risk contributing an idea, they may gradually gain the confidence to become valuable group members. In general, however, members of today's work force have grown up with a preference for egalitarian treatment and perform best in groups with a leader who can act as a facilitator, involving employees rather than prescribing to them. Facilitators are those who understand the value of group decision making and see their function as helping the group get started, establishing a climate of work, giving support to others, and keeping the group on track so that its objectives are achieved. The group's activities and the facilitator's attitude toward the group are based on respect for what can be accomplished through group discussion and fostering of a group climate where people feel comfortable and secure enough to contribute their ideas (38).

FACILITATOR PREPARATION

Facilitators' responsibilities begin prior to the discussion, in their preparation of the appropriate meeting environment. They must make sure that the room itself is comfortable, with adequate ventilation and lighting, and with a consciously arranged seating pattern. Sitting in a circle, for example, allows group members to see one another's faces, which tends to increase interaction among them. When people are arranged at long rectangular tables, persons tend to interact most with those in direct view and little with those on either side of them.

When meetings involve individuals who do not know one another, the facilitator should supply name tags or cards for everyone in the group. A sense of group spirit develops more quickly when people use one another's names as they interact. Allowing members time to introduce themselves is time well spent toward developing a comfortable climate. "Small talk" in groups is not a small matter. Just hearing one another allows the members to make some assumptions that help them to reduce anxiety. The individuals' tone of voice, dress, diction, and manner provide valuable clues to their character. Often, negative inferences disappear after the other's voice is heard and some information regarding the person's background is gathered.

GROUP FACILITATION SKILLS

The dietetics literature emphasizes the needs of nutrition counselors and educators to assist in group problem solving by further developing their roles as expert information disseminators, diagnosticians, team members, empathizers, and group facilitators (39, 40). Most practitioners will eventually need to direct others in groups and facilitate interaction among them. Effective facilitation requires training and discipline to stay in the role of guide and not become a participant. Described in the following paragraphs are specific skills that need to be practiced as one trains to develop group facilitation skills (40, 41).

Relieving Social Concerns

A tenet of group dynamics suggests that social concerns take precedence over "task" or work-related concerns. In other words, an individual's first concern is with being accepted and acknowledged as worthy. If individuals feel anxiety about being with unknown others, or others who may bear them ill will, they generally will not participate. One way a facilitator can attend to social concerns is to spend a few minutes at the beginning of each meeting,

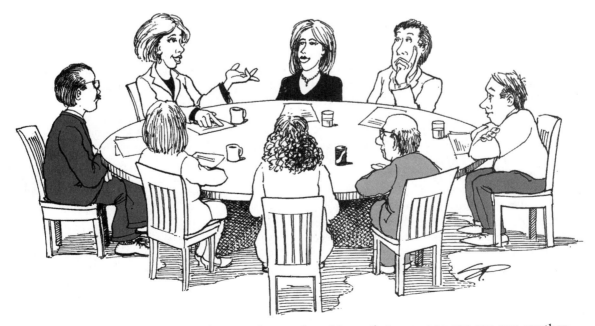

FIGURE 13.2.   Groups should be seated around a table so that everyone can see one another.

allowing people to interact socially, providing "open-time" to reestablish positive regard for one another. If ill will does exist among some of the participants, and the facilitator is aware of it, she can attempt to have the members resolve their conflict before the meeting or, if they are willing, at the meeting. Only after the members have had their social concerns met can they wholeheartedly participate in "task" concerns.

Tolerating Silence

After facilitators have made opening remarks, have made sure that everyone knows everyone else, have articulated the desire for everyone's participation, and have stated the reasons or purpose for the meeting, they might rephrase the topic in the form of a question and then invite someone to comment. Because members are frequently hesitant to express opinions with which their superior may disagree, they often wait to hear the supervisor's opinion first. There may be times when no one wants to initiate discussion and reduce the tension. Silence is likely to occur most during the early stages of an ongoing group. Once the group comes to understand that the facilitator truly does not intend to dominate, lead, or force opinions, members will begin to use the meeting time to interact with one another. For those first few meetings, however, the facilitator should repeat her intention not to participate, should encourage others to participate, and then should just sit patiently. Ordinarily, if the silence is tolerated long enough, someone will eventually take the responsibility for directing the discussion.

Guiding Unobtrusively and Encouraging Interaction

The facilitator guides indirectly, helping the members to relate better to one another and to complete the task. Facilitators should not allow themselves to become the focus. The facilitator can encourage interaction among the group members by looking away from speakers in the group as they attempt to make eye contact with him. Although this behavior may seem rude, the speaker will quickly get the idea and look to the other group members for feedback and response as the talk continues. The facilitator should resist the temptation to make a reply after others talk, instead wait for someone else to reply. If no one else makes a comment, however, the facilitator can ask for reactions. A question such as "Any reaction to that, Mary?" is preferred to "my reaction is . . . ."

Because facilitators wish to keep the focus on the group, they should remind group members during the first few minutes of the meeting that their purpose primarily is to get things started and then simply to serve as a guide. This assertion will eventually be tested. Most people have heard the same sentiment expressed by teachers and others and have learned that while some do mean it, the majority are paying it lip service only, want things done their way, and expect ultimately to be followed.

Knowing When and How to Resume Control

Just as a facilitator who rules and dominates in an authoritarian manner can stifle the group's creativity, facilitators who are too timid, uncertain, or frightened and who let the group wander can hinder the group's potential for synergy, i.e., for finding superior solutions. Facilitators need to determine if the group is capable of facilitating for itself. When it is, the facilitator's function is to remain on the sidelines. Only when there are no competent participants available to perform the necessary functions does the facilitator become an active member of the group.

Reinforcing the Multisided Nature of Discussion

The facilitator can reinforce the nondogmatic, multisided nature of discussion by phrasing questions so that they are open-ended. Examples include questions such as "How do you feel about that, Helen?" "Who in your opinion . . .?" and "What would be some way to . . .?" Facilitators need to think before asking questions in order to avoid closed and leading questions, questions that can be answered by only one or two words, or questions suggesting a limited number of alternative responses.

Exercising Control Over Loquacious Participants

The most common problem facilitators have is knowing what to say to someone who is overly talkative. There are, of course, many appropriate ways of handling this participant, and individual facilitators need to decide which techniques they personally feel most comfortable using, keeping in mind that when they interact with any single member of the group, all other participants experience the interaction vicariously. If the facilitator treats individual participants without respect, or humiliates or embarrasses them, all members will be affected by the experience.

Several techniques can be effective in dealing with the loquacious participant. The facilitator might interrupt the participant, commenting that the point has been understood, and begin immediately to paraphrase concisely so that the participant knows that he has been understood. While it is true that some group members talk excessively because they enjoy talking and because they believe that they are raising their status within the group through the quantity of their interaction, other talkative members often repeat themselves because of insecurity. They are not convinced that they have been understood. Usually, this kind of participant stops talking after being paraphrased. Of course, this process may need to be repeated several times during the course of the discussion.

A second problem arises with the participants who simply enjoy talking and do perceive increased status from it. These people do not stop talking after being paraphrased. They may need to be told that short, concise statements are easier to follow and that the group is losing the point from their extensive commentary. If that does not work, the facilitator may need to talk with the participant privately. Often, talkative group members are unaware that others are offended by their domination. The facilitator can point out to them that he has noticed others stirring and wanting to enter the discussion. It needs to be stressed to these participants that long-windedness cuts down on the time allowed for others to contribute to the discussion.

Recent studies are suggesting that "time-wasters" can also be controlled by establishing additional meeting guidelines on an *ad hoc* basis. The facilitator, for example, may say, "Because of the brief time remaining, we will no longer be able to permit interruptions" (42).

Encouraging Silent Members
For various reasons, including boredom, indifference, perceived superiority, timidity, and insecurity, there are usually some members who refuse to participate. The facilitator's action toward them depends on what is causing them to be silent. The facilitator can arouse interest by asking for their opinions of what a colleague has said. If the silence stems from insecurity, the best method is to reinforce positively each attempt at interjection. A smile, a nod, or a comment of appreciation for any expressed opinion is sufficient. Sometimes silent members "shout out" nonverbal signals. An overt frown, nod, and/or pounding fingers are all signals that should be interpreted as the silent member's willingness to be called upon to elaborate; however, if silent members have their heads down and blank facial expressions, it would be a mistake to force them into the discussion.

Halting Side Conversation
Generally, the facilitator should not embarrass members who are engaged in private conversations by drawing attention to them in the presence of the group. If the side conversation becomes distracting to other members of the group, those engaged in the conversation might be called by name and asked an easy question.

Discouraging Wisecracks
If someone in the group disrupts with too much humor or too many wisecracks, the facilitator needs to determine at what point the humor stops being a device to relieve tension in the group and starts to interfere with the group's interests. When facilitators believe that the humor is taking the focus off group issues and onto the joker, they need to interrupt, preferably smiling, with a comment such as "Now let's get down to business." If the comment needs to be made a second time, intense eye contact with the joker and no smile as the same remark is repeated usually halts the disruption.

Helping the Group to Stay on the Topic
When the group itself seems unable to stick to the agenda and wanders, a device underused by facilitators is a flip-chart to jot down points that have been agreed upon as a way to chart the group's progress. With a minimum of interaction, the facilitator can prod the group on by simply summarizing and writing down the points. Generally, the group's reaction is to go on to the next item on the agenda.

Avoiding Acknowledgment of the Facilitator's Preferences
Facilitators hinder the group when they praise the ideas they like and belittle those they dislike. It is particularly important that they avoid making comments that may be taken as disapproval, condescension, sarcasm, personal cross-examination, or self-approval. Once the group members know the facilitator's preferences, they will tend to incorporate these preferences in their own comments. Because the professionals are in a position to reward or punish subordinates, the group members quickly learn that if what the supervisors want is to be followed and not disagreed with, that is how they will behave toward them.

FACILITATOR/PARTICIPANT FUNCTIONS
In addition to the specific skills required of facilitators, there are numerous group skills that both participants and facilitators should possess. There is a mistaken notion that it is the facilitator's responsibility alone to see to it that the group's tasks are accomplished and that a healthy group spirit is maintained. In reality, these responsibilities belong to anyone who has the training and insight to diagnose the group's weaknesses and who has the skills to correct them. Because most people are used to being "led" in groups, the facilitator may need to reinforce verbally the functions that all participants are expected to perform. The following paragraphs describe some of these skills and functions that both facilitators and participants have a mutual obligation to develop in themselves:

1. Groups need members to propose new ideas, goals, and procedures. Individual members are expected to accept the responsibility of **initiating.** Any member who has the insight into what should be initiated and waits for someone else to do it is ignoring an obligation. The facilitator might also remind participants of the spate of behavioral literature that verifies the correlations between employee/participant involvement and superior decisions (43, 44).

2. Everyone shares the responsibility of **seeking information and opinions.** One does not have to have vast knowledge of the topic being discussed to be a valuable member. Asking the right questions and seeking information from others in the group who have knowledge are valuable functions.

3. **Clarifying** what others have said by adding examples, illustrations, or explanations is a major contribution. People are not all on the same "wavelength." Because of background, life experiences, education, natural intelligence, or environment, some people

tend to understand one another more easily than do others. Two people who have grown up under similar conditions, for example, have an easier time communicating than two people from different backgrounds. People who understand what someone else in the group is struggling to make clear and add examples and explanations to clarify the thoughts for the others have made significant contributions. Simply nodding in agreement and saying nothing is a disservice to the others.

4. Another function related to clarifying is **coordinating** relationships among facts, ideas, and suggestions. If one has the insight to understand how the ideas and activities of two or more group members are related and how they can be coordinated, the member serves a valuable function in expressing this relationship to the others.

5. **Orienting** is a name given to the function of processing for the group the pattern of its interaction and progress. The orienter clarifies the group's purpose or goal, defines the position of the group, and summarizes or suggests the direction of the discussion. Orienting by providing frequent internal summaries, for example, allows the group an opportunity to verify whether everyone is understanding the direction in which the group is going, and provides those who disagree or who have misunderstood with the opportunity to speak.

6. Perhaps the least understood and most valuable function one can perform for a group is being a **supporter.** Supporters are those who praise, agree, indicate warmth and solidarity, and verbally indicate to the others that they are in agreement with what is being proposed. It is a valuable function because without verbal support from others, good ideas and suggestions are often disregarded. If one person expresses an idea that the majority dislikes and that no one supports, the idea is quickly dismissed. Generally, if only one person supports the idea, the group will seriously consider the proposal. Frequently, a minority opinion can gain majority support because a single supporter agrees, causing the group to consider seriously the possible merits of the proposal. Support can be given by briefly remarking, "I agree," "Well said," "I wish I had said that," or "Those are my sentiments, too." Generally, one person alone cannot influence a group: one person with a supporter, however, has an excellent chance of doing so (45). This topic is developed further in the final section of this chapter.

7. **Harmonizing** is also a valuable contribution to the group. It includes mediating differences between others, reconciling disagreement, and bringing about collaboration from conflict. It is common for individuals to sit silently as they hear the valid arguments on both sides of an issue. One of the ways in which discussion differs from debate, however, is that discussion assumes that most issues are multisided, while debate tends to lend itself to two-sided issues only. The group member who verbally reinforces the positive aspects of the various factions and helps to suggest new and alternative solutions that include the best points of all sides is harmonizing.

8. Conflict, stress, and tension in groups are inevitable. When the stress or the tension mounts, it can enhance the conflict and the disagreement. Individuals who can find humor in the situation, reduce the formality or status differences among group members, and relax the others are called **"tension relievers."** A problem can occur when the tension reliever seeks recognition for himself and continues to joke, drawing the attention away from the issues. Relieving tension is valuable up to a point, after which it can be disruptive.

9. The final function in this discussion is **gatekeeping.** In gatekeeping, one notices which members have been sending out signals that they want to speak but have not had the courage or opportunity to enter the discussion. Gatekeeping ensures that all have an equal chance to be heard. As pointed out in the discussion of the facilitator's functions, there is a difference between people who are nonverbally signaling that they have strong feelings—by raising their eyebrows, tapping loudly, or grunting—and people who are silent. Group members become uncomfortable when they sense that other members might force them to talk. All members share the responsibility to protect others from being coerced into sharing opinions. Gatekeepers tend to say things such as "You look like you have strong feelings," or "I can tell by your face that you disapprove." Such comments are generally all the prodding the silent participant needs to enter the discussion.

Too often individuals believe that in the ideal group a single leader is responsible for each of the functions just discussed. In fact, all members—participants as well as facilitators—are responsible, and they need to be alert to or perform as many of the functions as they see a need for. Some people may be natural "harmonizers" or natural "orienters," or may be able to perform effortlessly some other valuable function; however, if the group needs a gatekeeper and none is present, the natural harmonizer who sees the need must exercise the gatekeeping function. One of the ways people familiar with group dynamics and with the skills needed to enhance the working of groups can detect members who have had training in the same area is by their willingness to act on their insight to correct a weakness in the group. As pointed out in a previous chapter, the mind operates several times as fast as the speed of human speech. While members of the group are talking, other sophisticated group members need to be reflecting on the dynamics of the group and on the needs at the moment. This process leads to an understanding of which functions need to be performed to help the group accomplish its task and maintain its healthy spirit.

Paradox of Group Dynamics

There is a paradox inherent in groups: they possess the potential, on the one hand, to stimulate creative thinking and to promote a decision or solution that is superior to that which any individual working alone could accomplish. On the other hand, groups possess the potential to stifle creative thinking and thus promote a quality of outcome inferior to that which individuals working alone might accomplish. Ordinarily, no one person is solely responsible for what happens in any given session; however, whether a group becomes a force to promote creative thinking and problem solving or a force that inhibits these functions depends primarily on the skills of its leader, and to a lesser degree, on the skills of the participants. There are specific behavior patterns that help a group to function effectively, and others that hinder the progress. Knowing how to facilitate positive behavior in groups and how to inhibit the negative behavior is an asset to dietetics practitioners.

SYNERGY

Professionals need to appreciate "group process" and to discover what can be done to stimulate their staff and/or client group so that they become a creative force that promotes synergy. Synergy refers to the phenomenon where the group's product (i.e., conclusion, solution, or decision) is qualitatively and/or quantitatively superior to what the most resourceful individual within the group could have produced by working alone (46). Today, much is understood about the phenomenon; however, it has not yet filtered into management practice. Although greatly influenced by the style of their facilitators, all groups possess the potential to be either a force for creative innovative thinking or a force that works to preserve the *status quo* and stifle new ideas (30). The purpose of this section is to offer suggestions on how to promote the former. The major variables that affect the group's potential for synergy are whether a single expert is available within the group, whether the group is heterogeneous or homogeneous, and whether the group and its facilitator are trained in the consensus-seeking process.

Facilitators should begin each meeting by stating their desire to promote a climate of acceptance and freedom of expression. Hearing the facilitator express this desire helps to set a group "norm" whereby everyone has a responsibility to participate. A norm is an unwritten rule to which the group adheres. Members "pick up" the code of appropriate behavior by noticing what the facilitator reinforces positively, ignores, tolerates, or rejects. Eventually, the facilitators' expressions of their desire for everyone to participate and the rights of each member

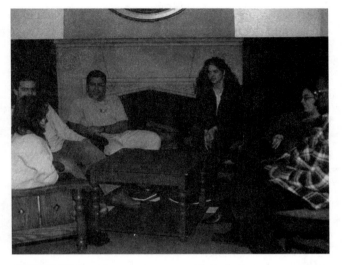

FIGURE 13.3. Groups can provide solutions superior to those of one individual.

to express subjective opinions without being abused by others will be tested. It is not enough to articulate norms; they must be enforced. If individuals are abused by others, told to be silent, embarrassed, humiliated, or insulted, for example, and the facilitator does not intervene to protect them, his articulated norm will be discounted and the actual behavior that has been tolerated will be considered the "real" norm. For that reason, it is critical that group facilitators realize the importance of their function to stimulate group interaction while protecting group members from being verbally abused or stifled. Realizing that synergy is most likely to occur in groups in which people can react authentically and are free to challenge the facilitator and the other participants, the dietetics practitioner needs to convince the group that they need to listen and respond honestly to one another's ideas.

As a rule, if a single expert is available and the rest of the group members are relatively ignorant of the matter being discussed, the expert should make the decision. In practice, however, there is usually no single expert available, and some group members are more informed than others, with a wide range of opinions being represented in the group. Under those conditions, the potential for synergy exists.

The variable of a heterogeneous versus homogeneous group of participants is more complicated. When group members are untrained in the consensus-seeking process and form a homogeneous group, they have less conflict and generally produce superior decisions to those produced by an untrained heterogeneous group. It is understandable that people who are similar in age, background, culture, life experiences, values, and the like have an easier time agreeing than with those with whom they have little in common.

The heterogeneous group that is untrained is likely to

respond in one of the following ways. If individuals in the group do not know one another, they will probably remain silent. Most people become anxious in the presence of strangers, whose response to them is unpredictable. Rather than risk sharing a contrary opinion and being insulted, humiliated, or embarrassed, they tend to go along with the opinions expressed by other members of the group. Decisions in such groups may appear to be produced by consensus, because there is no apparent disagreement, but in fact, consensus may not be present. Because there is no group commitment and cohesion, conflict presents a threat to the group's interpersonal structure. Members try to smooth conflicts rather than resolve them. When disagreement arises, the members make quick compromises to get along. They resort to conflict-reducing techniques, such as majority rule and trade-offs. The quality of decisions made in these groups tends to be low.

The other possibility is that a great deal of verbal conflict will occur among the untrained members in a heterogeneous group, with each member insisting on his own point of view, so that the group never arrives at a decision with which everyone can be satisfied. This tends to occur most often in *ad hoc* groups with high-power personalities.

The variable of training in the consensus-seeking process is the most critical of all for producing synergy. In studies conducted by Dr. Jay Hall, a social scientist, trained and untrained groups were measured; both types of groups produced synergy. In the trained groups, however, synergy occurred 75% of the time, while in the untrained groups, it occurred only 25% of the time (46). The implications are obvious: group leaders, facilitators, managers, supervisors, and all those who try to work with others in a participative manner need to understand the principles of training and instruct their groups in the process. A second conclusion was that under conditions of training, the heterogeneous groups performed better than homogeneous groups. In fact, the broader the range of opinions presented, the better the group's chances of arriving at superior decisions. The implication here is that a group of "lemons," group members who fight and cannot agree, can be turned into "lemonade" if the facilitator trains them in the consensus-seeking process.

GUIDELINES FOR SEEKING CONSENSUS

The training required to move a group from 25 to 75% efficiency in achieving consensus is based on a set of guidelines for group behavior; it is simple and not time-consuming. Professionals who decide to use this method with staff need to understand, however, that it may take several weeks of regularly reminding the group of the guidelines, and interrupting each time the guidelines are not followed, before the process becomes natural to the group. These guidelines for achieving consensus in groups are as follows:

1. All group members have the responsibility and obligation to share opinions.

2. After group members have expressed opinions on a particular issue, they have the right to ask others to paraphrase these comments to their satisfaction.

3. After being paraphrased, they may not bring up their perspective again unless asked to do so by another group member. Insisting on one's own point of view or blocking discussion is not allowed.

4. Everyone has the responsibility to understand the arguments and opinions of the other members, and may ask questions for clarification.

5. After all perspectives are understood, the group needs to arrive at a solution or decision with which everyone can be satisfied. In accomplishing this task, the group may not immediately resort to the stress-reducing techniques of majority rule, trade-offs, averaging, coin-flipping, and bargaining.

6. Differences of opinion should be viewed as natural and expected. Members need to be encouraged to seek them out so that everyone is involved in the decision process. Disagreements can help the group's decision because with a wider range of information and opinions, there is a greater chance that the group will develop superior solutions. Frequently, when the group members suspend their own judgment, new solutions emerge that no single individual would have been able to develop alone. These solutions tend to incorporate the best points of all views—of both the majority and the minority. Such solutions tend to be synergistic. At times, however, after considerable discussion, no new solution emerges. In those instances, alternative problem-solving techniques can be applied (47).

Alternative Problem-Solving Techniques

When a group is unable to agree on a solution, several other methods, each with its advantages and disadvantages, can be used. One method is for the leader to make the decision. The advantage is that the decision is arrived at quickly; the disadvantage is that those who dislike it may not support it. While leaders may feel that they have "won," others who feel that they have "lost" may attempt to subvert the decision or solution. Another possibility is for some members to accommodate others by no longer insisting on their preferred solution. This method will immediately relieve the group of conflict, but those who accommodated may later resent having done so and may not feel obliged to uphold the solution. Perhaps the most common method is compromise, each side giving in a little until both can agree. The problem with compromise is that often what is given up is sought back eventually. Compromise solutions tend to be short-lived. Other conflict-reducing techniques such as majority rule, trade-offs, and coin-flipping also tend to be short-lived because the members who gave up something to satisfy the immediate need for a solution feel no obligation to support the solution.

Group Participation in Decision Making

There are both advantages and disadvantages to participative decision making. The practitioner needs to be aware of them in order to decide, on a contingency basis, when this method is appropriate.

Advantages

1. When managers meet their team members one at a time, problems of communication and perceptual distortion may occur. Each time the manager discusses the issues on a one-to-one basis, the superior's manner and language vary, with each subordinate asking questions from a different perspective. Meeting together to discuss such matters as operational activities and politics provides an opportunity for everyone to hear the same descriptions at the same time, and to ask questions, which may clarify perceptions, so that everyone shares a common understanding.

2. Interpersonal relationship problems can be resolved, particularly when the staff is aware of the need for teamwork.

3. Motivation can be enhanced since the individuals involved in the decision may become more committed to it and may better understand how it is to be carried out. Resistance to change is lessened when individuals consider the alternative actions together and decide together on the goals and objectives for achieving change. They experience a greater commitment to changes that they themselves have either initiated or participated in developing.

4. The synergy of problem-solving can occur, allowing the group to arrive at solutions that are qualitatively superior to any that a single individual could arrive at alone.

Disadvantages

1. Group participation in decision making can be time-consuming; however, the time spent in goal setting, problem definition, and planning can result in more rapid implementation of the solution and less resistance to change.

2. Cohesive groups can become autonomous and work against management's preferences.

3. Groups can sometimes become a way for everyone to escape the responsibility for taking action, since each person may assume that someone else is ultimately responsible.

4. The goals and interests of employees and those of management may not be compatible.

5. Employees may not be qualified to participate. Participation requires not only a desire to be involved, but also an ability to communicate insights, reactions, and desires. Not everyone possesses these skills to the same degree, and some who have the desire, but not the ability, may need to be trained.

6. Individuals whose ideas are continuously rejected can become alienated.

7. Managers may use groups as a way to manipulate employees into making the decision that they, the managers, have already decided upon.

8. Work group involvement may raise employees' expectations that cannot always be met or that the manager did not intend, and once started, employees may want to be included in all decision making, whether or not their participation is appropriate.

9. The hazards of "groupthink" refer to the phenomenon of a group stifling individual creativity to preserve the status quo. It is the mode of thinking that persons engage in when seeking concurrences becomes more important in a cohesive group than a realistic appraisal of the alternative courses of action. The symptoms of groupthink arise when group members avoid being too harsh in their judgments of their leaders' or their colleagues' ideas for the sake of preserving harmony. All members are amiable and seek complete concurrence on every important issue to avoid conflict that might spoil the cozy, group atmosphere (47, 48).

Dr. Irving Janis, social psychologist, is the leading expert on the groupthink phenomenon. Below are some of the remedies he suggests to prevent its occurrence. Dietetics practitioners need to consider ways of adapting these practices to their own style of group facilitation with staff (47, 49).

1. At each meeting, the facilitator should verbalize the desire that all participants assume the role of "critical evaluator." Members need to be encouraged to look for the weaknesses in one another's arguments. The facilitator's acceptance of criticism from others is critical if the others are to continue the practice with her and with one another.

2. The facilitator should adopt from the start an impartial stance instead of stating preferences and expectations. Such a stance encourages open inquiry and impartial probing of a wide range of policy alternatives.

3. The organization should routinely set up several alternative policy planning and evaluation groups to work on the same policy question, with each group deliberating under a different leader. This practice can prevent the insulation of an in-group.

4. Before reaching a final consensus, the group members should discuss the issues with qualified associ-

ates who are not part of the decision-making group, and should then report back to the others the results of their informal surveys.

5.   The group should invite one or more outside experts to each meeting on a staggered basis and encourage the experts to challenge the views of the dominant group members.

6.   At every meeting of the group, whenever the agenda calls for an evaluation of policy alternatives, at least one member should be assigned to play the "devil's advocate," challenging the testimony of those who advocate the majority position.

7.   After reaching a preliminary consensus about what seems to be the best policy, the group should hold a "second-chance" meeting, during which time members express as vividly as they can all their residual doubts. This meeting gives everyone a last opportunity to rethink the entire issue before making a definitive choice (37).

MEETING MANAGEMENT

This section offers the professional several concise suggestions for exploring the "process variables" that affect staff as they work together in groups. There will be times when the manager senses tension among the staff but is uncertain of its cause. At these times, a department meeting can be called for the specific purpose of resolving and exposing work-related problems. Knowing how to assist the group in solving problems is a major responsibility of the professional. Enlightened supervisors recognize the value in calling the group together occasionally for "process meetings."

A process meeting is one called for the specific purpose of discussing the group as a group. The items discussed include the process variables mentioned at the beginning of this chapter: how the group functions internally, how the members relate to one another, which procedures the group follows, how members communicate among themselves, how they do their work as a group, and how they react to proposed changes. Dietetics professionals should initiate such meetings whenever they see a need; however, anyone in the department who sees a need for such a meeting should be encouraged to suggest it.

When supervisors decide to call the entire group together to share concerns about the dynamics in the work group, they should be sincere and candid in asking for assistance, and they should schedule the meeting at an appropriate time and place. The right time is when the staff is not preoccupied with other urgent problems and when they are being paid for their time. A group should never be given too brief a time limit when the task is to discuss the dynamics of their work group.

Until the staff becomes comfortable with them, the first process meetings may be slow in starting, with people asking, "Why are we here?" After the facilitator de-

scribes the reasons for inferring tension in the group, she should remain quiet until group members begin to offer their own subjective explanations for the tension. While process meetings are not yet common, supervisors who do hold them regularly find that they are able to short-circuit departmental problems by giving the staff members time to vent their feelings and to resolve conflicts with one another. An underlying assumption here is that the supervisor is already skilled in the techniques of conflict resolution and counseling.

A trend likely to continue through the early 21st century is the practice of taking an entire staff to an off-site planning retreat, process meeting, or problem-solving discussion. The alternative relaxed and casual environment with the extended open-ended time periods allows for optimal authentic interaction among the group and an ideal setting for extended process meetings (48, 50, 51).

A serious problem among administrators, department heads, and others who regularly need to depend on a staff for participative decision making is keeping group members motivated to participate, to follow through on assignments and tasks, and to be fully prepared before the meeting so that they can offer informed opinions. If there is a general problem with the group's not being prepared at meetings and the professional is not sure what the underlying causes are, she might consider distributing a survey. The survey could be passed out in advance, with members asked to remain anonymous. She could then tabulate the results and use the data as the basis for a process meeting. Usually, the professional acts as the group's facilitator and manages process meetings; however, from time to time she may wish to appoint another to moderate the meetings, especially if she observes herself talking too much or becoming defensive.

No two work groups are exactly alike or have identical problems and concerns. For that reason, facilitators should be creative in designing surveys that are tailored for their specific groups. The survey might be used to point out discrepancies between how people think the group feels about a particular work issue versus how it actually feels. The survey could also ask for opinions regarding the members' perceptions of the clarity of group goals, the degree of trust and openness within the group, the level of sensitivity and perceptiveness among group members, the amount of attention to group process, the ways in which group leadership needs are met, the ways in which decisions are made, how well the group's resources are used, and the amount of loyalty and sense of belonging in the group. As pointed out in Chapter 2, selective perception often leads individuals to motives and opinions that do not correspond with fact. Group discussion of survey results exposes the different perspectives existing subjectively within the group.

It may be that the group is satisfied with the status quo, and the supervisor is dissatisfied. Perhaps she objects to the fact that the staff members insist on deviating from the agenda, or that they ignore responsibilities they had agreed to at previous meetings, or that they are not prepared to discuss the issues on the agenda that had been sent to them to consider. When it is the facilitators who are dissatisfied, they should facilitate the process meeting, albeit very carefully. They need to reaffirm the norms they want, making sure that everyone understands the norms, and then the facilitators need to stop people any time a norm is violated.

Even among a group of individuals who see one another regularly and do not feel any need for a formal process meeting, there is still value in providing a time for them to relieve social concerns when they are called together for group meetings. It is a good idea for the supervisor to plan on giving the work group 5 to 8 minutes to settle in socially before they get down to business. Providing extra time requires that the business agenda be tailored accordingly. If 45 minutes of business have to be conducted, the facilitator needs to allow 55 minutes for the total meeting time. The group should be reminded regularly that those first minutes are intended to be social and not used as "grace time" for latecomers. Everyone is expected to arrive on time so that the social time is used for that purpose. The supervisor's arriving early to greet people provides an opportunity for individuals to discuss any special problems or concerns.

A common inference among work groups is that the "boss" is looking for a "rubber stamp" group and is not truly interested in what the members believe. Unfortunately, the "boss" or dietetics professional is usually the last to discover this inference. This phenomenon is called the "good news barrier to communication." An archetype common in the classic Greek tragedies of Aeschylus, Euripides, and Sophocles is that the messenger who brought the news to the king that his son had been killed in battle was then killed himself. The ancient Greek dramatists were tapping into a universal fear, which is alive and well today in the workplace. This unconscious fear causes negative situations to be described more positively to the supervisor and causes groups to fail to expose the "real" problems. It is to the practitioner's advantage to be informed of the most "truthful" and objective data available. A way to foster openness in groups of staff members is to be consistently supportive, relieving the anxiety that might accompany being candid in group discussions. The staff needs to be asked for input on how the meetings could be improved. Once their suggestions are understood, as many as possible should be implemented.

Often, a common complaint among administrators regarding staff meetings is that no one seems to have anything to say. The groups seem noncreative or unwilling to generate new ideas. Suggestions on how to solve this problem might include assigning members the task of writing brief reports before the meeting. Including their names on the agenda next to the report topic is usually enough to inspire them to gather their thoughts before-

hand. Of course, group leaders can stop the meeting at any time and dictate discussion questions to the group. After the group has been given 20 minutes to jot down some response, even in a personal shorthand, the meeting can be resumed. (Members should be reassured that no one else will read their answers.) In this way, everyone can have something to contribute. Another technique is to divide the group into small subgroups, allowing the individual hesitant to speak up in a large group to converse with one or two others. When the large group is reconvened, the subgroup, not the hesitant individual, can give a report on its conclusions. In that way, minority opinions that might not otherwise surface often obtain recognition within the group.

At the end of a meeting, assignments for the following meetings can be distributed. The supervisor can increase the likelihood of the group following through with their assignments by asking all members to paraphrase their responsibilities for the next meeting. The act of acknowledging responsibility in the presence of the others adds pressure on the participant to complete the assigned tasks. If members do come unprepared regularly, the supervisor should consider adjourning the meeting until they are ready. Usually, this needs to be done only once for members to get the point.

Several days before the meeting, the facilitator should have notes sent out with the agenda to remind participants of their obligations to report, read documents, have subgroup meetings, and the like. Placing names next to agenda items acts as a stimulus for members to be prepared to report at meetings.

Often, dietetics professionals assume that they must know how to handle all problems that may occur in the work groups and at staff meetings, mistakenly believing that they are expected to have the insight, expertise, and competence to correct all problems. What they actually need to have is the humility and courage to ask for help. Supervisors need to be conscious of the various resources in their work groups and be willing to use the talents of group members whenever possible. Allowing individuals who may be especially competent in a particular area to share their knowledge with the others, to manage individual group meetings, or to train subordinates involves more than just delegation. It involves showing respect for and raising the self-esteem of the individual subordinate. Supervisors must lead, but not always by leading. They can perform just as efficiently simply by seeing that the leadership takes place.

Supervisors must consider the possibility that they themselves are the cause of the group members' underlying tensions or of their being unable to "gel" at meetings. Some common pitfalls among supervisors include not allowing time at the end of meetings for people to comment on how meetings might be improved, making sarcastic remarks to participants during meetings, or becoming defensive when comments about the supervisor do emerge. Group members may be unable to participate optimally and may be frustrated with the facilitator if she neglects to do the following:

1. send out agendas

2. inform the group of the core topic for the meeting

3. give assignments to individuals

4. provide essential information to participants before the meeting

5. inform especially resourceful individuals of how they can participate

6. provide adequate time at meetings to discuss the topic fully

GROUPS AS SUPPLEMENT TO INDIVIDUAL COUNSELING

Group and individualized counseling may be used together. Even those persons who require intensive counseling can benefit by the examples, support, and ideas available in groups. When specialized and intense one-on-one dietary counseling does not produce the desired results, group counseling may be advantageous. When problems are mutual, the group can provide support, reinforcement, and all the advantages of synergy in solving problems. Groups also provide the resources for conducting role-playing and rehearsing actions for the real world.

As used in nutrition counseling, groups differ from group therapy. Group counseling is intended to be not a form of therapy, but a format to help people find solutions to dietary problems. These solutions can then be demonstrated, attempted, and evaluated with group support (52).

A primary goal in nutrition counseling is to promote self-sufficiency in clients. In groups where people learn basic change strategies by helping other group members design personal dietary change programs, and by encouraging mutual follow-through, this self-sufficiency goal is enhanced. Once the group understands the basic strategies, the practitioner can facilitate nondirectively, allowing the members to consult with one another.

Some consider group counseling impractical when it is limited to a single session. One-on-one counseling, however, is time-consuming. With the cutbacks in staff at some hospitals, any time saver, such as the use of groups, is helpful. Behavior change requires more than one session, but a single group session may be an efficient and time-saving way to give information to a group of patients or clients with similar problems. The practitioner is saved from having to explain basic concepts over and over. Being with others who share similar problems often encourages participants to change more than if they were counseled individually.

When the group is designed primarily for the professional to convey nutrition and dietary information, to teach principles of dietary change, and to encourage group members to use them, several principles should be incorporated into the teaching aspects of group sessions (52).

1. The number of major points covered per meeting should be limited. The dietetics practitioner should focus all efforts toward motivating the group to understand and use these main principles.

2. Since learning is a gradual process, teaching time in groups should be devoted to essential and necessary information. The intricate technicalities can be taught later.

3. The principles of education covered in other places in this book should be used: the goal of the session should be stated, examples should be given, and group discussion and problem solving should be stimulated. Participants should be encouraged to summarize the points learned and their intended applications of them.

4. The content should be presented and reinforced through a variety of means: written presentations, audiovisual media, role-playing, and demonstrations.

5. Group members should be required to write down or publicly verbalize short-term goals that are specific and "doable," so that they can be reviewed in the group the following week.

This chapter has stressed the necessity for practitioners to study group process and internalize the behaviors needed to participate in, facilitate, and model group interaction skills. Under proper leadership, groups can stimulate solutions and insights the individuals might not experience otherwise. Once they develop the skills needed to diagnose group needs and the ability to correct them by focusing on the group's resources, practitioners can function as change agents and as communication models for the other group members, while at the same time becoming more effective administrators.

REVIEW AND DISCUSSION QUESTIONS

1. What are the changes affecting the profession of dietetics?

2. What distinguishes the traditional style of leadership from the new style of leadership?

3. Why is a team approach superior?

4. How should a facilitator halt a side conversation?

5. Discuss the significance of the informal work group.

6. What is "synergy" and how can it be stimulated in groups?

7. Discuss several of the participant functions and how they either maintain the group's effectiveness or assist in accomplishing the group's task.

SUGGESTED ACTIVITIES

1. In groups of three, discuss the "best" small group experiences you have ever had. What occurred that

CASE STUDY

Betty Smith, RD, is planning a series of group meetings for her clients who are parents of children who have type I diabetes mellitus. Her concern today is planning for optimum group participation in the first session, which will be an hour long. She also wants to be sure to meet the needs of the group so that they will return for future sessions.

1. What suggestions do you have for the first session?

qualifies them as superior? Describe specific behaviors of both the group's leader/facilitator and the participants that seem to have made a difference. Time should be allotted for each group to share its insights with the others.

2. In groups of three, plan to meet in three different settings over the next 2 days, with different seating, room size, lighting, etc. Report your observations on the effects of the environment to the entire class. Notice whether different groups had simpler reactions and were influenced by the same factors. A simpler variation on this activity would be to hold a discussion for 10 minutes with the group arranged in a circle and then to continue the discussion with the group sitting in a straight row.

3. Make a list of at least three small groups in which you have been active, and describe the functions you performed in each. Compare your perceptions of yourself as a contributing group member with the perceptions that your friends or classmates had of you. Do you notice that you performed different functions in different groups? Do some functions overlap from group to group? Are your classmates in agreement with you regarding your functions within their group?

4. Thinking back to some recent experiences in group discussions, complete each of the following statements:
    A. My strengths as a group participant are . . . .
    B. My strengths as a group facilitator are . . . .
    C. What is keeping me from being more effective both as a participant and facilitator is . . . .
    D. What I plan to improve is . . . .

5. How do you determine if needed leadership and facilitative services are being provided during a discussion? Compare your observations with those of your classmates.

6. Write a question or description of a problem or issue, preferably from your own personal or professional experience, for which you do not have a solution. Present it to a small group and facilitate their discussion. Possible questions might include "Do people need to take vitamin supplements?" "What are the best food choices when eating at a fast-food outlet?" and "What recommendations should one give to someone who desires to lose weight or exercise more?"

7. Group together 4 to 5 people who have a common problem, such as needing to lose weight, needing to start eating breakfast, wanting to control excess consumption of snacks, needing to select nutritious meals, wanting to increase the fiber content of their diets, or wanting to exercise more often. State the problem and have the group attempt to solve it.

REFERENCES

1. McLaughlin M. The executive of the 21st century: a change of mind. N Engl Business 1989;11:42.
2. Goddard RW. Work force 2000. Personnel J 1989;68:64.
3. Conlin J. Conflict at meetings: come out fighting. Successful Meetings 1989;38:30.
4. Finn S. President's page: partnerships forge opportunity, innovation, and action. J Am Diet Assoc 1993;93:195.
5. Finn S. The power of teamwork. ADA Courier 1993;32:3.
6. Pace R. Dietetics leadership in the 21st century. J Am Diet Assoc 1995;95:536.
7. Montebello A. Teamwork in health care. Clin Lab Mgmt Rev 1994;8:91.
8. Hassell J, Games A, Shaffer B, et al. Nutrition support team management. J Am Diet Assoc 1994;94:993.
9. Lanza M. Total quality management. Clin Nurse Spec 1994;8:4.
10. Trnobranski P. Nurse-patient negotiation. J Adv Nurs 1994;19:4.
11. Hayes P. Team building. Nurs Mgmt 1994;25:5.
12. Scott J, Rantz M. Change champions at the grassroots level. Nurs Adm Q 1994;18:3.
13. Lustig A, Zusman S. Pharmacists as members of the healthcare team. Ann Pharmacother 1994;28:2.
14. Lenkman S, Gribbins R. Multidisciplinary teams in the acute care setting. Holist Nurs Prac 1994;8:3.
15. Davis L, Cox R. Looking through the constructivist lens. J Prof Nurs 1994;10:1.
16. McHenry L. Implementing self-directed teams. Nurs Mgmt 1994;25:3.
17. Sovie M. Nurse manager: a key role in clinical outcomes. Nurs Mgmt 1994;25:3.
18. Rice J. Team approach to charting. Leadership Health Serv 1994;3:3.
19. Goodale J. Effective teamwork and productivity conferences. Clin Lab Mgmt Rev 1994;8:3.
20. Blancett S. Self-managed teams. J Nurs Adm 1994;12:4.
21. Sundstrom E, DeMeuse IP, Futrell D. Work teams applications and effectiveness. Am Psychol 1990;2:120.
22. Tavantzis T, Krasnick C, Bender A. Introducing teamwork in physician groups. Med Grp Mgmt J 1994;41:2.
23. McKenzie L. Cross-functional teams in health care organizations. Health Care Supervis 1994;12:3.

24. Engelhardt D. A dynamic team approach to creating a dynamic practice. Compend Continuing Educ Dentistry 1995;16:12.

25. Coeling H. Understanding work group culture on rehabilitation units. Rehab Nurs 1996;21:1.

26. Fisher G, Opper F. An interdisciplinary nutrition support team improves quality of care in a teaching hospital. J Am Diet Assoc 1996;96:2.

27. Kappeli S. Interprofessional cooperation: why is partnership so difficult? Pat Educ Counsel (Ireland) 1996; 26:6.

28. Rich B, Hart B, Barrett A, et al. Peer consultation: a look at process. Clin Nurse Spec 1995;9:3.

29. Robbins S. Essentials of organizational behavior. Upper Saddle River, NJ: Prentice Hall, 1997.

30. Frey L. Innovations in group facilitation. Cresskill, NJ: Hampton Press, 1995.

31. Sinetar M. The informal discussion group—a powerful agent for change. Sloan Mgmt Rev 1989;29:61.

32. Koehler K. Managing change. Small Bus Rep 1989;14:15.

33. Breuer J. Orchestrating culture shock: what happens when companies must change. Inform 1989;3:46.

34. Carron A, Widmeyer N, Brawley L. Group cohesion and individual adherence to physical activity. J Sport Exer Psychol 1988;10:127.

35. Anonymous. Group decision making. Small Bus Rep 1988;13:30.

36. Dobbins GH, Zaccaro SJ. The effects of group cohesion and leader behavior on subordinate satisfaction. Grp Org Stud 1986;11:203.

37. Brilhart JK, Galanes GJ. Effective group discussion. 8th ed. Dubuque, IA: William C. Brown, 1995.

38. Schultz BG. Communicating in the small group. New York: Harper and Row, 1989.

39. Scope of practice for qualified professionals in diabetes care and education. J Am Diet Assoc 1996;96:606.

40. Baird LS, Schneier CE, Laird D. Training aid for dealing with special students. In: Baird LS, Schneier C, Russel C, et al., eds. The training and development sourcebook. Amherst, MA: Human Resource Development Press, 1994.

41. Patton BR, Giffin K, Patton EN. Decision-making group interaction. New York: Harper and Row, 1994.

42. Anonymous. How to control time eaters (without being rude). Working Woman 1989;14:110.

43. Bernard P, Hill N. Improving organization effectiveness through employee involvement. Bus Q (Canada) 1989; 53:58.

44. Watson WE, Michaelsen LK. Group interaction behaviors that affect group performance on an intellective task. Grp Org Stud 1988;13:495.

45. Watson RT, DeSanctis GP, Marschall S. Using a GDSS to facilitate group consensus. MIS Q 1988;12:463.

46. Hall J. Decisions, decisions, decisions. Psychol Today 1971;6:61.

47. Janis I. Groupthink. Psychol Today 1971;6:43.

48. Hargreaves J. How to make a workshop work. Industr Mkt Dig (UK) 1988;13:57.

49. Moorhead G, Montanari JR. An empirical investigation of the groupthink phenomenon. Hum Relat 1986;39:399.

50. Cronin F, Goodspeed SW. The planning retreat with the one-track mind. Healthcare Forum 1989;32:30.

51. Sipos A. Organizational climate and employee involvement. J Qual Participat 1988;11:62.

52. Rabb C, Tillotson J, eds. Heart to heart. Washington, DC: US Dept of Health and Human Services, 1983.

fourteen

DELIVERING ORAL PRESENTATIONS AND WORKSHOPS

A significant responsibility included in the day-to-day professional life of many dietetics practitioners includes making oral presentations and/or conducting workshops for groups of patients, for other professionals, for the general public, and for various other groups and organizations that wish to be educated in the areas of the individual's expertise. Being a good speaker can give one an edge over competition and lead to inferences of one's professional competence. Speaking and presentation skills may be as critical an indicator of one's career success as one's professional education (1). The presentation skills discussed in this chapter will serve the dietetics practitioner equally well in her teaching—both to students and/or patients (2). Like so many of the other skills discussed in this book, the skills needed to deliver a message orally and articulately cannot be learned by reading alone; one must be prepared to digest the information and then have the courage to R—I—S—K.

Although entire books are written on the broad and general subject of giving oral presentations, the purpose of this chapter is to develop and to discuss concisely the most salient principles occurring in the process of preparing and delivering oral presentations and workshops, dealing with the media, and talking in front of a hostile audience.

Following are suggestions for advance planning and organizing of a presentation, advance physical arrangements of the room, delivering the presentation, and post-presentation actions.

ADVANCE PLANNING AND ORGANIZATION FOR THE PRESENTATION

The key to holding the attention of an audience, particularly one with limited time to absorb the speaker's ideas, is to be coherent and to communicate simply; otherwise their minds will wander. The secret of conciseness and simplicity is for speakers to know their objectives before planning their talk. What do they want to accomplish? What changes do they want to take place in the attitude or behavior of the audience? Do they want them to perform a task or recall some information? A common mistake made among untrained presenters is to attempt to cover too much in the time allotted. Inexperienced speakers often feel the need to parade their expertise and overload the audience with information.

Unlike reading where one can go back and reconsider an idea, listening requires ongoing concentration. When the brain begins to feel overloaded and saturation sets in, it protects itself by shutting down. Has not everyone had the experience of pretending to be listening to an overly meticulous speaker as the imagination went elsewhere on holiday? Oral presentations need to be limited to a few major points that can be clearly explained and reinforced through details, examples, and a variety of media. Too much information and too many different points defeat the purpose. When listeners know where the presentation is going and are able to follow the presenter's reasoning, grasping examples with ease, they are much more likely to give their full attention.

Although presentations are often as brief as 10 minutes or as long as 90, presenters would do well to remember when adapting their goals to their group what the Reverend William Sloane Coffin said about the length of an effective sermon, "No souls are saved after 20 minutes." Once presenters have their general and specific goals tailored to their group, the next task is to organize them.

Introduction Critical to Speaker Credibility
Each of the three generally accepted divisions of a presentation (introduction, body, and conclusion) requires its own internal organization and serves a specific function. The introduction serves speakers by providing them the opportunity to establish credibility, to link themselves in some way to their audience, to let them know in what ways they will be better off as a result of having attended, and to describe for the audience in some serial fashion what they intend to cover.

Often when individuals are introduced to speak, their credentials are presented in advance; however, there will be times when no one is present to introduce the speaker or, when an "introducer" is available, she may neglect to mention important items related to enhancing the speaker's credibility. While self-serving comments delivered in a braggadocio manner may have a negative effect on audiences, audiences do, nevertheless, want to know that the person talking to them is worthy and knowledgeable. Practitioners, therefore, should subtly let listeners know during the introduction that they are qualified. For example, one might say, "... in an article I wrote last year for the *Journal of the American Dietetic Association* ...," or "of the several hundred patients I have worked with in the past ...."

Audiences tend to be more attentive when they believe that the person speaking to them is able to relate to their circumstances. During the introduction, whenever it is possible, speakers would do well to underscore any connection they may have with a particular group. For example, one might say, "I have lived in this community for 15 years ...," or "I was once 25 pounds overweight myself ...," or "I see we are all baby boomers and share many of the same sentiments about wellness." If one gives it some thought, almost all audiences have some traits with which the speaker can identify.

During the introduction speakers need to let the audience know how the topic relates to their needs; in other words, presenters should answer the unasked question in everyone's mind, "What is in this for me?" Abraham Maslow has synthesized the basic human needs into five areas: physiological; safety and security; belonging and social activity; esteem and status; and self-realization and fulfillment. When the professional announces that after listening to the speech, the listeners will in some way be better able to control their health, be more secure, be in a position where others think better of them or respect them more, think more of themselves, or feel they have the knowledge to develop latent potential in themselves, the audience "perks up" and prepares itself to attend to the forthcoming message. Not every human need can be related to every topic, but as many as possible and as appropriate should be suggested during the introduction. During the body and conclusions of the speech as well, the speaker should remind the audience how what is being discussed can be related to fulfilling their own needs.

Finally, the last critical component to be included in the introduction is a list of the topics that will be discussed. It might be presented something like this: "Today I intend to discuss three specific points. Number one, I will discuss the relationship of diet to heart disease; number two, I will discuss how to measure the fat and cholesterol content of foods, and number three, I will model how to order at a restaurant." As mentioned above, not only does this help the audience to listen to the talk with an expectation of what is to come, but the organization itself adds to the "halo effect" and increases the audience's perceptions of the speaker's credibility.

Three Key Objectives of the Body of the Presentation

The body of the presentation is the second major division and the place where the points mentioned in the intro-

duction are actually developed. Presenters need to have a rationale for the way they decide to organize this major section. The overall objectives generally are threefold: that the audience fully understands the message, that the audience believes, and that they are comfortable enough with the speaker to share their objections in the event that they are confused or wish to challenge the presenter.

To safeguard the first objective, understanding the message of the presenter, the speaker needs not only to construct the message clearly and concisely, but also to design visual aids, handouts, and/or participative experiences to enhance the audience's understanding. The second objective, content and speaker credibility, needs continuously to be reinforced throughout the presentation. The third objective, to develop a rapport with the audience to the extent that they dare challenge or question, is critical. When objections are unexpressed, presenters may infer falsely that the audience agrees and understands, causing the speaker to move too quickly from one point to another, leaving confused members behind.

A Presentation Can Be Concluded in More Ways Than One

Like the first two, the third division of the presentation, the conclusion, may be handled successfully in many different ways. The key is that all the ingredients be included somewhere. Ingredient one is for the audience to "feel" that the presentation is "winding down" and about to end. This needs to be done gradually and smoothly. It sounds nonprofessional and haphazard to end with remarks like "any questions," "that's all folks," or "thank you for your attention." Remember the presenter's credibility is influenced by the audience's perceptions of how well he is organized. Clues such as "In conclusion ...," "To summarize," "Before concluding, I want to leave you with one more thought," are helpful in letting the audience know that the presentation is about to conclude. If a summary is warranted, it should be given; if a final plea or pitch is warranted, that should be given; if a final quote, anecdote, or joke makes the point one more time, then that is appropriate.

One last word about conclusions is to be proactive in anticipating asking if there are any questions. Of course there are, but people are often hesitant to ask. The speaker should prepare a few for the audience, and then call on a participant who has been paying attention for a reaction. One might say, for example, "I noticed that you looked confused when I was discussing the fatty acid content of foods. What is it you would like further discussion of?" After responding to that first question generated by the presenter, it is often much simpler to get others to respond when the question is asked, "Are there any *other* questions or comments?"

Correlation Exists Between "Form" and Speaker Credibility

Although the discussion of the presentation's design is generally divided into the three areas of introduction, body, and conclusion, there is no one perfect way to organize. Speakers, each with varied styles, can be successful. There are, however, several points to consider when deciding upon a presentation's specific format. A fact that most people are not aware of is that the presentation's organization is critical, primarily because it relates to the presenter's credibility.

For example, if a speaker were to deliver a talk to two different audiences, giving one audience 10 bits of information in an organized way and giving the second audience the same 10 bits of information in a disorganized way, both audiences would retain about the same amount of information after hearing the talk, but only one audience would consider it seriously or possibly change their attitude toward the subject matter.

When an audience hears an organized speaker, one who gives the audience a sense of his knowing exactly where he is going, with a defined beginning, middle, and end, they are more likely to infer that he is competent in the area he is talking about. Many brilliant and qualified professionals, however, are not taken seriously when giving presentations because they sound too "loose," too unprepared, or too disorganized.

Media Format is Related to Inferences Regarding Presenter's Credibility

All media, and the way they are designed, presented, and utilized, are an extension of the speaker and, consequently, reflect directly on the speaker's credibility. Media include such things as handouts, blackboard, flipchart, pad/mock-ups, and so forth, as discussed in another chapter. A superior standard is inferred from media supplements that are obviously carefully put together. For example, a presenter whose overhead transparencies are executed with large print that can easily be read, as opposed to ordinary typewriter print, which cannot be easily read from a transparency, allows for the inference of an experienced and considerate presenter. Other signs include using stenciled letters in bold colors on posters, rather than sloppy printing or cursive writing. The condition of the poster itself leads either to positive or negative impressions of the speaker. Those that are discolored, bent, and old-looking suggest that the presenter does not care enough to add fresh aids for this group. Even the quality and color of the paper used in handouts can add or detract from the overall impression. If it is possible, the presenter is wise to try to coordinate all aids in colors that may be symbolic or meaningful. For example, a presenter giving a talk to an Italian-American Club could use the colors red, white, and green. This may sound superfluous but audiences do respond on an unconscious level to the extra care and preparation the speaker has made in tailoring a presentation on their behalf.

Language and Style of Oral Presentations Differ from Those of Written Presentations

The written text and the oral presentation are entirely different. There is no objection to a presenter writing out the entire talk, carefully organizing it according to topics, causes and effects, chronology, or whatever else seems appropriate. Once the talk is written, however, the speaker needs to recognize that the written manuscript represents the "science" of a presentation; the actual delivery represents the "art." Each time it is delivered,

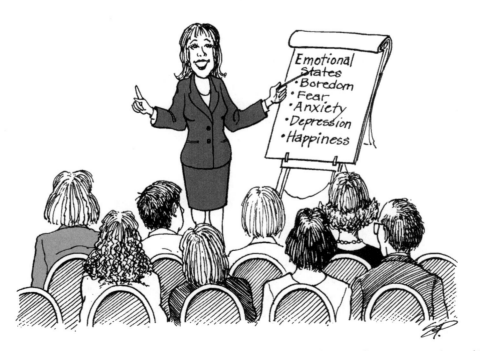

FIGURE 14.1.   In discussing emotional eating, the professional enhances her presentation with visuals.

it should be somewhat different, using different words, different examples, different anecdotes, and so forth to suit particular audiences and situations. The word choice too in the spoken language tends to be different from the word choice used in the written language. Sentences in oral speech tend to be simpler, shorter, and sound more conversational, including common words and contractions, while the written manuscript may be more erudite and academic. The only way for speakers to develop this "art" is to rehearse from a simple outline and not a manuscript, and to rehearse in front of real people who will react and comment, not in front of mirrors, walls, or car windshields.

Oral Presentations Should Never Be Read or Memorized

There are other good reasons for not rehearsing from a manuscript. The speech tends eventually to become memorized, and that can be deadly. Once a speech is memorized, speakers tend to become more "speaker-centered" than "audience-centered," which means that they tend to become more concerned about whether or not they can remember each line exactly as it is written on the manuscript and less concerned about whether or not the audience is enjoying, learning, listening, and understanding. Another problem that arises from manuscript speaking is that it is DULL! Because the facial expressions and vocal intonations are not spontaneous, the monologue tends to sound memorized and can easily become boring to listeners.

Advance Arrangements Need To Be Carefully Considered

Take control of seating the listeners before everyone settles down. It may be their boardroom, gymnasium, or meeting hall, but it is the presenter's "show." Conscious decisions should be made about whether or not to pull the group into a circle, half circle, rows, around tables, and so forth. When it is possible to know beforehand which persons are the most influential, their seats should be reserved and placed in the best position to see, hear, and appreciate any visual aids as well as the speaker. A final checklist for presentations is found in Table 14.1.

Creating Positive Impressions Begins the Moment the Presenter Enters the Room

Presenters are being "sized up" and adding to the presentation's ambiance from the moment they enter the room. They should, whenever possible, arrive early and make an effort to meet people. Their own self-confidence, whether real or feigned, will relax the audience and increase their perceptions of the speaker's desire to share information. Presenters should never volunteer any negative information regarding their own stress or fear of speaking. The audience wants to learn and enjoy, and when they are aware of the speaker's fragility or stage

---

TABLE 14.1.

Final Checklist

Attend to details and prepare a final checklist. Listed below are a few questions that the presenter might consider in order to avoid last minute problems.

Do I have my presentation notes?

Do I have all my supporting materials?

Have I enough copies for each of the attendees?

Will the facility be unlocked and open?

Are the tables and chairs arranged to suit my design?

Do I understand how to operate the lighting system?

Do I understand how to operate the ventilation system?

Do I know the location and operating condition of the electrical circuits?

Do I know how to work the projector?

Do I have an extra bulb, cassette, video, extension cords, etc.?

Will the projection screen be in place and adequate for this size group?

Do I have the type of sound system I require? Is it working?

Have arrangements been made to handle messages during the presentation?

Are there arrangements for hats and coats?

Will there be a sign to announce the place of the presentation?

Will someone be introducing me, and have I given her all the information I want shared with the group?

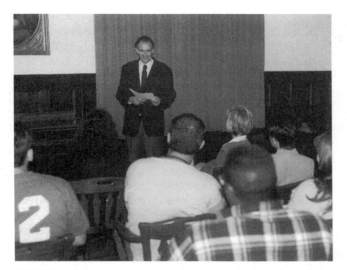

FIGURE 14.2. A presenter should visit the site of the presentation before the actual date.

fright, they tend to become nervous themselves in sympathy.

If the presenters are waiting to be introduced and are seated among the audience or on a stage, they should be aware that audience members who know they are the guest speakers will be watching their every move. That means that even before beginning the presentation, speakers must be careful to smile, look confident, and extend themselves to others. Once introduced, the way the speaker walks up to the dais is critical. During those first moments an initial impression is being created. The speaker should consciously walk confidently, looking and smiling toward the audience. Before uttering the first words to the audience, it is a good technique to spend a long 3 seconds just looking out at the audience, smiling and establishing eye contact with several individuals. This allows them to infer poise, confidence, and the speaker's desire to connect with them.

DELIVERING THE PRESENTATION
Never Share Internal Feelings of Fright or Anxiety
Speakers experience themselves in the situation from the inside out; the audience experiences them from the outside in. Simply, that means if asked whether they are nervous, anxious, etc., speakers should always answer "NO!" The audience is picking up the "tip of the iceberg" from their observations of the "outside" of the speaker; they do not actually feel the intensity of the speaker's anxiety and will probably be totally unaware of it, unless it is brought to their attention through one's own confession. One must act confident, even when one may not feel it internally.

One of the worst things presenters can do is to admit to an audience that they are scared, ill-prepared, missing material, or have done the presentation better in the past for other groups. The audience does not know what it might be missing, and is generally much less critical of speakers than the speakers are of themselves.

Stage Fright is a Vestige From Our Ancient Past
The feelings commonly referred to as stage fright may date back to the dawn of the human race, a time when our prehistoric ancestors had to survive by living in caves and sharing the food supply with other beasts. Faced by a predator, our ancestors had a genuine use for a sudden jolt of energy, which gave them the power to do battle or run, fight, or flee. The vestiges of this power, stemming from the secretions of the adrenal gland, still manifest themselves today when people sense danger. Who has not felt that ice block in the stomach while being reprimanded by the boss, or experienced the sweaty palms and racing heart while walking into a room full of strangers? Occasionally one still reads in the newspaper of accounts where individuals under conditions of fear or danger exhibit superhuman strength, the father, for example, who lifts the car off his child who has been pinned under the wheels. This is an example of the power that comes with the adrenaline jolt; however, when one is unable to fight, run, or in some other way use this surge, he may become overwhelmed by the internal feelings themselves. It is this feeling before and during a presentation that is commonly labeled stage fright.

The best safeguard against stage fright is adequate preparation and rehearsal. The more one practices in front of *live others,* the less nervousness one will have. Other ways of dealing with these feelings include being active during the presentation and "acting" calm and confident. If presenters know they are going to be full of extra energy because of their excess adrenaline secretions, they could plan on engaging in demonstrations during the presentation, passing handouts, using a pointer, or any other activity that involves motion. Motion is a release for the tension and anxiety and allows the audience to infer enthusiasm from the speaker's movement rather than fright, nervousness, or tension. It may not work for everyone, but many people can learn to control their public behavior if they visualize themselves as acting.

All movement should be meaningful. Do not pace. Presenters ought to look for opportunities to break the invisible barrier between themselves and their audience. Walking toward the audience, walking around the audience, walking in and out of the audience, walking among the audience are all acceptable ways of delivering a presentation. What is not acceptable is pacing back and forth, particularly with eyes down, as one pulls his thoughts together before uttering them. Movement into an audience is a communication vehicle in itself. When presenters penetrate that invisible barrier between themselves and the audience, they are nonverbally indicating their desire to connect, to be close, to better "sense" what it is the audience is feeling about the speakers and the content. In fact, as speakers walk among the audi-

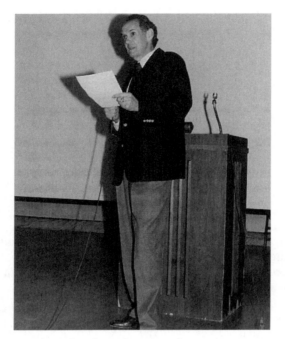

FIGURE 14.3. In a formal setting, the presenter may wish to leave the podium to have better rapport with the audience.

ence, the audience can begin to be seen from a different perspective, and one may gain new insights into how better to clarify particular points and issues from this experience.

Unnecessary Barriers Between the Presenter and Audience Should Be Omitted

Presenters do best when they omit all barriers between themselves and their audience. Avoid using a podium or lectern, even when one is provided by the sponsoring organization. Of course, there may be times when because of the quantity of material, a place to store things may be required. Even under this condition, using a table to set handouts and other materials on is preferred to a podium. A lectern should only be used when the speaker does not intend to move about; intends to lecture; and needs a stand to rest against and place notes upon. Adults generally do not learn optimally through the lecture method and unless the speaker is extraordinarily good, straight lecture behind a podium should be avoided. When one delivers the message standing in front of the group, without a barrier, one is more disposed to stop the talk to respond to the verbal or nonverbal feedback of listeners. Gestures and movement too can be expansive and visible without the lectern barrier.

Voice, Cadence, Pitch, Variation, and Rate Are Communication Vehicles

Vocal inflection and variation add interest and the impression of speaker enthusiasm. For some people controlling

this variation is simple and natural, but for others this is a challenge; nevertheless, the presenter needs to attend to voice modulation. The goal when speaking in front of a group is to sound natural and conversational; however, what sounds natural and conversational when one is standing in front of a large group of others is not the same as what sounds conversational in a small face-to-face group. "Natural and conversational" from the presenter's point of view is exaggerated. The highs need to be a bit higher and the lows need to be a bit lower. What may sound to the presenter's ear as "phony" and "theatrical" generally sounds far less so to the listener. The good news is that this trait can be fairly easily and quickly developed, even in those who recognize a problem in this area. It requires risking sounding foolish and exaggerated in front of trusting others, until adequate reinforcement has convinced the presenter that the increase in vocal variation is really to his advantage and allows him to be attended to more easily. In any case, a delivery that is of narrow range or monotone is difficult to attend to for more than a few minutes.

When talking in front of a group, generally the speaker should attempt to speak more slowly than in ordinary conversation. What is an appropriate rate in a small face-to-face discussion is probably too fast for a group presentation. For some reason, there seems to be a correlation between the speech rate of the speaker and the size of the audience. What might be easily grasped at a more rapid rate in face-to-face conversation, is not understood as quickly in large groups. Also the speaker's slower rate allows him to scan the audience better as he is speaking, to see if he is being understood, to see if some people need an opportunity to disagree, and to see if he needs to talk louder or increase his variation because some look bored.

Nonverbal Behavior, the Silent Language, Can Be Meaningful and Controlled

It is good practice to keep hands away from the body and from one another. Allow them to be free to gesture, and avoid holding anything in them while talking, unless it is a useful prop like a pointer or a visual aid. After 35 years of teaching presentational speaking to college undergraduates, this writer (R.J.C.) knows empirically that once speakers allow their hands to mesh together or to grasp one another behind the back, there is only a slight chance of their being released to gesture. Often people feel awkward with their hands hanging loosely at their sides. Perhaps if they could see themselves on videotape in this posture, they would realize that it is natural looking, but even more importantly, they would probably see that one tends not to stay in that position. As one talks with hands hanging loosely at the sides, eventually they begin to rise and gesture spontaneously to emphasize points the speaker feels important.

It is dangerous to begin a presentation holding a pen, paper clip, rubber band, or other instrument not directly related to the presentation. Unconsciously, the fingers begin to play with the instrument, and the audience becomes fascinated with watching to see what the speaker will do. A former student actually straightened out a paper clip and began to stab herself while talking. Needless to say, for the remainder of her presentation the class could not take their eyes off the mutilation scene, and missed the speaker's concluding points.

As One Speaks So Will One Be Judged

Professional speakers attend to their diction, particularly when pronouncing words like "for," "can," "with," "picture," "going to," and "want to." In ordinary conversation one is not likely to judge negatively a speaker who mispronounces common words and engages in sloppy diction, saying, for example, words like "fer," "ken," "wit," "pitcher," "gunna," and "wanna," for the words listed above; however, when that speaker is in front of an audience, these mispronounced words often stand out and lead to negative inferences regarding the speaker. If one thinks of well-known television anchorpeople, one will be unable to recall any who have faulty diction. Professionals who present themselves in front of groups must attend to their diction because they risk losing credibility if it is poor. Logical? No! True? Yes!

When individuals have decided to become conscious of their diction and decide to improve it, several steps are required. Step number one is to inform trusted others who are often around them to listen critically, and to stop them each time a diction error occurs. Only after individuals are made aware of their common errors, can they begin to train themselves to hear the errors. That is step two. Because the human mind operates generally at 5 times the rate of human speech, it is possible to listen critically to ourselves as we speak. Individuals attempting to rid themselves of poor diction or some other vocalized interference ("um," "ah," "and a," etc.) can train themselves to listen for the error and then to correct themselves. Like learning to ride a bicycle or to use a computer, this learning and training task is uncomfortable at first, but improvement comes quickly. Working on one's diction is an ongoing task. Professional speakers never stop listening to the way their words are coming out and planning ahead to pronounce them correctly.

The Visage Itself is a Communication Vehicle

Presenters need to train themselves to keep their faces animated, using a variety of facial expressions. For many of the same reasons expressed above, it is important that speakers use all the communication vehicles available to them in order to maintain the audience's attention. One's facial expression is itself a communication vehicle. When it is lively, animated, expressive, and changing regularly while the speaker reacts to the feedback coming toward him from the audience, it enhances the verbal message and allows the audience to go on unconsciously inferring the speaker's audience-centeredness. Because of their

natural dispositional personality, ethnic background, and so forth, this is easier for some people to do than for others; however, everyone can improve. Because it is not easy for one to "act" expressive does not mean that one cannot grow considerably in the ability to look expressive. Indeed one can.

Eye contact is a vehicle of communication. It should be used to see everyone and respond to the nonverbal feedback. It is surprising how many people seem to remember having learned some rule about being able to fool the audience into thinking that the speaker is seeing them while actually looking over the heads of the people in the last row. The point is that when speakers have the opportunity to present themselves and their ideas to an audience, they want the audience to understand them, to believe them, and to follow their recommendations.

One has the best chance of being successful in achieving those goals when one is able to interpret the audience's ongoing reactions to what is being said. Even though presentational speaking is generally considered a one-way communication situation, with the speaker talking at the audience as they listen, it is, in fact, a two-way situation with audience and speaker communicating with one another constantly and simultaneously.

Trained speakers see almost everything from their position in front of the room. If they are alert, they may see people who are beginning to fidget, and they can interpret and act on this feedback. They might decide consequently to give the audience a short break; they might liven their own movements to regain attention; they might engage in a new activity, one perhaps that involves audience participation; and so forth. They might see some people coming in late, looking awkwardly for a seat. This gives them the opportunity to publicly welcome them and ask others to move over to provide seating. They might see people who look angry. This gives them the opportunity to say, "You look angry. What has been said to offend you?" In other words speakers who use their eyes to connect with the audience make them a part of the presentation. The audience knows it, and will begin to send signals when they realize the speaker is sensitive to them.

Facial expressions are important. Presenters must remember to smile, and look like they are enjoying the experience of sharing information. Smiling can be rehearsed and may feel phony, but it needs to be built into the design of the presentation. Speakers do not need to be constantly grinning, but they do need to maintain an expression of gentleness, approachability, and nondefensiveness. The easiest way to convey these impressions is smiling often. Unfortunately, it is not easy to smile when one is unsure of the material. All the principles above can only be heeded after the speaker has sufficiently mastered the content and consciously, through rehearsal, developed skills.

Although individual situations may make this difficult, a general rule to remember is that when speaking for an hour or less, always plan on at least 10 minutes for some audience interaction. In talks of more than 45 minutes, actual audience participation activities should be planned whenever possible and appropriate.

POSTPRESENTATION

Remember to bring business cards and to remain afterwards for people who may want to talk. Speakers who have done a good job with eye contact, have smiled, and have prompted the inference of warmth will almost always have some audience members who wish to engage them in some consultation. This is frequently a source of additional speaking engagements, and it is, therefore, an opportunity for the best kind of public relations, face-to-face. When there is a long line of persons waiting to talk and time is limited, pass out business cards and tell everyone they are entitled to one call for free consultation. It is amazing how many people follow up on the offer.

WORKSHOPS

There are significant differences between a presentation and a workshop or training session. The differences are in the amount of time needed, the amount of audience participation recommended, and the goals of the leader. Presentations generally run no more than 90 minutes, while workshops may run from 90 minutes to several days. Audience participation and training are an integral part of workshop design, and the goals of workshops are generally to teach and train, while a presentation's goal often is to persuade the audience to accept a specific proposal. The following suggestions are particularly appropriate when designing workshops.

Workshop leaders should plan on using techniques that involve all participants and encourage open communication between themselves and the participants and among the participants. Ways to encourage participation include dividing the larger group into smaller groups, always giving them time in their small group to get to know one another, and then giving the small group activities related to the workshop topic. These small group activities may include such things as case studies, either real or hypothetical, role-playing, and questionnaire completion and discussion. Occasionally a group may be given a preworkshop assignment to complete a questionnaire, read material related to the workshop, or some other task. Reactions to these tasks can be processed among the participants in small groups.

Frequently, the most important point in determining the climate and direction of the workshop occurs during the first 20 minutes. Some suggestions for using the opening minutes to establish an open climate include using a group introductory activity to promote a relaxed and open atmosphere. When the group is small enough, generally 20 or less, spending time allowing participants to express themselves by identifying their major concerns and questions tends to promote this involvement. Work-

shop leaders can relieve participant anxiety by introducing themselves, sharing both personal and professional information, and giving a brief overview of their objectives for the workshop, the main topics to be covered, and their sequence and approximate time span. They should also reinforce that they do have expectations in terms of participants' cooperation and participation. Even when such introductory activities take as long as an hour, they are justifiable, because of the importance in establishing a common frame of reference with shared goals in a relaxed and receptive setting.

The leader should be aware of signals of fatigue or boredom from participants. These include identifying two or three participants whose behavior provides some type of clue to group climate, providing a variety of activities to break up the routine, and providing a change of pace. Most successful workshops are a blend of information-presenting activities with hands-on experiential type of activities. Another way to safeguard understanding and attention is regularly to summarize what has occurred, especially before moving on to a new topic. Continuity of training is promoted if there are purposeful and periodic reviews and summaries during the workshop. Leaders should note that it is not essential that they do the summarizing; in fact, having the participants do it for themselves provides feedback as to whether or not the group has grasped the important points.

Just as the introductory period to the workshop should not be rushed, so too should closure be carefully attended to. The amount of time spent in closing will depend on how much time is available for the entire workshop, of course, but in a full day's workshop of from 6 to 8 hours, allowing a full hour at the end for closure is appropriate. During this time loose ends are tied and the presenter has a final opportunity to verify if the group's original expectations have been met. Requiring the group to complete an evaluation of the workshop during the time provided for the workshop is the method most likely to get the largest return. These evaluations are most helpful to leaders who want to continue growing. They will process the evaluations and make changes in subsequent workshops based on the responses. The emphasis in a workshop is always on quality, not quantity. It is not how much the audience has heard; it is how much they have learned, will remember, and will use in the future that is the final measure of the workshop's success.

COMMUNICATING AND PRESENTING THROUGH THE MASS MEDIA

Increasingly, public health and dietetic interventions are dependent on effective health communication. Numerous studies have been done the past few years examining the influence of media politics, the accuracy of media reporting, use of media for health education and advocacy, the availability of training in media relations for staff members, and whether media interaction facilitated or impeded achievement of public health objectives (3–6).

The data are clear that the organization's image and credibility are most certainly influenced by both the manner and content of the organization's spokespersons as presented in the media. This portion of the chapter on presentation skills deals specifically with tips for presenting oneself or one's organization in the media and dealing with hostile audiences or audience members.

When one is given the opportunity to present information through the mass media, she needs to understand the power of the media to influence and the inferences listeners or viewers make based not only on the speaker's presentation and speaking skills but also on her manner. When one grasps the enormous persuasive power of mass media, she can train herself to use it to her advantage; however, if she is unaware and makes no special adaptations for the media, she may be unsuccessful—although the content is excellent. When communicating through the mass media, speakers need to remember that more than 50% of the listeners' interpretation of the message is influenced not by the content, but by the form—the speaker's manner, energy, level of enthusiasm, vehicles and media used for transmission, and so forth. Listed below are specific suggestions to assist the reader in preparing herself for media presentations. When one is given the choice of delivering a manuscript for someone else to read or showing up in person and presenting the information directly, without a manuscript, the second choice is preferred. People who may paraphrase or quote ordinarily will not have the same tone of confidence, integrity, passion, sincerity, etc. as the person speaking for herself will be able to demonstrate. In order to demonstrate passion, for example, the speaker will need to know the material thoroughly, have strong feelings about it, and allow herself to emote, and not read.

The following paragraphs offer specific suggestions for working with the media.

Air time is expensive and interviewers may interrupt or give signals to wind up the comments. When invited to be interviewed or share information through the mass media, speakers need to verify ahead of time how much time they will be allotted and plan accordingly. When time is limited, the speaker needs to decide ahead of time what points are most essential, have those highlighted, and express them first. If additional time is provided she can then elaborate or add additional information.

If one is accepting the invitation to be interviewed, she should offer to send questions to the interviewer ahead of time. Interviewers appreciate the gesture because it saves them time; more importantly, however, it gives the interviewee the opportunity to plan responses ahead of time.

If one is an alternative possibility for time on a news show, she will increase her chances of being selected if she submits videotape clips, slides, objects, pictures, etc. Television is a visual medium, and producers favor opportunities to provide multiple images.

Try always to accept invitations to be on the mass media, even when they are originally being produced for small audiences, esoteric cable programs, or minor rural stations. Once something is taped, there is no telling where else it may eventually be played or whom it will eventually reach.

Because time and talent are so expensive in the media, programs, even when being taped ahead of time, tend to run strictly on schedule. Guests should plan or arriving early but never late. That may mean verifying directions, bringing a cellular phone and the number of the station's direct line just in case, and reconfirming time and place.

Often radio and television interviewers do not have the time to become well informed regarding the specifics of their guest's causes. It would be a mistake to become offended or defensive by their ignorance. Being polite and kind will be interpreted by listeners as genuine human warmth; being short with an interviewer may well be interpreted as arrogance and reflect negatively on the speaker's cause.

Keep the message simple, not complicated. It would be wise to rehearse and tape answers and then listen carefully. Is the language clear and concise without sounding too erudite, jargonized, or technical?

There will probably be commercial breaks and when there are this should be viewed as a positive. If there are questions the interviewee wants to be asked or suggestions she wants to make, by all means, she should make them at this time.

Humor is a powerful communication vehicle, but not all people have the gift. Interviewees should be particularly careful about trying to be funny. It may make them look foolish unless they are confident they have the special gift. When, however, the material itself is genuinely funny and has been tried successfully in other audiences, the humor should be brought out.

Often television and radio programs conduct preinterviews to determine if the guest is articulate and interesting enough to hold the audience. This is the time to do one's best. Really try here! Because the host is being kind and polite, does not mean that he or she won't decide to omit the least interesting or articulate guests.

After one has seen or heard herself on mass media several times, she will eventually become adept at processing the experience while it is happening. Presenters need to develop a third eye to monitor themselves on the media and send back messages to themselves about how they are doing during the presentation or interview. Because the human mind whirls several times faster than the speed of speech, it is possible to see and hear oneself while talking and to modify accordingly. The rule generally is that on the mass media, natural behavior should be exaggerated somewhat bigger than life, but without being outrageous. Speakers need to behave in a way that generates inferences of self-confidence, sincerity, and even charisma.

Hand gestures on television should be carefully controlled. They tend to be distracting on the screen. Speakers need to sustain interest through their dynamic voice, cadence, inflections, pauses, tone, and facial expression. Although large expansive gestures generally don't work well, variety and variation do.

Very few nonprofessional presenters are able to improvise very long and come off looking professional. Answers to questions the interviewee expects to be asked should be rehearsed and not read from notes. If one is asked a question she can't answer, the smartest thing to do is admit it and offer to locate the answer and forward it to the appropriate people.

Part of the self-monitoring process should include the interviewee judging the length of her own answers. Long-winded answers or monologues should be avoided. They tend to get boring to listeners and irritate the interviewer.

Dress is a communication vehicle itself and should be attended to carefully when on the visual media. The best advice is to dress conservatively and in good taste, without being flashy or drawing attention to oneself through clothes. Busy ties, socks, plaids, or large jewelry are all inappropriate.

If one is representing her organization or making a book tour, she may find herself being asked the same questions over and over, day after day. Remember this is the first time this audience is hearing it; presentations need to sound fresh each time, even though it may be the speaker's twentieth time in two days answering the same questions.

Bored listeners and viewers change channels. Guest interviewees and presenters need to prepare themselves with interesting anecdotes and aphorisms. Personal experiences tend to hold attention. The deadliest mistake is to become too intellectual or abstract.

When several guests are on the same panel or are involved in a simultaneous interview, someone may attempt to dominate or interrupt. If this occurs it is easiest to bite one's lip and become angry but say nothing. If one does that, she will regret it later. One needs to be prepared to assert herself if this occurs. She can push herself back into the conversation and say something like, "Please let me finish my point," or "I'm almost finished, don't interrupt." This should be done with a smile and kind voice, but it should, by all means, be done. Listeners and viewers respect the person who stands up for herself—politely.

If one is offended publicly or has her feelings hurt, she needs to grin and bear it, rather than react emotionally. She can say "I don't agree" or "that feels unkind," but if she snaps back a retort, she risks being heard as weak or overly sensitive.

Because so much of what is produced for the media eventually gets repeated, speakers should avoid mentioning the time, place, or date of the live broadcast. If a piece isn't "dated," it has a better chance of being used at a later date by other affiliates who may need material.

There may be times when the speaker believes she is

being invited to talk about her cause and once she gets there the interviewer steers her on to other topics. When this occurs, it becomes the speaker's responsibility to get her message across even if the host isn't considerate enough to afford the right opportunities.

If the program is being pretaped, it would be a mistake to ask for a second chance. Generally second chances cost too much money and annoy the director. The guideline is to come prepared to do it right the first time. That may mean taking in a sheet of notes of key points. Prior to the program's conclusion, the speaker can glance at the notes and make sure she has said all that was critical.

If questions become inappropriate or are on topics the speaker would rather not discuss, she would do better simply to say, "I would rather not discuss that" than to waffle or "double-talk." Credibility is destroyed when listeners infer deception.

Never, never, never get defensive to a member of the audience or another panelist who takes the offensive angrily. The speaker should simply look to the moderator to move the program on.

Every show and moderator tends to have a unique style. Speakers should attempt to learn as much as they can about the format before their appearance. It will relieve their own anxiety and allow them to plan a strategy for ways to communicate their message best. They might also request to have 15 minutes alone with the interviewer before the broadcast to go over the questions. They may not get it, but if they don't ask, they most definitely won't get it.

Final impressions count, especially on the media. The speaker should use the final public moments to leave a positive impression of her as composed, assertive, and controlled. Privately, before leaving, she should look for the producer and director and thank them personally as well. A firm handshake and looking people in the eye while talking is a separate nonverbal message itself apart from the verbal one being expressed.

TIPS FOR DEALING WITH HOSTILE AUDIENCES

Whether on the mass media or in a classroom, the worst fear of most speakers is being verbally attacked by another publicly. This chapter will close with some final tips for dealing with hostile audiences or audience members.

When someone wishes to express an opinion directly contrary to the speaker's, rather than act attacked or become defensive, the speaker would do better to let the audience member know that while she disagrees, she understands why the individual has his opinion. Once people hear the other repeat their argument and admit that it has some merit, they are more willing to remain quiet and let the speaker go on.

If the speaker insists on having the audience decide that one person is right and one person is wrong, she risks alienating others in the audience who may have mixed feelings. When others express a different point of view, one of the best strategies is simply to allow it to exist. "Thank you; it is good to hear an alternative perspective" is an answer that allows both the attacker and the speaker to retain their dignity.

If the speaker is concerned about being sabotaged by audience questions, she can ask at the beginning that questions be submitted in writing and then field them herself, selecting those she is most comfortable answering.

When someone hostile in the audience is trying to use the time for his or her own platform, the speaker might suggest that before she yields the floor, she wants subsequent speakers to paraphrase her arguments before giving their own, and she can impose time limits as well. Irate angry people are often unable to paraphrase alternative views and expose their own narrow tunnel vision when attempting to explain the speaker's points. The argument works the other way as well. If the speaker wants to respond to a hostile member's comments, she too should begin with a paraphrase of the other's view. That way the rest of the audience knows she has, indeed, been listening and still feels differently.

When asked complicated questions of substance too long to be answered adequately in the time remaining, the speaker should admit that the question is both complicated and worthy. She could write the question down and ask for an address to respond but admit that the present time and place are inappropriate for detailed answers.

One way to defer antagonism is to ask if someone else in the audience wishes to respond. This tactic is especially effective if the majority is of the speaker's persuasion and the hostile member represents a minority.

Most things in life are not either black or white. The speaker who reminds the audience that she prefers to work toward collaboration rather than a win-lose solution sounds "reasonable." Talking to others as if they are adversaries increases tension and anxiety among the listeners.

If one is going to be speaking in front of hostile audiences, she should invest in professional training. A coach, for example, who role-plays with the presenter, asking hostile questions, provides an opportunity to rehearse responses and assists the speaker in developing appropriate tone, gesture, and facial expression to compliment her diffusing comments.

It is to one's advantage to know before hand if she is entering into a forum with a hostile audience. This can be determined with a brief survey or interview among audience members before the presentation. When one knows the majority of the audience is likely to be hostile, she can preface with comments to short-circuit some of their remarks. She can highlight, for example, those points on which they agree; she can anticipate criticism and include a rebuttal before being challenged; she can

present alternative solutions that overcome the minority objections; and so forth.

When there is a moderator present or an emcee, the speaker should mention before the program that she wishes him to intervene if the discussion gets too "hot." A good moderator will know to displace the hostility for the guest, but some need to be reminded. The important thing for the speaker to do is smile and hear herself say things like, "I understand your position" and "I respect your right to have a different opinion." Winning the battle by way of a microphone and platform can lose the speaker the war if she is rude and unfeeling toward the audience member who is attacking. She needs to appear magnanimous.

The speaker should anticipate having the last word by bringing a printed handout to leave the audience. If the situation is emotional and a few dominate, she will know that those who wanted to learn the facts were at least able to take them home in print.

Sometimes audience members ask unreasonable questions similar to the "Have you stopped beating your wife?" variety. No matter what the answer, the respondent looks bad. If this occurs, the speaker need only remain calm and point out how any answer reflects badly, and then move on to another question. Engaging in debate with a hostile member who is out to make the speaker look bad is not a good use of the audience's time.

Shakespeare's Mark Antony in the play *Julius Caesar* begins his speech with "Friends, Romans, and Countrymen," and he was talking to a hostile audience. The point is that persuasive speakers know to exaggerate all the things about themselves that the audience can relate to as similar. It is less easy to attack someone who is similar to oneself.

If one wants the audience to think of all the reasons why the speaker's plan is best, it may be a good idea to begin with a list of the weaknesses. Once those are out and accounted for, the hostile members can relax, and everyone can think together about the advantages. If the speaker were to begin with a discussion of the advantages, those opposed would be unable to think because their minds would be countering with the negatives.

When hostile members are quoting inaccurate facts and figures that demean the speaker's arguments, rather than telling them they are wrong, she would do better to say something like, "I have different figures. Here is my source and date. What is yours?"

When tough questions are asked of a speaker, she should be grateful for the opportunity to confront issues. Keeping the conversation only on the positive doesn't change any minds. For people to have their opinions changed, they need to hear arguments refuted. Skillful persuaders encourage coherent criticism and thank people for exposing their objections. Market surveys, for example, show that customers who complain are far more likely to continue doing business with the offending organization than those who are upset but hesitant to com-

CASE STUDY

Joan Stivers, RD, works in a corporate wellness program. She has noticed that some of the employees who eat in the employee cafeteria make less than optimum food choices for lunch. Others go out to a nearby fast-food restaurant. She was asked by management to give a 30-minute presentation on healthy, nutritious lunches.

1. What should she do in the introduction?
2. What are the objectives of the body of the presentation?
3. What approaches would you recommend with this audience?
4. How should she handle the conclusion?

plain. Let people vent, just remember to control the time and not to get defensive.

The reader is reminded in conclusion that the suggestions provided in this chapter need to be practiced rather than memorized for an examination. Developing presentation skills and handling the myriad of problems that can occur with media, interviewers, and hostile audiences is a process that occurs over time. One gets better and better with each subsequent opportunity to practice.

REVIEW AND DISCUSSION QUESTIONS

1. What are the three generally accepted divisions of a presentation?
2. What should an introduction provide?
3. What are the three key objectives of the body of the presentation?
4. Why is it important for presenters to proofread all their materials, including handouts, flip-charts, posters, and transparencies?
5. What does it mean to be audience-centered?
6. How can presenters avoid stage fright?
7. Why are a presenter's facial expressions important?
8. What is the difference between a presentation and a workshop?

SUGGESTED ACTIVITIES

1. Presentation I: Design and deliver a 10-minute presentation on some issue related to foods, nutrition, or dietetics, such as safety of the food supply, a new food product, fiber in foods, reduced fat or calories in foods, snacks, restaurant meals, or sodium.
2. Presentation II: Design and deliver a presentation intended for a group of parents of obese children. A minimum of two visual aids is required, transparencies and posters. Included in the 20-minute presentation should be 5 full minutes of audience-speaker interaction. "Are there any questions?" at the conclusion is not acceptable.
3. Presentation III: Design and deliver a 30-minute presentation intended for a group of people who have

recently learned they have diabetes. A minimum of three visual aids is required, including flip-chart and handout material. Plan on at least 8 minutes of interaction with the audience; this should be prompted by the speaker's perceptions of the nonverbal feedback emanating from the audience.

4. Presentation IV: Design and deliver a 60-minute presentation intended for a group of people who have paid to be taught and/or trained by you in an area related to your specialty in the area of dietetics. Develop whatever aids seem appropriate.

If possible all presentations should be videotaped. Presenters should provide reaction sheets to the audience and later write a critique of the taped presentation, responding to their own subjective reactions, the critique sheets of the audience, and the instructor's comments.

REFERENCES

1. Naughton D. Make your words count. Washingtonian 1996;3:78.
2. Roach R, Pichert J, Stetson B, et al. Improving dietitians' teaching skills. J Am Diet Assoc 1992;92:1466.
3. Gellert D, Higgins K, Farley W, et al. Public health and the media in California. Public Health Rep 1994;109:284.
4. Gellert G, Higgins K, Lowery R, et al. A national survey of public health officers' interactions with the media. JAMA 1994;271:1285.
5. Szeinback S. Image development for health care firms. Med Interface 1994;7:124.
6. Larson D, Anderson R, Maksud D, et al. What influences public perceptions of breast implants. Plast Reconstr Surg 1994;94:318.

ADDITIONAL SOURCES

Bertrand K. Speak now, or . . . Bus Mkt 1990;75:68.
Fletcher L. How to design and deliver a speech. New York: Harper Collins, 1995.
Mandel S. Technical presentation skills. Los Altos, CA: Crisp, 1989.
Raines R. Visual aids in business. Los Altos, CA: Crisp, 1996.
Robbins L. The business of writing and speaking. New York: McGraw-Hill, 1996.
Nowling B. Keep it short and simple. J Am Diet Assoc 1994; 94:972.

fifteen

PLANNING, SELECTING, AND USING MEDIA

Educational media include all teaching aids that appeal to a learner through the senses, i.e., sight, sound, taste, smell, and touch (1). There are many advantages to using media. Using media correctly and effectively enhances one's professional image. When making a presentation, for example, attractive slides with bulleted points, charts, and graphs also help to make one's points understandable to the audience. Trainers who use visuals are "perceived as better prepared, more professional, more persuasive, more credible, and more interesting" (2). This chapter examines the types of media most commonly available, offers suggestions for use, and discusses the advantages, limitations, and evaluation.

BENEFITS OF MEDIA
"A picture is worth 1000 words" is an old adage that is true. The use of media greatly benefits the audience. Four pictures, therefore, are worth 4000 words. The more information the educator wants to get across, the more that media are helpful. When people can see things, rather than merely hear them or read about them, they remember more. Media are especially helpful to low-income groups with limited reading ability and cultural and ethnic groups who speak little English. The professional should bear in mind that just because one is talking is no guarantee that anyone is listening. This fact has major implications as professionals plan educational presentations for patients, clients, employees, other professionals, and the public.

How much do people learn from media? Following is one estimate on the amount of learning using the senses:

People learn **10%** from listening. People learn **80%** from what they see (3).

What about recalling information later? People remember **20%** of what they hear. But they remember **50%** of what they both see and hear (3). It is obvious that giving the audience something to see helps learning and remembering. Lecturing alone, therefore, such as about nutrition to a group of pregnant women, about low-fat diets to men with hypercholesterolemia, or about sanitation to employees, is not going to get the results one desires.

Which of the following is more meaningful, the description in words or the visual description? The word description is as follows:

Four lines are printed on a flat surface. Two lines are

1-inch long on either end of a figure, and two lines are 2-inches long at the top and bottom of the figure. The four lines are joined end-to-end to each other at 90 degree angles to enclose a space.

Here is the same information described visually:

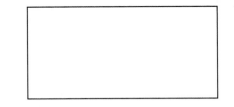

Today's audiences grew up with television and tend to relate more quickly to pictures than to words. The data show that 98.3% of households own television sets with an average of 2.2 sets per home (4). According to one estimate, the average American family spends 7.5 hours daily watching television, more time than any other activity except sleep and work (5). They also rent videos. Visual images bombard us daily in everything from media advertising to T-shirts with messages and pictures. Some people read fewer books and newspapers and may dislike the concentrated effort that reading requires. If this describes one's clients or employees, the professional needs to ask what can be done to present information visually. Individuals may be inattentive to lectures because they lack what television offers—motion, color, sound, visual effects, music, and drama.

Visual methods are not the total answer to presenting information. There is no guarantee that seeing a visual automatically ensures learning from it. After all, how much do people remember of their hours in front of the television set? Media, however, are part of the instructional input. Visuals enhance written and oral communication methods and make them more interesting. Pictures and sounds have the power to compel attention, to enhance understanding, and to promote learning in a shorter time frame than by using solely verbal explanations. A study of nutrition education on a low-fat, low-cholesterol diet to patients in a clinical setting, for example, compared three methods: individualized instruction for 30–45 minutes, a slide/verbal classroom presentation for 45 minutes, and a videotape presentation with a 15-minute follow-up visit by a dietitian. The videotape method proved to be just as effective as measured by a test of comprehension, and considerably more time efficient (6).

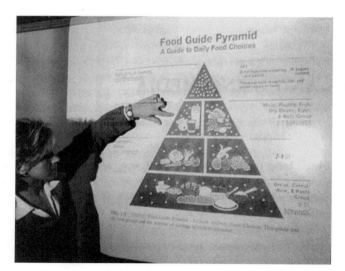

FIGURE 15.1.   A picture is worth 1000 words.

When media quality is high, one's total presentation looks more professional, better prepared, more credible, interesting, and persuasive as one appeals to individuals through their senses—sight, sound, touch, taste, and smell (2). Of course, the reverse can be true. The presenter should be sure to check spelling, for example.

PLANNING MEDIA

Media need to be planned carefully in conjunction with the overall program or learning situation. Answers to the following seven questions will help one's thinking (3):

1.   What are the objectives of the session? What should the person learn or be able to do?

2.   What methods or activities (lecture, discussion, individual counseling, and the like) enhance learning besides media? Where can media fit into these plans?

3.   Who is the audience? What are the characteristics of the learner, such as age, sex, educational level, and cultural or ethnic group. People with low literacy skills, for example, may need different approaches than college graduates.

4.   What is the learner's current level of knowledge of the topic? A presentation to a lay group, for example, would need different visuals than one to a group of professionals. And new employee training may need a different approach than that for long-term employees.

5.   What purpose(s) does the media serve? Is it to generate interest in the subject; to affect attitudes, emotions, or motivation; to entertain; to present information; to attract and hold attention; to involve the learner in mental activity promoting learning; or some combination of purposes?

6.   How can one concisely organize and sequence the points being made and emphasize them with visuals?

7.   How will one evaluate the effectiveness of the media presentation as well as the total presentation?

CRITERIA FOR SELECTION

It is possible to purchase ready-made media or to make one's own. In deciding which to use, the following 10 questions may be considered:

1.   What is the cost to purchase media versus to make one's own? This may be an overriding factor in selection decisions.

2.   Is it appropriate to the objectives of the presentation? This is especially important when purchasing ready-made materials.

3.   What is the length of time to show the material, such as a video?

4.   What equipment is available in the room of the presentation?

5.   What is the setting? Is the speaker in front of a long, narrow room where people in the back may not be able to see? Or is the room square?

6.   What is the size of the audience? Ten, fifty, one hundred, or five hundred?

7.   What is the preference of the presenter for media? What is one comfortable using?

8.   What is the preference of the audience for media? Is it visual, auditory, reading material, or a combination?

9.   How much time will it take to prepare one's own media? What people with technical expertise in design and production are available to assist?

10.   Is anyone available at the presentation to assist with showing overhead transparencies or to distribute handouts?

It is important to evaluate media as one uses them. Eventually, one wants to know what proves most effective in the shortest time frame in learning and retention, thus providing efficiency.

KINDS OF MEDIA

After considering what needs to be communicated and thinking about the audience, the dietetics professional may select the appropriate media for the purpose. Any one or several may be applicable. Table 15.1 outlines the possibilities. This section discusses the types of media to consider from real objects to multimedia presentations.

Real Objects

Nothing is more realistic that showing actual foods or food packages. A lesson on food labeling, for example, may include a variety of food packages so that the audience can participate "hands-on" with actual products in learning to read and understand the label. To avoid audience distraction, it is well to keep items covered or out-of-sight when they are not being used. Passing things

TABLE 15.1.

Types of Media

Real Product	Printed Media
Foods	Handouts
Food packages	Brochures/
Food models	newsletters
Food service equipment	
	Projected Visuals
Audio Formats	Overhead
Audiotapes	transparencies
Compact discs	Slides
Phonograph records	Filmstrips
Display Media	Graphics
Chalkboard	Diagrams
Flip-chart	Charts
Bulletin boards	Cartoons
Photographs	Clip art
Pictures	
Moving Images	
Videos	
Films	
Multimedia	

around may also be a major distraction. Making recipes to be tasted in group sessions when teaching about nutrition or modified diets is another suggestion. An individual with heart disease, for example, who has seen the dietetics professional prepare a tasty recipe, sampled it, and received the recipe is more likely to try it at home. In a series of classes, audience members may assist and provide recipes.

A tour to the grocery store is another possibility. A nutrition intervention study based on the American Heart Association's grocery store tour taught adults to read food labels so they could decrease the risk of coronary heart disease by selecting foods lower in total fat, saturated fat, and cholesterol (7). The tour was provided in three formats: an actual tour of a grocery store, an American Heart Association video, and a home study program. Results showed that those who took the actual tour reported that they learned an extreme amount, were likely to make at least one food purchasing change, and liked the delivery format more than those who participated in the other two formats. Even though the actual tour was more effective in promoting behavioral change, the educators preferred the video because it demanded less of their time and was the easiest format with which to recruit participants.

When discussing portion control of beverages, how many people have 4- and 8-ounce glasses at home any-

more? One may need a variety of sizes and shapes as well as disposable cups from fast-food restaurants when portion size is important.

In training employees, it is preferable to train them using the real object, such as a meat slicer, dishwashing machine, cash register, or other equipment. Actual "hands-on" experience is preferable.

Advantages
Realistic.

Hands-on learning and audience participation enhance motivation and retention.

Limitations
Some foods are perishable.

May not have cooking facilities available.

Not suitable for groups larger than 15–20.

Food Models
Food models are representations of the real objects. Many professionals maintain an inventory of three-dimensional plastic food models. They are helpful in estimating client portion sizes, for example, during an assessment of food intake, and in teaching portion sizes on controlled caloric intakes. Besides the visual stimulation, putting the model in the person's hands makes a more active experience using another of the senses—touch. Plastic, life-sized food models may be purchased from sources, such as Nasco Nutrition Teaching Aids in Fort Atkinson, WI.

Advantages
Are realistic and colorful.

Are portable.

Shows portion sizes.

Limitations
Cannot be seen in large groups.

Pictures/Packages
Pictures from magazines or catalogs or clip art may be displayed on posters or bulletin boards. The National Dairy Council has life-sized cardboard photographs of foods, for example. It is preferable to select a neutral background color on a bulletin board, and various materials may be used as background to add interest, such as wrapping paper, construction paper, fabric, and foil.

To enlarge a picture for display, one can place the picture on an overhead projector and project it onto a chalkboard or wall. After taping a piece of paper onto the board, one may use a marker to outline the projected image. One can move the projector closer to reduce the size or further away to make it larger (3).

Sample packages and containers of recommended foods may be displayed. To discuss a "Nutrition Facts"

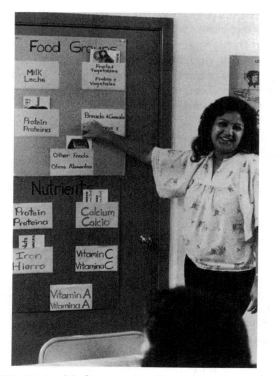

FIGURE 15.2. Media must be adapted to the audience.

label or ingredients labeling with a client, it is helpful and realistic to have actual ones available. Labels may be removed from packages and mounted on cardboard or into a book for display. One may desire to have different collections, for example, when teaching about healthy snacks, low-fat food choices, low-calorie foods, and the like.

Advantages
Colorful and eye catching.

Inexpensive.

Packages are portable.

Limitations
Lacks motion.

Some people do not look at bulletin boards.

Can be overdone unless the message is focused.

Photographs
The professional may take photographs or have them done professionally. They can be enlarged to any size desired. They may be used on bulletin boards, for example, or in individual or very small group discussions. If one is photographing people, such as employees and clients, a signed form releasing the use of the photographs without limitation is advisable.

Advantages
Inexpensive.

Limitations
Distracting to pass them around in groups.

Charts/Posters
Information may be presented in charts or on posters one makes or purchases. The U.S. Department of Agriculture's graphic design of dietary recommendations in the Food Guide Pyramid is an example. Numerical data can be presented in bar charts, pie-shaped charts, or in line graphs.

Have you ever seen a poster board set on the chalk tray of a classroom only to have it fall off in the middle of a presentation? While the audience may find this amusing or feel embarrassed for the ill-prepared speaker, it may hinder credibility considerably. The presenter needs a tripod or easel to attach it to while explaining its significance. It is not necessary to read word-for-word from a visual. At most, one may tell why it is significant or paraphrase the content. If possible, it should be removed from audience view after discussing it.

Posters are also a medium for sharing research findings and other information at professional meetings. Often the posters are divided into specific segments that are prepared on separate sheets. They are attached onto mounting boards at the meeting site (8).

Advantages
Inexpensive.

Portable short distances only.

Limitations
Cannot be seen except in very small (15–20) groups.

Homemade charts may be overcrowded with content.

Get worn with repeated use.

Flip-Charts
When a chalkboard is unavailable, a flip-chart with a display easel may substitute. A number of large sheets of paper are fastened together. One can write or draw with crayon or black or colored felt-tip pens, being sure to select ones that do not bleed through the paper. Writing should be large and bold, at least 1-inch high or more for every 30 feet of audience space, to be seen. Inexperienced presenters may want to ask someone to do the writing for them (9).

Each sheet is turned at the top after completion. Finished sheets can also be torn off and attached to a wall or chalkboard. When one needs a record of points made by the audience, a flip-chart is preferable to a chalkboard because the sheets can be carried from the meeting. Alternately, one can prepare the sheets in advance and reveal them sequentially while standing facing the audience. This allows for the creative use of color, clip art,

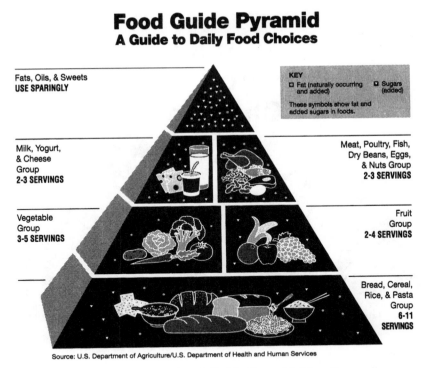

FIGURE 15.3. Food Guide Pyramid (visual).

glitter, fabric, and other materials (9). It is advisable to leave a blank page when the audience focus should be on the presenter.

Advantages
Informal and inexpensive.

Limitations
Awkward to carry very far.

Cannot be seen in larger groups.

Requires good handwriting.

Requires practice to write quickly while speaking.

May be too informal for some purposes.

Chalkboard
Everyone has seen the chalkboard used and misused. If one writes legibly and large enough to be seen, it may be a good supplement to a presentation.

Major pitfalls occur if one is a poor speller and if one turns one's back to the audience and talks to the board while writing. One needs to avoid standing with one's back to the audience. If this is a problem for the presenter, overhead transparencies are preferable.

Advantages
Inexpensive.

Easy to use.

Limitations
Requires good timing so that one does not talk to the board.

Not good in large groups.

Poor spelling and handwriting.

Overhead Transparencies
When an overhead projector is available, transparencies are a great visual complement to a presentation. The speaker stands, not sits, facing the audience beside the projector, being careful not to block the view of the screen. Have you ever attended a presentation where the speaker does not know how to turn on the projector? Or where the audience notes that the print is too small to read or out of focus?

The professional may ask someone else to change the transparencies as the presenter talks from a position elsewhere in the room. One may point to items while talking, or progressively disclose the contents by covering with paper or cardboard the portions that one does not want seen yet. Some speakers like to have a title or other visual on the projector as the audience assembles. To assist the audience, it is advisable to number the points on the transparency in the order in which one is discussing them and in order of importance. If all items are of equal importance, bullets (•) are more generic. When not in use, the projector should be turned off so that people are not staring into a bright, blank screen.

It is possible to mark on the clear or colored plastic film while talking, such as underlining items or checking them off. Felt-tip pens designed for transparencies come

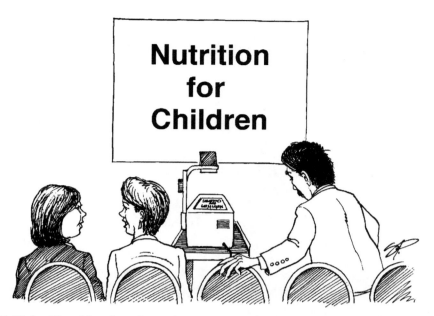

FIGURE 15.4. The title of one's presentation may be displayed as the audience gathers.

in various colors. The water-based ones may be removed later with a damp cloth, or the permanent ones, with lighter fluid.

It is well to bear in mind that the average projector surface is 10 by 10 inches, transparencies are 10 by 12, and most paper is 8.5 by 11, so the actual message area is about 7.5 by 9.0 to 9.5 inches (3, 10). A border needs to be left around all edges. Write legibly and large enough that material can be seen at the rear of the room.

A more professional look may be obtained by typing the information. Large type must be used, since regular typewriter size will not be readable. About 30 points or one-quarter inch is good, but one needs to check the room size to be sure (10). See Table 15.2 for samples. When the page is prepared, there are certain transparencies that can be placed in the paper bin and fed through a photocopier to produce the transparency. Some computer programs will prepare them, also. Special transparency film is available for the printer, and color ink-jet or laser printers are capable of producing full-color transparencies (11).

Graphs or charts from scientific and professional journals, enlarged cartoons, and other data may be presented easily in this form. Photographs do not reproduce well unless one has a digital camera that will place pictures into a computer graphics file to be printed on a transparency. For repeated use, it is advisable to mount the transparencies in cardboard frames. This avoids the problem of static electricity with the transparencies sticking to one another.

Advantages
Easy to use and inexpensive.

Can maintain eye contact with the audience, which helps to control attention.

Uses normal room lighting.

Can write on them while talking.

Limitations
In a large, deep room, may not be seen in the back.

Easy to overcrowd information.

Bulb may burn out; carry an extra.

Print Handouts
Health care professionals tend to give patients and clients a great deal of information verbally, thinking people can remember it all. By the time they get home, most have probably forgotten at least half of it or more. Trainers may do the same with new employees.

Putting things in writing that clients, patients, employees, and other audiences can refer to later solves this problem. For modified diets, for example, oral counseling is frequently supplemented with written materials including the foods to eat and those to limit or avoid, recipes, and the like. Print materials are effective in reinforcing individual counseling sessions and group classes. When planning employee training, the presenter may consider giving an outline of the content with space for note taking, or a list of the main points to be remembered. When using an overhead transparency with a lot of information, people will be writing instead of listening unless one distributes copies of the information on the transparency.

In teaching about normal nutrition, for example, the Food Guide Pyramid and/or the Dietary Guidelines for Americans may be distributed. Government agencies and private organizations produce print materials for wide-ranging audiences or one can make one's own.

For written materials, it is advisable to assess the readability or grade level since some adults have low literacy

TABLE 15.2.

Type Styles, Fonts, and Print Sizes

10 point type
12 point type
14 point type
18 point type
24 point type
36 point type
48 point type

Times Roman
Chicago
Courier
Helvetica
Monaco
Signet Roundhead
New York
Commercial Script

skills. It is estimated that as many as 23 million adults are functionally illiterate (12). About 24.8% of adults are not high school graduates (4). Some are low-income individuals or recent immigrants with limited ability in English. Print materials in other languages may be needed. Educational materials must be understandable to people for whom they are intended. Nutrition educators need to select and/or develop print materials that are comprehended to be effective.

Several readability formulas are available to help assess the readability or grade level both as software programs and in print. The SMOG, FOG, Flesch, Raygor, and Fry tests are examples. Readability tests examine the linguistic and structural qualities of written materials. Owing to the scientific and technical nature of health communications, vocabulary and wording of patient education materials may be incomprehensible to many adults unless readability formulas are used to assess the approximate educational level a person must have in order to understand the material.

A study of WIC participants with a self-reported educational level of 11.8 years, for example, found a mismatch between reading and comprehension skills levels on the 1990 Dietary Guidelines for Americans, portions of which were written at the college level according to a computerized readability analysis program. It is well to consider that an individual's reading skill level may be as much as five grades below the highest grade completed in school (12).

In a study of the readability levels of 38 print materials on cholesterol education available from various sources, both the SMOG and FOG Grading formulas were used. They revealed that the average reading grade level was close to grade 11, a difficult level (13). Another study surveyed 209 nutrition education pamphlets that might be used with low literacy adults. Using the Flesch, Raygor, and Fry tests, results showed that there were few materials for those with limited literacy skills. Sixty-eight percent of the materials were written at the ninth grade level or higher and only 11% were at the sixth grade level or below (14). Manuals are available to assist professionals in writing for individuals with limited reading skills (15, 16).

When giving a talk to a small lay group, one may give as a handout a short preassessment of multiple-choice and completion questions. One never mentions the word "test" to adults, of course, since it may conjure up unfavorable memories of past schooling. It is a self-assessment or series of questions around which to frame the presentation. The questions elicit a lot of audience participation, discussion, and additional questions. This approach is valuable because it recognizes that adults come with many answers from their past experience. One finds out what the audience already knows, compliments them on their knowledge, and presents information at their level. The presenter can use the audience handout to write the additional points to be made, thus avoiding switching back and forth from the handout to notes for the presentation.

Print materials may be personalized using word processing and desktop publishing software. If writing a longer pamphlet, focus groups are a valuable tool in planning, pretesting, and evaluating print materials (17).

Advantages
Audience can refer to it later at home or at work.

Good when information has to be remembered.

Helps the person to focus attention and follow points.

Limitations
People may never look at it again.

Time spent in preparing materials.

Audiotape Recordings
Recordings may be more appropriate for individual listening than for a group presentation. If they are long, an outline or work sheet may be needed to assist the individual's listening and learning. If preparing one's own, an informal, conversational tone of voice with slow, clear enunciation is needed. Cassettes are available in various lengths. A C-60 cassette, for example, can record a total of 60 minutes using both sides of the tape.

Advantages
Inexpensive and easy to use.

Portable.

Limitations
No guarantee of retention or learning.

No guarantee that hearing includes careful listening, comprehension, or understanding.

Slides
Slides may be computer generated using such programs as Microsoft's PowerPoint, Lotus's Freelance, or ASAP WordPower. The program's output goes to a digitizing camera that can convert the images into film that can be developed into slides. In a few cases, slides are available for purchase and may come with an audiotape accompaniment. A 35-mm camera of one's own will make satisfactory 35-mm slides of a standard 2- by 2-inch dimension.

With a remote control projector, the presenter can advance the slides while talking and turn off the projector at appropriate times so that the audience focus returns to the presenter. Professionals begin and end with a black slide to avoid the white glare of the screen without a slide. If a very short part of the presentation does not include the use of a slide, a colored slide can be inserted

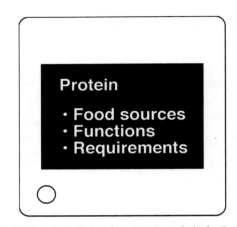

FIGURE 15.5. A dark background with light lettering is preferred for slides.

there instead of turning the projector off and on. If the room is not completely dark, some colors may be affected. Presenters may need to inquire about lighting in advance.

If one has a lot of slides, the presenter can easily change their sequence for various presentations. Slides are a good place to introduce humor with cartoons or other pictures. It is advisable to number and label all slides as well as mark the upper right-hand corner with a dot where the thumb drops the slide into the tray correctly, which is upside-down (10). The old wooden pointer with the rubber tip is being replaced by a simple, electronic point of light that points to the screen. One should practice with the pointer before the presentation.

Advantages
Small and easy to carry along in trays.

Can change the sequence as appropriate.

Good for both large and small groups.

Limitations
May be out of order if not checked.

May be projected upside-down or backwards if not checked.

With dim room lighting, one cannot note the audience reactions. If the presentation is after lunch, some audience members may be dozing.

Filmstrips
Filmstrips are a series of 35-mm still pictures in a continuous strip. Some may be available for purchase and may come with an audiocassette accompaniment requiring special equipment for use. Most people are now using slides instead.

Advantages
Includes both sight and sound stimulation.

Relatively low cost.

Limitations
Expense of special equipment.

Material purchased may not match your objectives.

Videos/Motion Pictures

The combinations of sight and sounds from videos and films are pleasing to most people, but video is rapidly replacing film for most educational purposes. Purchased or rented videos should be previewed to check for appropriateness and a dated look of hair styles and dress. Many groups, such as the American Dietetic Association, American Heart Association, American Diabetes Association, National Dairy Council, the Educational Foundation of the National Restaurant Association, drug companies, government agencies, and private media companies offer visual materials. A video cassette recorder (VCR) and monitor are necessary for audience viewing. Because audiences tend to view passively, they should be told what to look for prior to viewing and preplanned activities or discussion questions should follow. A video may be viewed alone at the learner's own pace or viewed repeatedly to enhance learning. The presenter may pause a video in the middle for discussion.

Many employee programs for orientation and training use video formats, sometimes with printed workbooks or learner's guides. If the employee views a video alone, discussions with the instructor should follow to explain the relationship of the video to the job (18). Interactive video is a video inscribed on a disc that plays on a video-disc player. With an interlinked computer program the learner watches the video, which is interrupted periodically with various questions to be answered.

One may be able to make videotapes with a camcorder, but keep in mind that today's audiences are sophisticated viewers who may not respond well to amateur productions (19). They may have seen professionally made programs. If one has an idea for a video, a storyboard may be used to outline the shots for each scene in roughly sketched pictures (3). It should include the audio and production techniques for each shot, the director, camera person, actors, props, behind the scenes crew, costumes, makeup, and lighting. If taping clients or employees, a written release of use without limitations is advisable.

Advantages
Realistic, enjoyable, and dramatic.

Includes both sight and sound stimulation.

If it tells a story, people retain it better.

For learning, someone can view it repeatedly.

Can have an emotional impact and help to change attitudes.

Limitations
May not fit the purpose and objectives.

May be expensive.

Requires equipment.

Complex issues may be misinterpreted unless discussed.

Computer Graphics

One may have available a computer program that produces media in the form of graphs of numerical data, charts, illustrations, diagrams, and overhead transparencies. If so, professional looking materials may be made rather easily.

Computer-Based Multimedia

The chalkboard and eraser with an occasional slide presentation are going the way of the dinosaur. Today's educator is faced with understanding electronics. Multimedia means user-controlled delivery of a variety of media forms by computer (11). Computer-based multimedia can integrate several media sources, such as text (words and graphs), sound (speech, music, and sound effects), and visuals (still pictures, video, and animation) (20, 21). Presentation software can transform static material into colorful animation. To keep readers abreast of the latest products, the journal *Media & Methods* presents product information and technological advancements (22). Scanners are devices that allow one to place electronically either pictures or text into a computer. Special programs and equipment are necessary in conjunction with established computer systems.

Presentation software packages allow the professional to design and customize presentations using text, color, motion, animation, and sound, if one has a sound card. Computer driven presentation may be developed with such programs as Microsoft PowerPoint, Lotus Freelance, Aldus Persuasion, and WordPerfect Presentations. Special equipment and appropriate computer memory are necessary.

Computer nutrition communication may be either stand-alone or on-line (21). Stand-alone programs are available on floppy disc, CD-ROM (compact disc-read only memory) disc, or laserdisc with accompanying floppy discs. They may be used at stand-alone kiosks in health clinics, community centers, schools, businesses, and homes. A WIC program used a multimedia nutrition education program for clients in a freestanding kiosk (23). On-line applications are programs that run connected to a network, modem, satellite, or other electronic communications technology (21). Nutrition educators may find that their clients are well informed about food, nutrition, and health information if they are receiving information over a network.

Advantages
Gain attention and interest.

Colorful and bold.

Increased comprehension.

Limitations

Expensive hardware and software.

Time-consuming to prepare.

Time-consuming to learn to use.

Combinations

The dietetics professional should consider using more than one of the above visuals in a presentation. She may have handouts, for example, along with overhead transparencies or slides. Alternatively, one may use actual foods, handouts, and the chalkboard. Many combinations are possible.

ART AND DESIGN PRINCIPLES

The quality and effectiveness of media may depend to a great extent on art and design principles. One does not have to be a great artist. But some understanding of simple principles will improve results.

Simplicity/Unity

The presenter should try to convey only one idea at a time since too many ideas confuse the audience. Decide what should be at the center of attention or interest and then build around it. This may need to be the largest sized item for the audience to focus on it immediately.

Margins

To look professional, visuals need a margin in the same way that pictures need a frame. Overhead transparencies, for example, need an inch on all sides. Posters, charts, and bulletin boards also need margins. It is not advisable or attractive to write all of the way to the edge or to crowd visuals.

Wording/Lettering

It is important to be concise and use the fewest words possible. Working on conciseness of visuals should help to organize the thoughts that the presenter wants to get across. Titles and labels are placed at various locations. Headings or headlines need to clarify the emphasis and should be in larger print.

Standardizing the size of the lettering and the kind of lettering or fonts makes a more professional appearance. Times Roman is more readable than some stylized scripts. See Table 15.2 for examples of fonts (10, 24). The size must be large enough to be read. A rule of thumb on the size of lowercase letters projected on overhead transparencies, for example, is that they are one-half inch high for each 10 feet of viewer distance (3). So someone standing 20 feet away should be reading 1-inch-sized letters. A study of 38 print materials on cholesterol education found print size that was too small for many older adults (13). Colored lettering may be used, but do not go overboard. If one does not print well, sheets of stick-on letters or a stencil may be purchased. Bold type stresses importance (Table 15.2).

The number of words should be limited to 20–36. Raines recommends the "rule of six," which is to use not more than six lines and not more than six words per line (10). Capital letters are appropriate for short titles of 5–6 words or less, but a combination of capital and lowercase is preferable for longer titles, allowing space for readability. (A Combination of Uppercase and Lowercase Letters Is Preferable. ALL CAPS ARE MORE DIFFICULT TO READ.) One may wish to number lists or use bullets (•), underline words for emphasis, or add stars to key points.

Generally it is advisable to keep paragraphs short. Some find a narrow column of 40–45 characters easier to read than longer lines.

In individual counseling sessions, the author discovered that some clients do not get out their eyeglasses until asked to respond to something in print on the handout being discussed. Of course, some do not read well at all, so simple visual presentations are even more important for them.

Color

Color can enhance visuals and demand attention. Everything does not have to be black and white, but colors should be used sparingly, one to three at the most. One may combine colors that are pleasing aesthetically, and not clashing. It is best to decide the focus of the visual and select the color for that first. Colors have meanings to people. In most western countries, red and orange are considered "hot," for example, while green, blue, and violet are considered "cool" colors (3). The presenter should start by considering the background color. If it is light, any bright colors may be used. With a dark background, lighter shades are needed and print has to be larger to be read.

Pictures/Art Work/Graphics/Layout

The dietetics professional should consider the layout and its effect on the audience's understanding. Is it too crowded? Confusing? Pleasing? Is it serving its purpose? Color, arrows, yarn, clip art, underlining, and boxing in information to separate it may draw the viewer's attention.

Balance

There are two kinds of balance, formal and informal. Informal balance is asymmetrical and more attention getting and interesting. Formal balance occurs when one has the mirror image of the other half. Bear in mind that our society reads from left to right and top to bottom, so that is the way your audience will view any visual (Fig. 15.6).

USING MEDIA

After preparing both the presentation and the media, several practices are critical to success. During practice, one may find that a few changes need to be made. Can the

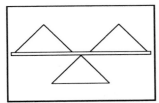 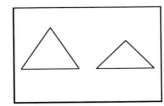

Formal balance   **Informal balance**

FIGURE 15.6. Formal and informal balance.

writing on charts or transparencies, for example, be seen from all areas in the room? If not, modifications are needed.

The presenter needs to practice with the slides, overheads, or other media. One may practice at home with a friend or colleague present to obtain feedback. If no one is available, practice in front of a mirror is a possibility, although that is not as good. Preferably one should practice in the actual setting of the presentation. If this is not possible, the presenter should arrive 30 minutes in advance to check on things and give instructions to anyone assisting. One needs to know, for example, how to run the equipment and lower the lights in the room.

For maximum impact, words should be delivered at the same moment as the visual message. People are then seeing and hearing the same thing.

EVALUATING RESULTS

Educational evaluation is treated in detail in another chapter. It is important to obtain feedback not only on one's presentation, but also on the media used. Some educational programs use written evaluation forms. If not, one may inquire about audience reactions afterward. Any suggestions may be used as a basis for revising and improving the materials. While it probably is not possible for novices, experienced presenters can watch the audience for nonverbal reactions during the presentation.

The following questions may be asked:

Were the media effective in fulfilling their purpose?

What did the audience learn from them?

Could they be improved?

How much time did they take? Was it worth it?

Were the materials cost effective?

There is no doubt that media enhance learning and retention from presentations and educational sessions as well as having the potential to enhance one's professional image. If not using at least 5 to 8 visuals, one may be 5000–8000 words short.

REVIEW AND DISCUSSION QUESTIONS

1. What benefits does the use of media provide in presentations?

2. What should be considered in planning media?

3. What are the criteria for selecting media?

4. Why should the readability of print materials be assessed?

5. Why is it important to evaluate media as one uses it?

6. When training employees, why is it preferable to train them using the real object, such as meat slicer, dishwashing machine, cash register, or other equipment?

7. What are some advantages of using video formats for training and education?

8. What is the "rule of six"?

9. Why should a presenter arrive at the presentation 30 minutes before it starts?

SUGGESTED ACTIVITIES

1. Think about your earliest experiences in school. Can you remember any visual materials used by a teacher? Describe as much as you can remember and your age at the time.

2. Prepare a chart, poster, or bulletin board depicting one idea. Write a description of your objectives and intended audience. Write a critique of your visual explaining how you used art and design principles to enhance quality.

3. Prepare overhead transparencies by hand, by using a photocopier machine, and with a computer program, if available.

4. If a camcorder is available, plan a media presentation using the storyboarding technique. Prepare a video of a new employee process or something the employee needs to learn about, such as kitchen sanitation, food handling, hand washing, and the like. Or tape a recipe preparation for a modified diet or a session on normal nutrition.

5. If a 35-mm camera is available, take a series of slides that tell a story.

6. If equipment is available, videotape an oral presentation that includes media. Alternatively, an audiotape recording will show how one sounds.

7. Assign one student or a group of students to learn to use various types of equipment (overhead projector, slide projector, videocassette recorder (VCR), movie projector, etc.). Each should write a task analysis (see Chapter 12) for the equipment and then train others in its use.

8. Select a commercially prepared video. Evaluate it in terms of its intended audience, objectives, effectiveness, art and design principles, cost, and the like with an evaluation form from the instructor.

9. Think of a real object or model you could use in teaching. Write a description of how you would use it including your objective and intended audience.

10. View an educational program on television. Evaluate it using an evaluation form from the instructor.

CASE STUDY

At 9:00 am Julie gathered her flip-chart and Magic Markers and headed for her office door. She was conducting an employee training session that began at 9:00 am. As she entered the training room, she said to the 20 participants, "Oh well, I'm here. Let's begin by watching a short video."

As Julie inserted the video into the VCR, she realized that the carriage was broken and she would not be able to show it. Frustrated and embarrassed, Julie said, "Nothing in this company works right. I guess I'll have to ask them to bring me another VCR."

After calling Media Services to obtain another VCR, Julie turned to the group and said, "I was in a hurry this morning and I forgot my handouts for the session. It will just take me a few minutes to go back to my office to get them."

1. What should Julie have done to create a more positive image of herself and to improve this training session?

---

11. Find two food advertisements. Write a critique of each according to art and design principles.

12. Select two educational pamphlets. Critique the content using a readability formula if available. Critique the visuals as well.

REFERENCES

1. Read DA, Greene WH. Creative teaching in health. Prospect Heights, IL: Waveland Pr, 1989.
2. Johnson V. Picture-perfect presentations. Train Dev 1989;43:45.
3. Heinich R, Molenda M, Russell JD, et al. Instructional media and technologies for learning. 5th ed. Englewood Cliffs, NJ: Prentice-Hall, 1996.
4. The American Almanac: Statistical abstract of the United States, 1995–1996. Austin, TX: Reference Press, 1996.
5. Kamalipour Y. The brain drain: what television is doing to us. Chicago Tribune, May 2, 1994.
6. Brandao JJ, Brademan GM, Moore CE, et al. Effectiveness of videotaped dietary instruction for patients hospitalized with cardiovascular disease. J Am Diet Assoc 1992;92:1268.
7. Carson CA, Hassel CA. Educating high-risk Minnesotans about dietary fats, blood cholesterol, and heart disease. J Am Diet Assoc 1994;94:659.
8. Coulston AM, Stivers M. A poster worth a thousand words: how to design effective poster session displays. J Am Diet Assoc 1993;93:865.
9. Doyle SL. Ten tips for fabulous flips. Train Dev 1993;47:18.
10. Raines C, Williamson L. Using visual aids: a guide for effective presentations. Rev ed. Menlo Park, CA: Crisp, 1995.
11. Teague FA, Rogers DW, Tipling RN. Technology and media: instructional applications. Dubuque, IA: Kendall/Hunt, 1994.
12. Busselman KM, Holcomb CA. Reading skill and comprehension of the dietary guidelines by WIC participants. J Am Diet Assoc 1994;94:622.
13. Glanz K, Rudd J. Readability and content analysis of print cholesterol education materials. Pat Educ Counsel 1990;16:109.
14. Dollahite J, Thompson C, McNew R. Readability of printed sources of diet and health information. Pat Educ Counsel 1996;27:123.
15. Shield JE, Mullen MC. Developing health education materials for special audiences. Chicago: American Dietetics Assoc, 1992.
16. National Cancer Institute. Making health communication programs work. Bethesda, MD: NIH pub. No. 89-1493, 1989.
17. Trenkner LL, Achtenberg CL. Use of focus groups in evaluating nutrition education materials. J Am Diet Assoc 1991;91:1577.
18. Rae L. Training 101: choose your method. Train Dev 1994;48:19.
19. Utz P. Camcorders: the heart of video production. Media Meth 1994;30:14.
20. Beerman KA. Computer-based multimedia: new directions in teaching and learning. J Nutr Educ 1996;28:15.
21. Kolasa KM, Miller MG. New developments in nutrition education using computer technology. J Nutr Educ 1996;28:7.
22. Verrecchia FP. Spotlight on AV and presentation equipment. Media Meth 1993;30:16.
23. Carroll JM, Stein C, Byron M, et al. Using interactive media to deliver nutrition education to Maine's WIC clients. J Nutr Educ 1996;28:19.
24. King WL. Training by design. Train Dev 1994;48:52.

Counseling Guidelines—Initial Session

STEP	TOPIC	QUESTIONS TO ASK	QUESTIONS TO AVOID

1	Candidly review the problems of dietary change.
	  1. Review overall rationale and objectives for recommended diet.
	  2. Acknowledge difficult nature of dietary change.
	  3. Listen to patient's concerns about the recommended diet.
		What are your thoughts and feelings about this diet?	Do you have any opinion about this diet?

2	Build some commitment to solve problems.
	  1. Indicate your willingness to work with patient.
	  2. Clarify to patient that he must assume primary responsibility for making dietary changes.
	  3. Propose program of frequent meetings for next 3 months, close self-observation of diet, phone contact.
	  4. Emphasize slow but steady approach to change.
	  5. Obtain patient's verbal commitment to meet any of your proposals.
		What aspects of this program are you willing to try now?	Do you want to try anything now?

3	Plan some specific changes in diet during coming month.
	  1. Emphasize good points of 3-day record.[a]
	  2. Look on record for ideas on dietary changes.
	  3. Probe patient for more ideas.
	  4. Pinpoint *one* aspect of diet pattern to change.
		What do you see that could be changed or improved?	Do you see anything to change?

STEP	TOPIC	QUESTIONS TO ASK	QUESTIONS TO AVOID
	5. Acknowledge patient's desire for radical and fast changes in diet, but reemphasize that the most successful approach is slow and steady.		
	6. Help patient set realistic dietary change goals (e.g., one meatless evening meal per week, substitution of a salad bowl for usual main entree at one lunch per week).	What is a realistic goal for you?	Is this a realistic goal?
4	Plan how to make a change successful.		
	1. Identify problems that are likely to interfere with achieving goal. Consider problems in the following areas:	What problems are likely to interfere with your plans?	Are any problems going to interfere with your plans?
	a. Physical environment (e.g., what foods are available in house, snacking in front of TV in evening, absence of reminders on refrigerator or dining table)	What can you change in your home, office, or car that will help you achieve your goal?	Do you need any reminders?
	b. Social environment (e.g., influential people, such as spouse, children, business associates, whose approval and support or criticism can affect achievement of dietary change goal)	Who can help, what can they do, and what can I do to help during the next few weeks?	Do you need any help?
	c. Cognitive or private environment (e.g., what patient says to himself when confronted with personal thoughts such as the following: What others will say about his planned behavior; thoughts of failure or disappointment when he is not perfect in his behavior)	What encouraging things can you say to yourself when confronted with these inevitable thoughts?

Other's approval.

Potential failure. | Will you give yourself encouragement? |
| 5 | Plan how to keep track of progress. Devise an unobtrusive and convenient way for patient to keep a record of the desired or target behavior (e.g., count egg cartons, measure side of vegetable oil container, attach pencil *and* paper to refrigerator, table, wallet, etc.) | How are you going to keep track of (target behavior)? | Can you keep track of (target behavior)? |

STEP	TOPIC	QUESTIONS TO ASK	QUESTIONS TO AVOID
6	Plan counseling continuity and support.	When is it convenient for me to call and discuss your progress? When can we schedule our next appointment?	Do you want me to contact you sometime?
7	Make certain that spouse, if present, is involved in answering questions, providing ideas, and discussing potential problems and solutions.		

Reprinted with permission from Wilbur CS. Nutrition counseling skills. Audio cassette series 5. Chicago: American Dietetic Assoc, 1980.
[a] Before initial counseling session, patient should be given materials and instructions for completing a 3-day food diary.

appendix B

Counseling Guidelines—Follow-Up Sessions

STEP	TOPIC	QUESTIONS TO ASK	QUESTIONS TO AVOID
1	Review patient's progress. Emphasize the positive and check commitment.[a]	What thoughts do you have about this approach to lowering your cholesterol?	Do you have any thoughts about this approach to counseling?
2	Discuss the problems that interfered with achieving the goal and how patient attempted to solve them.	What problems did you face?	Did you have any problems?
3	Plan next specific change in diet for coming month. 1. Look at old food record for ideas. 2. Probe patient for ideas. 3. Pinpoint one aspect of diet pattern to change. 4. Reacknowledge patient's probable desire to make fast, radical changes, but reemphasize the importance of slow but steady approach. 5. Set a realistic behavior change goal. 6. Include plans for patient to continue with the changes he accomplished last month.	What do you see that could be changed or improved?	Do you see anything to change?
4	Plan how to make change successful. 1. Identify problems that are likely to interfere with achieving goal. Consider problems in the following areas:	What problems are likely to interfere with your plans?	Are any problems going to interfere with your plans?

STEP	TOPIC	QUESTIONS TO ASK	QUESTIONS TO AVOID
	a. Physical environment (e.g., what foods are available in house, snacking in front of TV in evening, absence of reminders on refrigerator or dining table)	What can you change in your home, office, or car that will help you achieve your goal?	Do you need any reminders?
	b. Social environment (e.g., influential people, such as spouse, children, business associates, whose approval and support or criticism can affect achievement of dietary change goal)	Who can help, what can they do, and what can I do to help during the next few weeks?	Do you need any help?
	c. Cognitive or private environment (e.g., what patient says to himself when confronted with personal thoughts such as the following:	What encouraging things can you say to yourself when confronted with these inevitable thoughts?	Will you give yourself encouragement?
	What others will say about his planned behavior;	Other's approval.	
	Thoughts of failure or disappointment when he is not perfect in his behavior;		
	Negative feelings of hunger or irritability that will accompany behavior change;	Negative reactions to change.	
	Feeling goal not as important as once thought, usually 4–5 days after counseling session)	Devaluation of goal over time.	
5	Plan how to keep track of progress. Devise an unobtrusive and convenient way for patient to keep a record of the desired or target behavior (e.g., count egg cartons, measure side of vegetable oil container, attach pencil *and* paper to refrigerator, table, wallet, etc.)	How are you going to keep track of (target behavior)?	Can you keep track of (target behavior)?

STEP	TOPIC	QUESTIONS TO ASK	QUESTIONS TO AVOID
6	Plan counseling continuity and support.	When is it convenient for me to call and discuss your progress? When can we schedule our next appointment?	Do you want me to contact you sometime?
7	Make certain that spouse, if present, is involved in answering questions, providing ideas, discussing potential problems and solutions.		

Reprinted with permission from Wilbur CS. Nutrition counseling skills. Audio cassette series 5. Chicago: American Dietetic Assoc, 1980.
[a] Be prepared to handle *either* the patient's success *or* failure in achieving previous goal.

Index

References in italics denote figures; those followed by "t" denote tables